Jose L. Pascual • Timothy G. Gaulton
Editors

Opioid Use in Critical Care

A Practical Guide

Springer

Editors
Jose L. Pascual
Professor of Surgery and Neurosurgery
Perelman School of Medicine
Clinical Associate, School of Nursing
University of Pennsylvania
Philadelphia, PA
USA

Timothy G. Gaulton
Department of Anesthesiology and Critical Care
Perelman School of Medicine, University of Pennsylvania
Philadelphia, PA
USA

ISBN 978-3-030-77398-4 ISBN 978-3-030-77399-1 (eBook)
https://doi.org/10.1007/978-3-030-77399-1

This Springer imprint is published by the registered company Springer Nature Switzerland AG
The registered company address is: Gewerbestrasse 11, 6330 Cham, Switzerland

Contents

Contributors

Ramani Balu Division of Neurocritical Care, Department of Neurology, Perelman School of Medicine, University of Pennsylvania, Philadelphia, PA, USA

Edward A. Bittner Department of Anesthesia, Critical Care and Pain Medicine, Massachusetts General Hospital, Boston, MA, USA

Harvard Medical School, Boston, MA, USA

Christina Boncyk Department of Anesthesiology, Division of Anesthesia Critical Care Medicine, Vanderbilt University Medical Center, Nashville, TN, USA

Daniel R. Brown Department of Anesthesiology and Perioperative Medicine, Mayo Clinic, Rochester, MN, USA

Kyle Bruns Department of Anesthesiology, Division of Anesthesia Critical Care Medicine, Vanderbilt University Medical Center, Nashville, TN, USA

Meghan M. Caylor Department of Pharmacy, Hospital of the University of Pennsylvania, Philadelphia, PA, USA

Anthony Chau Department of Anesthesia, BC Women's Hospital, Vancouver, BC, Canada

Department of Anesthesiology, Pharmacology & Therapeutics, University of British Columbia, Vancouver, BC, Canada

Jessica R. Crow Department of Pharmacy, The Johns Hopkins Hospital, Baltimore, MD, USA

Stephanie L. Davis Department of Pharmacy, The Johns Hopkins Hospital, Baltimore, MD, USA

Amy L. Dzierba Department of Pharmacy, NewYork-Presbyterian Hospital, New York, NY, USA

Lillian Emlet Departments of Critical Care Medicine & Emergency Medicine, VA Pittsburgh Healthcare System/University of Pittsburgh Medical Center, Pittsburgh, PA, USA

Marie-France Forget Department of Medicine, Division of Geriatric Medicine, Centre hospitalier de l'Université de Montréal, Montréal, QC, Canada

Université de Montréal, Faculty of Montréal, Montréal, QC, Canada

Timothy G. Gaulton Department of Anesthesiology and Critical Care, Perelman School of Medicine, University of Pennsylvania, Philadelphia, PA, USA

Nicholas Goodmanson Department of Medicine, University of Illinois at Chicago/ Advocate Christ Medical Center and Advocate Lutheran General Hospital, Champaign, IL, USA

Christina J. Hayhurst Department of Anesthesiology, Division of Anesthesia Critical Care Medicine, Vanderbilt University Medical Center, Nashville, TN, USA

Mary Ann Hernando Perelman School of Medicine at the University of Pennsylvania, Philadelphia, PA, USA

Internal Medicine, Columbia University Irving Medical Center, New York, NY, USA

Christopher G. Hughes Department of Anesthesiology, Division of Anesthesia Critical Care Medicine, Vanderbilt University Medical Center, Nashville, TN, USA

Andrew S. Jarrell Department of Pharmacy, Oregon Health & Science University, Portland, OR, USA

Sandra L. Kane-Gill University of Pittsburgh School of Pharmacy, Department of Pharmacy and Therapeutics, Department of Biomedical Informatics, Pittsburgh, PA, USA

Lewis J. Kaplan Corporal Michael J Crescenz VA Medical Center, Surgical Services, Surgical Critical Care, Philadelphia, PA, USA

Perelman School of Medicine, University of Pennsylvania, Department of Surgery, Division of Trauma, Surgical Critical Care and Emergency Surgery, Philadelphia, PA, USA

Kunal Karamchandani Department of Anesthesiology and Pain Management, UT Southwestern Medical Center, Dallas, TX, USA

Jane Keating University of Connecticut, Department of Surgery, Hartford, CT, USA

Ashish K. Khanna Department of Anesthesiology, Section on Critical Care Medicine, Wake Forest School of Medicine, Wake Forest Baptist Medical Center, Winston-Salem, NC, USA

Outcomes Research Consortium, Cleveland, OH, USA

Andrew Kim Department of Anesthesiology and Critical Care, Hospital of the University of Pennsylvania, Philadelphia, PA, USA

Arthur Kitt Department of Anesthesiology and Critical Care, Hospital of the University of Pennsylvania, Philadelphia, PA, USA

Niels D. Martin Perelman School of Medicine at the University of Pennsylvania, Department of Surgery, Division of Traumatology, Surgical Critical Care & Emergency Surgery, Philadelphia, PA, USA

J. A. Jeevendra Martyn Harvard Medical School, Boston, MA, USA

Shriners Hospitals for Children, Boston, MA, USA

Massachusetts General Hospital, Boston, MA, USA

Mark E. Mikkelsen Perelman School of Medicine at the University of Pennsylvania, Philadelphia, PA, USA

Division of Pulmonary, Allergy, and Critical Care Medicine, Perelman School of Medicine at the University of Pennsylvania, Philadelphia, PA, USA

Athir H. Morad Departments of Anesthesiology and Critical Care Medicine, Johns Hopkins University School of Medicine, Baltimore, MD, USA

Justin Muir Department of Pharmacy, NewYork-Presbyterian Hospital, New York, NY, USA

Matthew Niehaus Department of Emergency Medicine, University Hospitals Cleveland Medical Center/Case Western Reserve University, Cleveland, OH, USA

Akhil Patel Department of Anesthesiology, Cooper University Hospital, Cooper Medical School of Rowan University, Camden, NJ, USA

Mark R. Pedersen Department of Anesthesia, University of Iowa, Iowa City, IA, USA

Teresa Poon Department of Pharmacy, NewYork-Presbyterian Hospital, New York, NY, USA

Charles Prior Department of Anesthesia, BC Women's Hospital, Vancouver, BC, Canada

Dane Scantling Perelman School of Medicine at the University of Pennsylvania, Department of Surgery, Division of Traumatology, Surgical Critical Care & Emergency Surgery, Philadelphia, PA, USA

Rachel Steinhorn Department of Anesthesia, Critical Care and Pain Medicine, Massachusetts General Hospital, Boston, MA, USA

Harvard Medical School, Boston, MA, USA

Robert D. Stevens Departments of Anesthesiology and Critical Care Medicine, Johns Hopkins University School of Medicine, Baltimore, MD, USA

Departments of Neurology, Johns Hopkins University School of Medicine, Baltimore, MD, USA

Departments of Neurosurgery, Johns Hopkins University School of Medicine, Baltimore, MD, USA

Departments of Radiology, Johns Hopkins University School of Medicine, Baltimore, MD, USA

Han Ting Wang Department of Medicine, Division of Internal and Critical Care Medicine, Hôpital Maisonneuve-Rosemont, Montréal, QC, Canada

Faculty of Medecine, Université de Montréal, Montréal, QC, Canada

Chapter 1
The Epidemiology of Opioids in Critical Illness

Timothy G. Gaulton

Introduction

Since its establishment over five decades ago to manage cases of respiratory failure from poliomyelitis [1], intensive care medicine has evolved into a multidisciplinary field that cares for acutely ill patients presenting across a range of diagnoses and complexities. In the United States (US), over a quarter of hospital discharges each year involve a stay in the intensive care unit (ICU) [2]. This accounts for nearly four million ICU admissions a year and close to half of total hospital charges. Globally, it is estimated that annually, between 13 and 20 million patients undergo mechanical ventilation and 15–19 million individuals are diagnosed with sepsis, one of the leading causes of admissions to an ICU [3]. These numbers are expected to increase over the next several decades. The number of ICUs varies significantly among countries, with nearly 6000 in the US and 319 in Canada. Similarly, ICU bed numbers and availability also vary widely across US states and other countries. The burden of disease from critical illness worldwide is extensive and associated with significant morbidity, mortality, and cost.

Intensive care services are essential to support the health of any population, whether it is dealing with the consequences of an aging population, managing acute injury and illness in times of conflict and pandemics, or dealing with public health crises such as the opioid epidemic. The goals of critical care are multifaceted including, first and foremost, the need to sustain life through rapid diagnosis and stabilization in ill or injured patients. Yet, of equal importance, is the goal of preventing harm and treating patient and family suffering. In the ICU, nothing is as ubiquitous and distressing as pain. The appropriate management of pain is a fundamental

T. G. Gaulton (✉)
Department of Anesthesiology and Critical Care, Perelman School of Medicine, University of Pennsylvania, Philadelphia, PA, USA
e-mail: timothy.gaulton2@pennmedicine.upenn.edu

J. L. Pascual, T. G. Gaulton (eds.), *Opioid Use in Critical Care*,
https://doi.org/10.1007/978-3-030-77399-1_1

component of compassionate medical care; however, despite its importance, patients continue to experience pain and suffer from the unintended consequences of its treatment.

The interaction between critical care medicine, pain, and opioids is complex, challenging, and evolving. First, as mentioned, pain is common in the ICU and opioid analgesics represent the mainstay of acute pain therapy. Second, numerous studies have demonstrated that deep levels of sedation are associated with adverse patient outcomes. Consequently, opioid administration has become fundamental to strategies aimed at keeping patients awake and minimizing sedatives. Third, ICUs are common places for individuals that have suffered a terminal illness and are receiving end-of-life care. And finally, the opioid epidemic has led to an increase in the incidence of opioid overdose admissions to the ICU.

Opioid Use in the General Population

The opioid epidemic is a public health emergency that has placed tremendous burden on families, communities, and public health systems. Millions of Americans suffer from an opioid use disorder, defined as a problematic pattern of opioid use leading to significant impairment or distress [4]. Since 1999, over 11 million Americans have misused prescription opioids and nearly 400,000 people have died from an opioid overdose [4, 5]. Alarmingly, over 130 deaths from an opioid overdose are estimated to occur each day in the US [5]. The increase in deaths from opioid overdoses has been described in three distinct waves: (1) overdose deaths from prescription opioids that began to increase around 1999, (2) overdose deaths from heroin starting in 2010 as tighter restrictions were placed on prescription opioids, and (3) overdose deaths from synthetic opioids such as fentanyl beginning in 2013 [6]. Worldwide, the use of prescription opioids has more than doubled from 2001 to 2013 and use now accounts for over 7.3 million daily doses [7]. The growth of prescription opioids has occurred mainly in North America and western/central Europe and has been associated with an increase in opioid misuse, diversion, and harm. In the US, these increases were in part a response to multiple efforts labeling inadequate pain control, including non-cancer pain, as a gap in the quality of health care. In 1995, the American Pain Society launched "Pain is the Fifth Vital Sign" campaign that championed an expansion of the use of opioids for analgesia [8]. This campaign was later adopted by various governing health bodies including the Veteran's Health Administration and the Joint Commission [9]. Eventual policy efforts in the US linked patients' ratings of pain intensity to hospital reimbursement through Medicare's Hospital Value Based Purchasing Program [10]. Overall, the institution of stricter standards for pain management resulted in a larger reliance on opioids for analgesia and a resultant increase in their prescriptions by providers. Furthermore, pharmaceutical companies used targeted marketing campaigns to reduce the public awareness to the risks of opioids and even labeled practices that recommended that opioids not be prescribed for pain as potentially inhumane. As an example, Oxycontin, an extended release formulation of oxycodone, was marketed for its lower probability of abuse. Sales of Oxycontin increased from 670,000 to 6.2

million from 1997 to 2002 [11]. In light of growing concerns about the adverse effects of opioids and misleading marketing campaigns, multiple US states have brought lawsuits against Purdue Pharma, the manufacturer of Oxycontin.

Strategies to reduce the inappropriate prescribing of opioids and their subsequent adverse effects have since occurred at the patient-, hospital-, and government-level. Important research has been done in an attempt to reverse misconceptions of acute pain treatment. Several common practices have been explored and questioned. For example, in one observational trial, the amount of opioids prescribed at the time of hospital discharge following surgery or a caesarean delivery did not have any correlation with pain scores or patient satisfaction [12, 13]. Efforts have been multidimensional and have included shared decision making, patient and provider education, the use of enhanced recovery programs that involve opioid sparing approaches to analgesia, while increasing patient psychiatric support for known associations between depression, pain, and opioid use. In 2016, the CDC published guidelines on the prescribing of opioids for chronic pain [14]. In response, several states imposed limitations on the allowable duration of first-time opioid prescriptions. Moreover, nearly all states have implemented Prescription Drug Monitoring Programs (PDMPs) [15]. PDMPS contain information on controlled substance prescriptions and are accessible to prescribers, pharmacies, and law enforcement officials. Due to low initial rates of utilization, several states have now legally mandate prescribers to query PDMP prior to writing a prescription. The implementation of PDMPs has been associated with reductions in opioid prescribing.

Encouragingly, the majority of policies targeted to prevent opioid abuse are supported by the public [16]. Over 50% of Americans think that increasing pain management training for medical students and physicians would be a very effective strategy. A majority think that other policies such as offering public education and awareness programs and monitoring of physicians' prescribing habits would be somewhat effective. Less than 50% however supported limiting the amount of opioids that providers could prescribe with nearly 55% being concerned that guidelines would make it more difficult for legitimate opioid analgesic recipients to receive adequate prescriptions. These guidelines may not be appropriate for all patients. In particular, patients with illnesses associated with high rates of mortality and low quality of life such as cancer and dementia have a high prevalence of concurrent acute and chronic pain. In such populations, opioid prescriptions may be needed for proper palliation; more research and education are thus necessary to avoid underrecognizing patient needs and developing appropriate opioid prescription approaches.

Intersection of the Opioid Epidemic with Intensive Care Services

ICUs have not been spared from the health burden caused by the opioid epidemic (Fig. 1.1). Adult ICU admissions for opioid-related overdoses, including those from prescription opioids, synthetic opioids, and heroin, increased 0.6% per month from 2009 to 2015 in a study of 162 hospitals from 44 different states [17]. There was

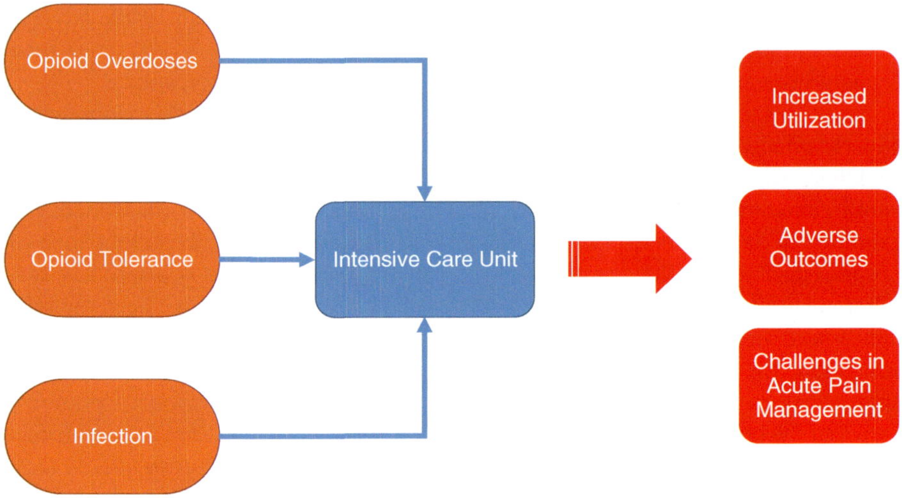

Fig. 1.1 Impact of the opioid epidemic on intensive care services

marked variation in admissions by state. For example, the rate of ICU admissions for opioid overdose nearly doubled in Pennsylvania as opposed to Texas where it remained stable over the same time period. A quarter of admitted patients experienced aspiration pneumonia, 8% had evidence of anoxic brain injury, and 15% developed rhabdomyolysis; 1 in 10 patients required mechanical ventilation and 1 in 16 required renal replacement therapy. The average cost of an ICU overdose admission has also increased dramatically over the past decade. Of concern, the mortality of these opioid-related overdoses admitted to ICUs has also increased, from 7.3% in 2009 to 9.8% in 2015. Moreover, opioid use is associated with an increase in healthcare utilization even in cases not involving overdoses. This is more common with intravenous drug use which can cause serious systemic infections from endocarditis, hepatitis C, and human immunodeficiency virus (HIV). However, opioids may increase the risk of an infection even independent of the route of administration. In 25,392 participants of the Veterans Aging Cohort Study, moderate and high doses of prescribed opioids were associated with increased susceptibility to pneumonia, particularly in individuals with HIV on immunosuppressive medications [18].

Furthermore, opioid users may have an increased risk of poor outcomes after critical illness. In trauma patients, preinjury use of opioids was associated with longer ICU and hospital length of stays [19]. Munch and colleagues found that 1-year mortality after a non-surgical admission to the ICU was significantly higher in patients who were current opioid users (34.8%) as compared to non-users (20.6%) [20]. It remains unclear however how association exists and what the relative contributions are from the direct effect of opioids, such as immunosuppression, or from the indications for opioid use such as pain from a malignancy that may influence long-term outcomes. Nonetheless, it is imperative for providers to recognize that users of opioids are at high risk of becoming acutely ill and suffering complications from acute illness.

As will be discussed in later chapters, patients who are tolerant of opioids, particularly those with an opioid use disorder (OUD), can pose a management challenge for ICU providers and likely suffer from significant stigma. Opioid tolerance, as defined by the US Food and Drug Administration, is the intake for at least a week of the equivalence of 60 mg per day of oral morphine [21]. According to Boudreau and colleagues, age-sex standardized prevalence rates of opioid use for chronic pain ranges from 39.2 to 46.8 per 1000 individuals [22]. Rates of opioid use are even higher in certain populations such as trauma patients where preinjury use is present in up to 1 in 6 patients. [23]. Opioid-tolerant patients can develop central sensitization, tolerance, and opioid-induced hyperalgesia which makes it more difficult to manage their acute pain and places them at higher risk of inadequate pain control. Providers may be unfamiliar with opioid-equivalent doses and conversions. They may also fear causing adverse effects when using the higher dose of opioids required in these patients or worry about causing relapse in patients with a history of addiction. Few guidelines exist on the management of acute pain and sedation in patients with opioid tolerance and opioid use disorders. Only 7% of US ICUs surveyed reported having a guideline to address the sedation and pain management of patients with opioid use disorder [24]. Moreover, less than half of surveyed hospitals had available outpatient resources for these patients after discharge. General recommendations typically involve a multimodal and multidisciplinary approach to analgesia. Yet, given the high rate of complications in patients who are opioid tolerant, significantly more research is needed to define best practices in this population.

Epidemiology of Pain in Critical Illness

The prevalence of pain in patients with critical illness varies by subpopulation (e.g., medical, surgical). However, on average, it is estimated, from surveys of ICU survivors, that 50–80% of patients experience moderate to severe pain during their ICU stay, with percentages higher when invasive procedures occur [25]. Pain can derive from many sources whether it is the reason for ICU admission (e.g., surgery), invasive procedures (e.g., intravenous lines), invasive devices (e.g., mechanical ventilation), immobility or even routine nursing care (e.g., turning and repositioning). In a multinational cohort of ICU patients, Puntillo and colleagues identified chest tube removal, wound drain removal, and arterial line insertion as the three most painful procedures commonly performed in the ICU [26]. In this study, positioning and mobilization were associated with mild pain on average. In general, demographic and comorbid conditions associated with the presence of pain include younger age, depression, anxiety, and female gender. Acute pain, particularly when it is not adequately treated, can have significant short- and long-term physiologic and emotional consequences, mediated primarily by inflammatory, sympathetic, and neuroendocrine activation. Downstream physiological effects include increased work of breathing, tachycardia, hypertension, persistent catabolism, agitation, and delirium, among others. Additional detriment can occur by delaying mobility or inducing emotional distress that can lead to post-traumatic stress disorder. Importantly, inappropriately treated pain is one of the biggest concerns raised by ICU patients [27].

Given the high prevalence of pain and its adverse effect on patient outcomes, it is recommended that pain be routinely monitored in all adult ICU patients using validated pain assessment tools [28]. Guidelines advise against using vital signs alone to quantify pain, instead suggesting they should simply be cues to prompt a formal pain evaluation. Instead, it is recommended to use behavioral pain scales such as the Behavioral Pain Scale and the Critical Care Pain Observation Tool (see Chap. 2) in those unable to participate in a pain assessment. Effective and timely management of pain is the first component of ICU liberation strategies, the most publicized being the ABCDEF bundle (Assessing and treating pain, Both Awakening and Breathing Trials, Choice of appropriate sedation, Delirium monitoring and management, Early mobility and Exercise, and Family Engagement) that has been globally adopted by ICUs. The goals of pain management in the ICU are to first alleviate patient discomfort and are highly individualized with vigilance given to the prevention of adverse effects of administered analgesics.

Opioid Use in Acute Hospital Settings

As compared to outpatient prescribing, opioid use in inpatient settings has undergone less scrutiny and empirical evaluation despite standards by the Joint Commission implicating inpatient pain management as in the rise of outpatient opioid use [29]. In a study of 1.14 million non-surgical admissions in 286 acute care facilities across the US, Herzig and colleagues found that opioids were used in 51% of these admissions [30]. The mean daily dose in oral morphine equivalents was 68 mg and 23% of those patients received more than 100 mg. Moreover, opioid use was not without significant risk – hospitals with higher rates of opioid use had higher relative risks of severe opioid-related adverse events compared to hospitals with lower rates of opioid use. Donohue and colleagues performed further work to characterize the patterns and settings of opioid administration in the hospital and their associations with post-discharge use [31]. Within 12 community and academic hospitals in western Pennsylvania, they found that at least one opioid dose was administered in 48% of admissions. The patients in this study were previously opioid naïve yet received opioids on nearly 70% of the days they spent in the hospital. Predictors of inpatient opioid use included younger age, female gender, having Medicaid, and being admitted for a surgical procedure. Patients with comorbid musculoskeletal pain and depression were also more likely to receive opioids while those with alcohol use and mental health disorders had lower rates of opioid use. Notably, non-opioid analgesics were used prior to opioids in less than a quarter of patients and only used at any time during the hospital stay in 22.6% to 54.2% of admissions. The authors further reported that inpatient opioid use was associated with a 2.07 higher relative risk for a composite outcome of opioid use, death, or readmission at 90 days after hospital discharge. This is in line with growing evidence from surgical patients that has correlated the administration of opioids after surgery with a number of opioid-related outcomes that include prescription opioid misuses, the development of opioid use disorder, opioid diversion, and new prolonged opioid use [32, 33].

Opioid Use in Critical Care Settings

The use of analgesics in intensive care has been influenced by guidelines that were introduced in the early 1990s. In 1992, the Agency for Health Care Policy and Research recommended that for acute mild to moderate pain, patients should be treated with a non-steroidal inflammatory drug but if in moderate to severe pain they should be treated with an opioid [34]. The Society of Critical Care Medicine (SCCM) released the first recommendations for pain and sedation management of adult patients in the ICU in 1995 and gave support to primary role of opioids in pain control, preferentially recommending the use of morphine unless hemodynamically instability was present [28]. These guidelines were updated in 2018 with similar recommendations for intravenous opioids as the first-line therapy for non-neuropathic pain, noting that all opioids would be equally effective when targeting to specific pain endpoints. Importance is given to using the lowest effective dose of opioids necessary in order to reduce the incidence of adverse effects.

Opioids now have a more prominent role in sedation practices. SCCM guidelines have recommended that light levels of sedation, daily awakening trials, and the minimization of benzodiazepines be used to improve short-term clinical outcomes. Evidence has shown that benzodiazepines and deeper levels of sedation increase the risk of delirium along with other adverse outcomes such as ICU length of stay and duration of mechanical ventilation [28] (see Chap. 9). It has now become evident that not all mechanically ventilated patients require sedation and that agitation and anxiety often reflect under treated pain. In a randomized controlled trial of 140 mechanically ventilated patients, Strom and colleagues showed that patients who received no intravenous sedation spent fewer days on mechanical ventilation than patients who received intravenous sedation [35]. The minimization of sedation is a key component of ICU liberation strategies, notably the ABCDEF bundle, where its adoption has been associated to improved survival and lower delirium rates [36, 37]. This has led to a shift in sedation practices where pain assessment is prioritized and analgesics are prioritized (most commonly opioids) to achieve desired sedative and wakefulness goals. The term analgo-sedation has been colloquially adopted to reflect the analgesia-first sedation practice.

Studies on the use of opioids in intensive care have shown that the majority of patients receive opioids during their ICU stay, although practices vary significantly across institutions (Table 1.1) [38]. In 2014, Burry and colleagues identified that 84.8% of patients on mechanical ventilation received opioids. Fentanyl

Table 1.1 Characteristics of opioid analgesic use in the ICU

Prevalence of Use	50.6–90%
Route of Administration	1. Intravenous Infusion 2. Enteral 3. Intravenous Bolus Only
Type	4. Fentanyl 5. Morphine 6. Hydromorphone

was the most commonly used opioid (54.3%) followed by morphine (35.0%) and hydromorphone (7.7%). Intravenous infusions were the most common route of administration, used in 83.6% of patients, compared to 8.6% who received intravenous bolus dosing only and 21.3% of patients who received enteral opioids. This high rate of opioid use is consistent with reported use that approached 90% in a randomized controlled trial of daily sedation interruption in mechanical ventilated patients conducted by Mehta and colleagues in 2012 [39]. In this study, patients who received protocolized sedation and interruption received an average of 550 mcg/day of fentanyl equivalents compared to 260 mcg/day in patients who received protocolized sedation only. Notably, Burry and colleagues found that a pain scale was only used in 19.1% of patients in this study. Factors associated with opioid use were increased duration of mechanical ventilation, use of physical restraints, use of a pain scale, and treatment at a university hospital compared to community hospital. In a study of 43 ICUs in France, Payen and colleagues in 2007 reported that 90% of patients received an opioid [40]. Sufentanil and fentanyl were the most commonly used opioids followed by morphine. Similar to Burry et al., intravenous infusion was the most common route of administration. Opioids were primarily given for ventilator synchrony and patient comfort. Only a quarter of patients received an opioid bolus prior to a painful procedure being initiated and pain scales were used in a minority of patients (40%). In adults aged 65 years and older, Jung and colleagues used a national claims database in Korea and found that 50.6% of these patients were administered an opioid [41]. Of these patients, less than half were concurrently administered a non-opioid analgesic. Opioids were administered for an average of 3 days and patients received an average of 23.8 mg in oral morphine equivalent doses. Opioid use does seem to vary with concurrent use of intravenous sedation. Wunsch and colleagues in 2009 found that over two-thirds of patients on an infusion of a benzodiazepine received an opiate infusion in contrast to less than a quarter of those on a propofol infusion [42]. Furthermore, opioid administration does not seem to vary by time of day. In a study of older adults in a medical ICU, no clear temporal relationship was demonstrated between fentanyl dose and whether it was a day, evening, or night shift [43]. This is in contrast to haloperidol and lorazepam administration where use of these drugs increased significantly during evening and night shifts. These epidemiologic studies show that opioid use in the ICU is ubiquitous, intravenous infusions are the most frequent route of administration, and pain scales are not used routinely.

Other synthetic opioids have been used in the ICU for analgesia and to attenuate opioid tolerance and hyperalgesia. Examples include remifentanil and methadone and while they have potential advantages compared to other opioids, they are yet to become a common part of clinical practice. Remifentanil is a derivative of fentanyl that has a rapid onset and short duration of action. It is metabolized by plasma esterases and importantly, does not accumulate in the presence of hepatic and/or renal dysfunction. Due to these drug characteristics, it offers many potential advantages for use in the ICU. Compared to other intravenous analgesics such as fentanyl or intravenous sedatives such as propofol, remifentanil has been shown in randomized controlled trials to reduce the time that a patient spends on mechanical ventilation [44, 45]. However, remifentanil is associated with significant cost and possible opioid induced hyperalgesia, more so than other opioids, which has limited its widespread adoption [46].

Methadone has also been increasingly used and studied in critical illness as a way to prevent potential opioid withdrawal and hyperalgesia. It is a synthetic opioid commonly used for addiction treatment that acts as an antagonist at the N-methyl-D-aspartate (NMDA) receptor. Wanzuita and colleagues performed a randomized controlled trial of 75 ICU patients in Brazil and found that administration of enteral methadone increased the probability of successful weaning from mechanical ventilation [47]. Yet, similar to remifentanil, this practice has not been widely adopted in adult ICUs, in part due to methadone's prolongation of the QTc interval and a potential risk of cardiac arrhythmia. Lastly, some parenteral opioids are avoided in the ICU due to their side effect profile and safety concerns. For example, meperidine can have neurotoxic effects including seizures related to its metabolites which can accumulate in renal insufficiency, a common ICU condition.

Opioid Use in End-of-Life Care

Many individuals spend the final days of their life in the ICU. In the US, 1 in 5 people who die are admitted to an ICU at or near the time of their death [48]. Of Medicare recipients, more than 1 in 10 spend greater than 7 days in an ICU in the last 6 months of their lives [49]. End-of-life care is an integral responsibility of an ICU that challenges its providers and staff. The trajectory of critical illness is dynamic and often unpredictable and deteriorations, despite efforts to resuscitate and monitor, can be profound and at times, unexpected. Unfortunately, detailed discussions on patient wishes often do not occur when a patient is healthy but rather occur around the time of acute illness when a patient may be incapacitated and unable to express their desires. Therefore, decisions regarding end-of-life care should be shared with surrogate decision makers. As described previously, interventions designed to sustain life such as a mechanical ventilation may be a source of pain and discomfort. As it is in other ICU contexts, pain is a common and distressing symptom that is especially feared by patients who are approaching the end of their life. In the final 3 days of life, nearly 40% of hospitalized patients reported moderate to severe pain [49]. When a decision is made to transition to comfort care, the ICU team should develop a plan for evaluation and treatment of pain and other distressing symptoms. Intravenous opioids can be administered as continuous infusions to provide a basal level of pain relief and may be less disruptive to the family than intravenous bolus administration. However, bolus dosing will be required to reach a steady state and to maintain adequate control of symptoms. The amount of opioid medication required may be much higher than what was given in prior phases of critical illness, particularly if opioids have been given previously and tolerance has developed. Individual patient responses are variable and reevaluation is paramount. Although an extended decision algorithm is outside the scope of this chapter, opioid infusions used for terminal illness are administered within the principle of double effect where the intent of palliation and symptom alleviation may shorten the time to death.

Epidemiology of Opioid Adverse Effects

Opioid Withdrawal

Given the frequent use of opioids in the ICU, acute withdrawal from opioids is likely common in patients recovering from their critical illness. However, few studies currently exist to characterize the epidemiology of opioid withdrawal in the ICU. Concurrently, validated assessment tools to define withdrawal in critical ill adults are lacking [50]. Furthermore, it can be challenging to differentiate withdrawal from opioids from other analgesics and sedatives, such as benzodiazepines, that are commonly co-administered. Using the Diagnostic and Statistical Manual fifth edition (DSM-V) criteria for opioid withdrawal, Wang and colleagues reported an incidence of opioid withdrawal of 17.6% in 54 adult patients in the ICU who received opioids for more than 72 h [51]. Cammarano and colleagues reported an incidence of acute withdrawal using expert consensus criteria of 32% among 28 patients who had been discharged from the ICU after a stay of greater than 7 days [52]. However, these data were identified retrospectively and there was a higher concurrent incidence of benzodiazepine use. Regardless, both studies showed strong correlation between the amount of opioids administered and the development of withdrawal. Patients who developed withdrawal were more likely to have been heavily sedated, received mechanical ventilation for longer durations, and spent longer stays in the ICU compared to patients who did not develop withdrawal. Adjunct medications such as ketamine, clonidine, and dexmedetomidine may help prevent and treat withdrawal yet require further study before their routine use can be recommended. As patients recover from critical illness, it is important to recognize that opioid withdrawal may be common.

Opioid Use After Critical Illness and Chronic Intensive Care Related Pain

Data on opioid prescribing at the time of hospital discharge after an ICU stay have recently become more available. Karamchandani and colleagues reported that 4.1% of veterans who underwent surgery and were admitted to the ICU after the procedure developed new persistent opioid use [53]. Reassuringly, the odds of persistent opioid use decreased by 39% in the 3 years after 2013 when the Veterans Health Administration Opioid Safety Initiative was introduced along with the release of the American College of Critical Care Medicine Guidelines on Pain, Agitation, and Delirium. This decrease was not limited to patients in the ICU, but rather reflected in all veterans. This points to the fact that the decrease in rates of persistent opioid use may be more a reflection of system-wide efforts across the VA to reduce opioid prescribing rather than improved pain management in the ICU, yet further study is warranted. Other studies have shown that prescriptions for opioids can be common on discharge after an ICU stay, ranging from 12% in older adults admitted for respiratory failure or shock to 30.6% in patients who had been placed on enteral opioids (e.g., methadone, oxycodone) while in the ICU [54, 55]. For older adults, opioids are the most common medication inappropriately prescribed on hospital discharge [55].

Relatedly, chronic pain can develop in survivors of critical illness. Termed chronic intensive care related pain (CIRP), it is highly prevalent and a source of ongoing emotional distress. CIRP is defined as persistent pain that is present at least 6 months after ICU admission and was not present before admission [56]. In a study of 295 medical and surgical ICU survivors, 77% and 74% of patients reported persistent pain at 3 and 6 months, respectively [57]. This pain commonly interfered with daily life, as reported in nearly 60% of patients who experienced pain. Higher doses of opioids used in the ICU were not associated with post-ICU pain however while increased age and sepsis were predictors. Chronic pain is a notable component of the post-intensive care syndrome that has been more recently described in patients recovering from critical illness and part of the ongoing challenge faced by survivors. Unfortunately, the effective strategies to prevent and treat CIRP have not been defined.

Conclusion

Intensive care services are fundamental to public health and well-being. This is particularly relevant in the face of an aging population and a greater prevalence of chronic illness. ICUs are a critical touchpoint for the opioid epidemic on multiple fronts. First, opioid use is associated with increased ICU utilization, principally from opioid overdoses that often require life-support. Habitual narcotic users also have poor outcomes from critical illness in general. Second, pain and opioid administration are ubiquitous in the ICU. It is therefore critical for ICUs to understand the safe and effective use of opioids yet not be overly restrictive in their administration. Third, survivors of critical illness have high rates of pain and can become persistent users of opioids, suggesting that there are long-term consequences to acute illness and ICU care. Overall, the intersection of opioids and intensive care is complex and dynamic and requires continual understanding and vigilance to maintain safe practice.

Financial Support None.

Disclosures The author reports no financial or other potential conflicts of interest exist.

References

1. Weil MH, Tang W. From intensive care to critical care medicine: a historical perspective. Am J Respir Crit Care Med. 2011;183(11):1451–3.
2. Barrett ML, Smith MW, Elixhauser A, Honigman LS, Pines JM. Utilization of intensive care services, 2011. HCUP Statistical Brief #185. December 2014. Agency for Healthcare Research and Quality, Rockville, MD. http://www.hcupus.ahrq.gov/reports/statbriefs/sb185-Hospital-Intensive-Care-Units-2011.pdf
3. Adhikari NK, Fowler RA, Bhagwanjee S, Rubenfeld GD. Critical care and the global burden of critical illness in adults. Lancet. 2010;376(9749):1339–46.
4. Dart RC, Surratt HL, Cicero TJ, Parrino MW, Severtson SG, Bucher-Bartelson B, et al. Trends in opioid analgesic abuse and mortality in the United States. N Engl J Med. 2015;372(3):241–8.
5. Hedegaard H, Warner M, Miniño AM. Drug overdose deaths in the United States, 1999–2016. NCHS data brief, no 294. Hyattsville: National Center for Health Statistics; 2017.
6. Centers for Disease Control and Prevention. Opioid Overdose - Understanding the Epidemic. (2017). Available online at: https://www.cdc.gov/drugoverdose/epidemic/index.html. Accessed 1 December 2019)
7. Berterame S, Erthal J, Thomas J, Fellner S, Vosse B, Clare P, et al. Use of and barriers to access to opioid analgesics: a worldwide, regional, and national study. Lancet. 2016;387(10028):1644–56.
8. Campbell JN. 1995 APS presidential address. Pain Forum. 1996;5:85–8.
9. Baker DW. History of the joint Commission's pain standards: lessons for today's prescription opioid epidemic. JAMA. 2017;317:1117–8.
10. Thompson CA. HCAHPS survey to measure pain communication, not management. Am J Health Syst Pharm. 2017;74:1924–6.
11. Hwang CS, Chang H-Y, Alexander GC. Impact of abuse-deterrent OxyContin on prescription opioid utilization. Pharmacoepidemiol Drug Saf. 2015;24(2):197–204.
12. Lee JS, Hu HM, Brummett CM, Syrjamaki JD, Dupree JM, Englesbe MJ, et al. Postoperative opioid prescribing and the pain scores on hospital consumer assessment of healthcare providers and systems survey. JAMA. 2017;16(317(19)):2013–5.
13. Bateman BT, Cole NM, Maeda A, Burns SM, Houle TT, Huybrechts KF, et al. Patterns of opioid prescription and use after cesarean delivery. Obstet Gynecol. 2017;130(1):29–35.

14. CDC Guideline for Prescribing Opioids for Chronic Pain — United States, 2016. MMWR Recomm Rep [Internet]. 2016 [cited 2019 Dec 11];65. Available from: https://www.cdc.gov/mmwr/volumes/65/rr/rr6501e1.htm
15. Haffajee RL, Jena AB, Weiner SG. Mandatory use of prescription drug monitoring programs. JAMA. 2015;313(9):891–2.
16. Blendon RJ, Benson JM. The public and the opioid-abuse epidemic. N Engl J Med. 2018;378(5):407–11.
17. Stevens JP, Wall MJ, Novack L, Marshall J, Hsu DJ, Howell MD. The critical care crisis of opioid overdoses in the United States. Ann Am Thorac Soc. 2017;14(12):1803–9.
18. Edelman EJ, Gordon KS, Crothers K, Akgün K, Bryant KJ, Becker WC, et al. Association of prescribed opioids with increased risk of community-acquired pneumonia among patients with and without HIV. JAMA Intern Med. 2019;179(3):297–304.
19. Cannon R, Bozeman M, Miller KR, Smith JW, Harbrecht B, Franklin G, et al. The prevalence and impact of prescription controlled substance use among injured patients at a level I trauma center. J Trauma Acute Care Surg. 2014;76(1):172–5.
20. Munch T, Christiansen CF, Pedersen L, Sørensen HT. Impact of preadmission opioid treatment on 1-year mortality following nonsurgical intensive care. Crit Care Med. 2018;46(6):860–8.
21. Federal Drug Administration. Joint Meeting of the Drug Safety and Risk Management (DSaRM) Advisory Committee and Anesthetic and Analgesic Drug Products Advisory Committee (AADPAC). 2019. https://www.fda.gov/media/127780/download. Accessed 1 Dec 2019.
22. Boudreau D, Von Korff M, Rutter CM, Saunders K, Ray GT, Sullivan MD, et al. Trends in De-facto long-term opioid therapy for chronic non-Cancer pain. Pharmacoepidemiol Drug Saf. 2009;18(12):1166–75.
23. Pandya U, O'Mara MS, Wilson W, Opalek J, Lieber M. Impact of preexisting opioid use on injury mechanism, type, and outcome. J Surg Res. 2015;198(1):7–12.
24. Reichheld AM, Hills-Evans K, Sheehan JK, Tocci NX, Tandon M, Hsu D, et al. A national survey of approaches to manage the ICU patient with opioid use disorder. J Crit Care. 2019;54:42–7.
25. Chanques G, Sebbane M, Barbotte E, Viel E, Eledjam J-J, Jaber S. A prospective study of pain at rest: incidence and characteristics of an unrecognized symptom in surgical and trauma versus medical intensive care unit patients. Anesthesiology. 2007;107(5):858–60.
26. Puntillo KA, Max A, Timsit J-F, Vignoud L, Chanques G, Robleda G, et al. Determinants of procedural pain intensity in the intensive care unit. The Europain® study. Am J Respir Crit Care Med. 2013;189(1):39–47.
27. Turner JS, Briggs SJ, Springhorn HE, Potgieter PD. Patients' recollection of intensive care unit experience. Crit Care Med. 1990;18(9):966–8.
28. Devlin JW, Skrobik Y, Gélinas C, Needham DM, Slooter AJC, Pandharipande PP, et al. Clinical practice guidelines for the prevention and management of pain, agitation/sedation, delirium, immobility, and sleep disruption in adult patients in the ICU. Crit Care Med. 2018;46(9):e825.
29. Baker DW. History of the joint commission's pain standards: lessons for today's prescription opioid epidemic. JAMA. 2017;317(11):1117–8.
30. Herzig SJ, Rothberg MB, Cheung M, Ngo LH, Marcantonio ER. Opioid utilization and opioid-related adverse events in non-surgical patients in U.S. hospitals. J Hosp Med. 2014;9(2):73–81.
31. Donohue JM, Kennedy JN, Seymour CW, Girard TD, Lo-Ciganic W-H, Kim CH, et al. Patterns of opioid administration among opioid-naive inpatients and associations with postdischarge opioid use. Ann Intern Med. 2019;171(2):81–90.
32. Shah A, Hayes CJ, Martin BC. Factors influencing long-term opioid use among opioid naive patients: an examination of initial prescription characteristics and pain etiologies. J Pain. 2017;18(11):1374–83.
33. Neuman MD, Bateman BT, Wunsch H. Inappropriate opioid prescription after surgery. Lancet. 2019;393(10180):1547–57.
34. Acute Pain Management Guideline Panel (1992a). Acute pain management: Operative or medical procedures and trauma. Clinical Practice Guideline No. 1. AHCPR Publication No.

92–0032. Rockville, MD: Agency for Health Care Policy and Research, U.S. Department of Health and Human Services, Public Health Services.
35. Strøm T, Martinussen T, Toft P. A protocol of no sedation for critically ill patients receiving mechanical ventilation: a randomised trial. Lancet. 2010;375(9713):475–80.
36. Barnes-Daly MA, Phillips G, Ely EW. Improving hospital survival and reducing brain dysfunction at seven California community hospitals: implementing PAD guidelines via the ABCDEF bundle in 6,064 patients. Crit Care Med. 2017;45(2):171–8.
37. Girard TD, Kress JP, Fuchs BD, Thomason JW, Schweickert WD, Pun BT, et al. Efficacy and safety of a paired sedation and ventilator weaning protocol for mechanically ventilated patients in intensive care (awakening and breathing controlled trial): a randomised controlled trial. Lancet. 2008;371(9607):126–34.
38. Burry LD, Williamson DR, Perreault MM, Rose L, Cook DJ, Ferguson ND, et al. Analgesic, sedative, antipsychotic, and neuromuscular blocker use in Canadian intensive care units: a prospective, multicentre, observational study. Can J Anaesth. 2014;61(7):619–30.
39. Mehta S, Burry L, Cook D, Fergusson D, Steinberg M, Granton J, et al. Daily sedation interruption in mechanically ventilated critically ill patients cared for with a sedation protocol: a randomized controlled trial. JAMA. 2012;308(19):1985–92.
40. Payen J-F, Chanques G, Mantz J, Hercule C, Auriant I, Leguillou J-L, et al. Current practices in sedation and analgesia for mechanically ventilated critically ill patients A prospective Multicenter patient-based study. Anesthesiology. 2007;106(4):687–95.
41. Jung S-Y, Lee HJ. Utilisation of medications among elderly patients in intensive care units: a cross-sectional study using a nationwide claims database. BMJ Open. 2019;9(7):e026605.
42. Wunsch H, Kahn JM, Kramer AA, Rubenfeld GD. Use of intravenous infusion sedation among mechanically ventilated patients in the United States. Crit Care Med. 2009;37(12):3031–9.
43. Pisani M, Bramley K, Vest M, Akgün K, Araujo K, Murphy T. Patterns of opiate, benzodiazepine, and antipsychotic drug dosing in older patients in a medical intensive care unit. Am J Crit Care. 2013;22(5):E62–9.
44. Dahaba AA, Grabner T, Rehak PH, List WF, Metzler H. Remifentanil versus morphine analgesia and sedation for mechanically ventilated critically ill patients: a randomized double blind study. Anesthesiology. 2004;101(3):640–6.
45. Wanzuita R, Poli-de-Figueiredo LF, Pfuetzenreiter F, Cavalcanti AB, Westphal GA. Replacement of fentanyl infusion by enteral methadone decreases the weaning time from mechanical ventilation: a randomized controlled trial. Crit Care. 2012;16(2):R49.
46. Beers RA, Calimlim JR, Uddoh E, Esposito BF, Camporesi EM. A comparison of the cost-effectiveness of remifentanil versus fentanyl as an adjuvant to general anesthesia for outpatient gynecologic surgery. Anesth Analg. 2000;91(6):1420–5.
47. Angus DC, Barnato AE, Linde-Zwirble WT, Weissfeld LA, Watson RS, Rickert T, et al. Use of intensive care at the end of life in the United States: an epidemiologic study. Crit Care Med. 2004;32(3):638–43.
48. Mularski RA, Osborne ML. End-of-life care in the critically ill geriatric population. Crit Care Clin. 2003;19(4):789–810. viii
49. Connors AF, Dawson NV, Desbiens NA, Fulkerson WJ, Goldman L, Knaus WA, et al. A controlled trial to improve care for seriously III hospitalized patients: the study to understand prognoses and preferences for outcomes and risks of treatments (SUPPORT). JAMA. 1995;274(20):1591–8.
50. Chiu AW, Contreras S, Mehta S, Korman J, Perreault MM, Williamson DR, et al. Iatrogenic opioid withdrawal in critically ill patients: a review of assessment tools and management. Ann Pharmacother. 2017;51(12):1099–111.
51. Wang PP, Huang E, Feng X, Bray C-A, Perreault MM, Rico P, et al. Opioid-associated iatrogenic withdrawal in critically ill adult patients: a multicenter prospective observational study. Ann Intensive Care. 2017;7(1):88.

52. Cammarano WB, Pittet JF, Weitz S, Schlobohm RM, Marks JD. Acute withdrawal syndrome related to the administration of analgesic and sedative medications in adult intensive care unit patients. Crit Care Med. 1998;26(4):676–84.
53. Karamchandani K, Pyati S, Bryan W, Pepin M, Lehman EB, Krishnamoorthy V, et al. New persistent opioid use after postoperative intensive care in US veterans. JAMA Surg. 2019;154(8):778–80.
54. Kram B, Weigel KM, Kuhrt M, Gilstrap DL. Discharge prescribing of enteral opioids after initiation as a weaning strategy from continuous opioid infusions in the intensive care unit. J Opioid Manag. 2018;14(1):35–42.
55. Morandi A, Vasilevskis E, Pandharipande PP, Girard TD, Solberg LM, Neal EB, et al. Inappropriate medication prescriptions in elderly adults surviving an intensive care unit hospitalization. J Am Geriatr Soc. 2013;61(7):1128–34.
56. Baumbach P, Götz T, Günther A, Weiss T, Meissner W. Prevalence and characteristics of chronic intensive care-related pain: the role of severe sepsis and septic shock. Crit Care Med. 2016;44(6):1129–37.
57. Hayhurst CJ, Jackson JC, Archer KR, Thompson JL, Chandrasekhar R, Hughes CG. Pain and its long-term interference of daily life after critical illness. Anesth Analg. 2018;127(3):690–7.

Chapter 2
Assessment of Pain in the Intensive Care Unit

Athir H. Morad and Robert D. Stevens

Pain in the Intensive Care Unit

The pain response is one of the most important phylogenic adaptations in evolution [1]. The extreme rarity of a congenital insensitivity to pain (e.g. autosomal recessive SCN9A gene mutation) underscores the importance of an intact pain response for maintaining tissue integrity and survival of the organism from early infancy [2]. Critically ill patients are exposed to a wide range of painful stimuli—including primary disease, organ failure, surgery, instrumentation and devices, and confinement to bed. It follows that effective pain management is a fundamental priority in intensive care medicine. However, the intensive care unit (ICU) presents many challenges to effective assessment and treatment of pain. Patients may have impaired capacity to communicate pain due to intubation, sedation, induced paralysis, or brain dysfunction. Overmedication with analgesics can mask symptoms of life-threatening processes, while insufficient analgesia can overwhelm patients and distract from the diagnosis of concurrent and potentially significant

A. H. Morad (✉)
Departments of Anesthesiology and Critical Care Medicine, Johns Hopkins University School of Medicine, Baltimore, MD, USA
e-mail: morada@jhmi.edu

R. D. Stevens
Departments of Anesthesiology and Critical Care Medicine, Johns Hopkins University School of Medicine, Baltimore, MD, USA

Departments of Neurology, Johns Hopkins University School of Medicine, Baltimore, MD, USA

Departments of Neurosurgery, Johns Hopkins University School of Medicine, Baltimore, MD, USA

Departments of Radiology, Johns Hopkins University School of Medicine, Baltimore, MD, USA
e-mail: rstevens@jhmi.edu

J. L. Pascual, T. G. Gaulton (eds.), *Opioid Use in Critical Care*,
https://doi.org/10.1007/978-3-030-77399-1_2

illness or injuries. Additionally, growing concerns over opioid safety and the harms of addiction, discussed throughout this book, underscore the need for prudence in prescribing opioids. The cornerstone to effective management of pain is to measure it. In this chapter, we review different instruments used for the assessment of pain in the ICU.

Neuroanatomy of Pain

A comprehensive account of spinal cord dorsal horn integration and modulation of nociceptive signals is beyond the scope of this chapter. The mechanisms underlying reflex withdrawal from a painful stimulus have been elucidated in some detail. When peripheral nociceptors are activated by a noxious stimulus, neural signals reach the dorsal ganglia adjacent to the spinal column and enter the dorsal horns of the spinal cord. Interneurons transmit the signals to motor neurons within the anterior horn of the spinal cord to trigger an immediate, reflexive, motor response to deflect from the nociceptive source (Fig. 2.1). The spinal cord segment network also projects to cortical pain centers via the spinothalamic tract which conducts signals from the dorsal horn to the thalamus and then to the cortex where the perceptual and emotional responses to pain are generated. The cerebral cortex in turn modulates pain signaling in the spinal cord via descending pathways (Fig. 2.2) [3]. In addition to nociception from somatic structures throughout the periphery, visceral afferent stimuli caused by stretching, spasm, ischemia, or inflammation of pelvic, abdominal, thoracic, and cervico-facial organs can also be transmitted via the dorsal horn of the spinal cord to elicit a pain response.

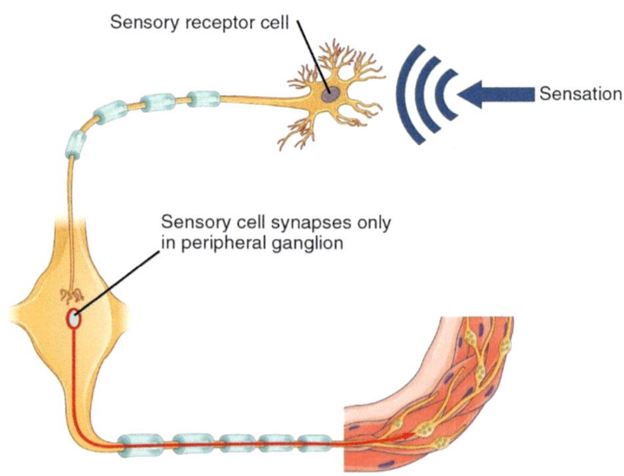

Fig. 2.1 Pain Reflex Arc (Modified Source: "1507 Short and Long Reflexes. jpg," by OpenStax College, https://upload.wikimedia.org/wikipedia/commons/6/68/1507_Short_and_Long_Reflexes.jpg, Licensed under the Creative Commons Attribution 3.0, https://creativecommons.org/licenses/by/3.0/deed.en)

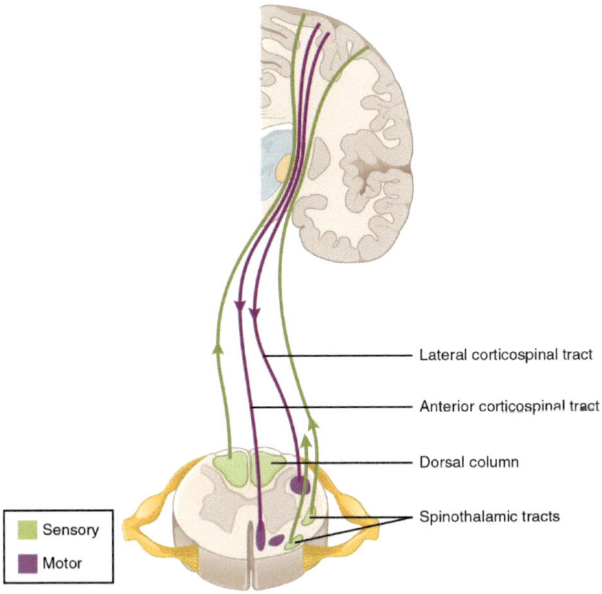

Fig. 2.2 Spinothalamic tract. (Source: 1615 Locations Sinal Fiber Tracts.jpg by Open Stax College. https://upload.wikimedia.org/wikipedia/commons/4/40/1615_Locations_Spinal_Fiber_Tracts.jpg. Licensed under the Creative Commons Attribution 3.0, https://creativecommons.org/licenses/by/3.0/deed.en)

Categories of Pain in the ICU

The main categories of pain are acute pain, chronic pain, and neuropathic pain.

Acute pain refers to a predictable physiological response to a chemical, thermal, or mechanical injury caused by surgery, trauma, or acute illness [4]. While the term "acute" suggests a brief duration, persistent nociceptive signaling may perpetuate acute pain for up to 6 months [5]. Therefore, the acute terminology refers to the type and initiation phase of the pain response rather its duration. The precise location of acute somatic pain is readily identifiable and may be described as sharp or stabbing. Acute visceral pain is generally more difficult to localize and can even trigger a "referred pain" phenomenon whereby the perceived location of pain is remote from the actual source for pain. For example, myocardial infarction may be experienced as shoulder or jaw pain. Visceral pain is typically perceived a dull ache, tightness, or cramp sensation.

Chronic pain is defined as pain that is sustained beyond the period of tissue injury and healing. In this situation, abnormal signaling from peripheral somatic or visceral nociceptors persists in the absence of direct stimulus, a phenomenon attributed to maladaptive neuroplasticity within the CNS. Definitions for the minimal duration for chronic pain vary from 3 months to beyond 6 months. Patients who experience chronic pain often develop associated anxiety and depression [6]. The symptomatology in chronic pain may have somatic, visceral, or neuropathic features. In addition, patients may experience symptoms of *allodynia*, whereby a non-noxious stimulus is perceived as pain, or *hyperalgesia* in which there is an exaggerated response to a noxious stimulus. Hyperalgesia becomes especially problematic when patients who have preexisting chronic pain syndromes experience acute pain, a phenomenon described as "acute on chronic pain" [7, 8].

Neuropathic pain results from direct injury to nerves in the peripheral or central nervous system. Neuropathic pain is described as burning or tingling in nature. Neuropathic pain can be acute or chronic. Since healing of nervous tissues occurs more slowly than in other tissues, neuropathic pain is often associated with a more sustained or chronic course. In contrast to somatic and visceral chronic pain which occur in the absence of stimulus, neuropathic pain resulting from persistent peripheral nerve injury may be considered chronic in nature [9].

Causes of Pain in the ICU

Pain experienced by patients in the intensive care unit (ICU) can be categorized as non-procedural or procedural. Non-procedural pain is the unprovoked discomfort experienced in over half of critically ill patients [10]. Procedural pain is discomfort that results from interventions which are commonly performed in the ICU. Examples include phlebotomy, invasive brain monitoring, central venous catheter placement, arterial catheterization, intubation, mechanical ventilation, naso- or orogastric tube placement, different endoscopic procedures in the lungs or gastrointestinal tract, tracheostomy, paracentesis, and chest tube insertion (reported to be the most painful of all procedures in the ICU). Additionally, routine and necessary provider care such as physical examination as well as nursing care such as bathing, turning, and bed manipulation may be extremely painful to the critically ill patient. Compared to pain at rest, procedural pain is generally more severe, estimated on average to have twice the intensity of non-procedural pain [11]. In aggregate, procedural and non-procedural pain are extremely common in the ICU and may be underreported, particularly by patients with impaired communication such as those who have brain injury or are undergoing sedation or mechanical ventilation.

A subpopulation of critically ill patients with a high likelihood of impaired communication are patients with acute brain injury. Pain in these patients may be underreported due to often lacking documentation by providers on pain assessments and/or the withholding of treatment with potentially sedating analgesics [12]. Oversedation can mask and potentially delay the diagnosis of acute neurological changes. While this may provide a rationale to avoid analgesics, the unintended consequence is an inadequate accounting of pain and thus a high risk of insufficient analgesia in brain-injured patients [13–15].

Conversely, another common obstacle to effective assessment and treatment of pain in the ICU is excessive sedation. While the potential harms of over-sedation and immobility are outside the scope of this chapter, overmedication with sedatives may mask pain rather than effectively treat it. Differentiating between clinical states associated with sedation and analgesia is a challenge for clinicians in the ICU. In one study, investigators evaluated postoperative patients with sedation and pain scores at set intervals. Patients who were susceptible to the sedative effects of opioids and more somnolent postoperatively reported higher pain scores than non-somnolent patients when aroused and queried, and they recalled higher postoperative pain on the following day than patients who experienced less sedation postoperatively. This study highlights the fact that behavioral evidence of sedation, even as a side effect of opioids, does not necessarily correlate with analgesia [16].

Differentiation Between Pain and Other Behavioral Syndromes

A fundamental clinical challenge for the ICU clinician is the potential for overlap between the signs of pain and other neurobehavioral states commonly encountered such as delirium, anxiety, and agitation. A comprehensive review of these topics is addressed in a recent expert consensus statement issued by the Society for Critical Care Medicine [17]. These guidelines discuss the available evidence for distinguishing these complex behavioral syndromes in order to facilitate more accurate diagnosis and treatment.

There are five criteria for the diagnosis of delirium according to the American Psychiatric Association Diagnostic and Statistical manual of Mental Disorders, fifth edition [18]. The first is a disturbance in attention. The second is that the disturbance develops over the course of hours or days and fluctuates throughout the day. The third criterion involves a change in cognition such as difficulty with memory, orientation, or language. The fourth is that the condition cannot be explained by another preexisting or developing neurocognitive disorder. The last criterion is that the condition is the result of a medical condition, substance intoxication or withdrawal, medication side effect, or due to multiple etiologies. Different screening tools are utilized clinically to assess for delirium in the ICU, the most widely implemented of which is the Confusion Assessment Method (CAM) and the Confusion Assessment Method in the ICU (CAM-ICU). According to one estimate, the CAM-ICU had a sensitivity of 83% and a specificity of 100% in detecting delirium when compared against the DSM-V as a standard (Table 2.1, Fig. 2.3) [19].

Anxiety is defined as a state of apprehension, agitation, increased motor attention, autonomic arousal, and fearful withdrawal [20]. Several diagnostic instruments have been validated to assess anxiety. Among the tools are the State-Trait Anxiety Inventory (STAI), the Profile of Mood States (POMS), the Positive and Negative Affect Schedule (PANAS), and the Visual Analog Scale (VAS-A) [21]. Unlike the widely used CAM-ICU instrument, the routine adoption of anxiety assessment tools in the ICU has been quite limited. According to one study, patients on mechanical ventilation reported variable degrees of anxiety throughout their ICU

Table 2.1 DSM-V diagnostic criteria for delirium [40]

1. A disturbance in attention
2. The disturbance develops over the course of hours or days and fluctuates throughout the day
3. A change in condition such as difficulty with memory, orientation, or language
4. The condition cannot be explained by another preexisting or developing cognitive disorder
5. The condition is not the result of a medical condition such as acute intoxication, medication side effect, or withdrawal from a medication or substance

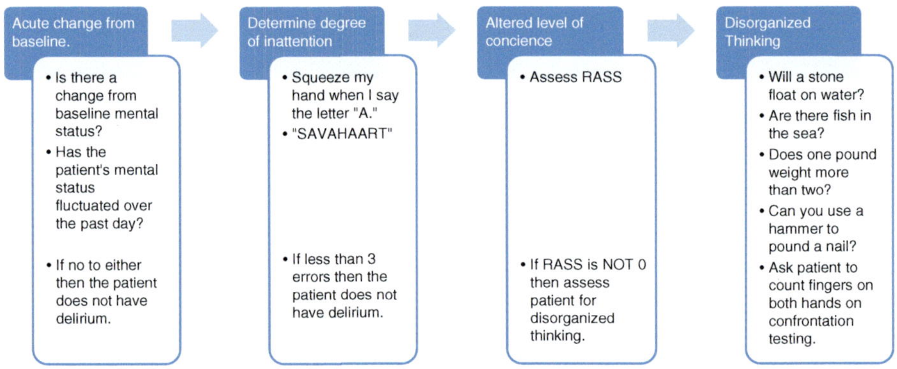

Fig. 2.3 CAM-ICU survey [41]

length of stay, without a clear pattern of resolution [22]. Recent longitudinal cohort studies of post-ICU survivors suggest an association between anxiety states in the ICU and the development of long-term post-traumatic stress disorder (PTSD) [23].

Agitation is a behavioral phenotype of dramatically increased motor activity which may be observed in a subset of critically ill patients with or without pain. The Richmond Agitation Scale (RASS) is a 10-point scale ranging from +4 indicating combative behavior, a score of 0 representing a calm alert state, and a score of −5 assigned to unarousable sedation [24]. The RASS score is a global indicator of neurobehavioral status and should not be regarded as a measure of pain.

History of Pain Scales

Initially intended as investigative tools for experimental psychology, pain scales attempted to quantify the subjective experience of pain in a burgeoning field of study called quantitative sensory testing (circa mid twentieth century). The original studies evaluated pain thresholds of test subjects by determining the amount of stimulation a human could tolerate before calling for the termination of the stimulus. Subsequently, standardized descriptors of pain were developed by investigators to fit within various categories of pain that were being characterized. One example is the McGill Pain Questionnaire that incorporates a large selection of terms to describe pain [25]. (Table 2.2) Pain scales began to proliferate thereafter from simple four-point scales (no pain, mild, moderate, severe pain) to the 11-point numerical rating scale (NRS) (0–10) commonly used in medical practice today. By the 1960s, the visual analog scale (VAS) had been proposed to allow for the non-verbal reporting of pain. The Wong-Baker FACES® Pain Rating Scale, arguably the best known pain measurement tool, was developed for pediatric patients (Fig. 2.4). This scale was developed in the early 1980s to help children express the degree of pain they experienced irrespective of their ability to communicate verbally or abstract ability to understand the visual analog scale. Variations of the scale were subsequently applied to adults.

Table 2.2 McGill pain questionnaire descriptive terms [25]

Flickering	Tugging	Fearful	Tight
Quivering	Pulling	Frightful	Numb
Pulsing	Wrenching	Terrifying	Drawing
Throbbing	Hot	Punishing	Squeezing
Beating	Burning	Grueling	Tearing
Pounding	Scalding	Cruel	Cool
Jumping	Searing	Vicious	Cold
Flashing	Tingling	Killing	Freezing
Shooting	Itchy	Wretched	Nagging
Pricking	Smarting	Blinding	Nauseating
Boring	Stinging	Annoying	Agonizing
Drilling	Dull	Troublesome	Dreadful
Stabbing	Sore	Miserable	Torturing
Lancinating	Hurting	Intense	PPI
Sharp	Aching	Unbearable	No pain
Cutting	Heavy	Spreading	Mild
Lacerating	Tender	Radiating	Discomforting
Pinching	Taut	Penetrating	Distressing
Pressing	Rasping	Piercing	Horrible
Gnawing	Splitting		Excruciating
Cramping	Tiring		
Crushing	Exhausting		
	Sickening		
	Suffocating		
Brief	Rhythmic	Continuous	
Momentary	Periodic	Steady	
Transient	Intermittent	Constant	

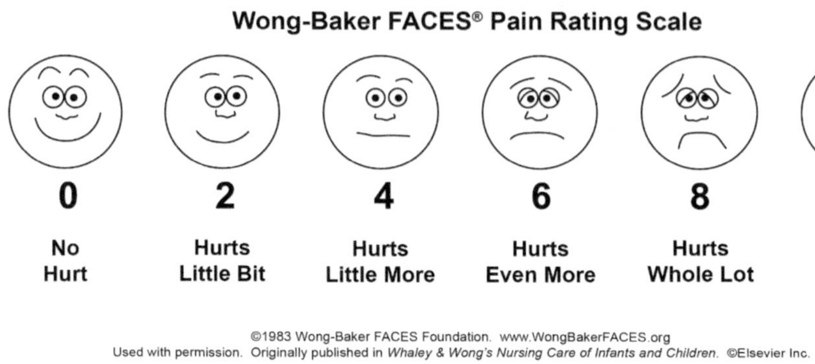

Fig. 2.4 Wong-Baker FACES (Wong-Baker FACES Foundation (2020). Wong-Baker FACES® Pain Rating Scale. Retrieved [2/25/2020] with permission from http://www.WongBakerFACES.org)

Pain Scales in Current Practice

Several tools have been validated for the assessment of pain in the intensive care unit (ICU). These tools can be divided into two categories. Self-report scales are intended for patients who are able to communicate. Behavioral assessment tools are used in patients who are unable to communicate. Protocol-based pain surveys in the ICU have been associated with reductions in pain scores, opioid requirements, duration of mechanical ventilation, and ICU length of stay [26].

The most direct means of assessing a patient's pain is through verbal communication. When patient and provider share the same language, pain can be communicated and measured with the Visual Analog Scale (VAS), the Verbal Descriptor Scale (VDS), and the Numeric Rating Scale (NRS) [27] (Fig. 2.5). The VAS is administered by showing the patient a 10-cm line that is labeled with no pain on the left and worst imaginable pain on the right. On confrontation testing, the patient is asked to mark the point on the line that represents their pain. The most commonly administered VDS in the ICU attempts to categorize the spectrum of pain by offering five degrees of pain to choose from. The pain categories are typically aligned in the same direction as the VAS and include no pain, mild pain, moderate pain, severe pain, and extreme pain. The NRS covers a more granular spectrum of pain scores, typically 0 (indicating no pain) to 10 (worst pain). The VAS requires visual interaction and can be administered to patients who are intubated, while the VDS and the NRS can be administered in writing or verbally to patients who are not intubated. The verbally communicated scales offer the added benefit that they can be administered on the telephone following hospital discharge for long-term studies [28].

Behavioral assessment tools are reserved for patients who are unable to accurately or reliably report the pain they experience. The two most utilized pain scales are the Behavioral Pain Scale (BPS) for intubated and non-intubated patients and the Critical-Care Pain Observation Tool (CPOT) [29, 30]. Since the validation of these scales, several other modified scales have been reported. The Behavioral Pain Scale (BPS) was one of the original instruments intended to assess pain in non-verbal, mechanically intubated patients [29]. It evaluates three behavioral categories

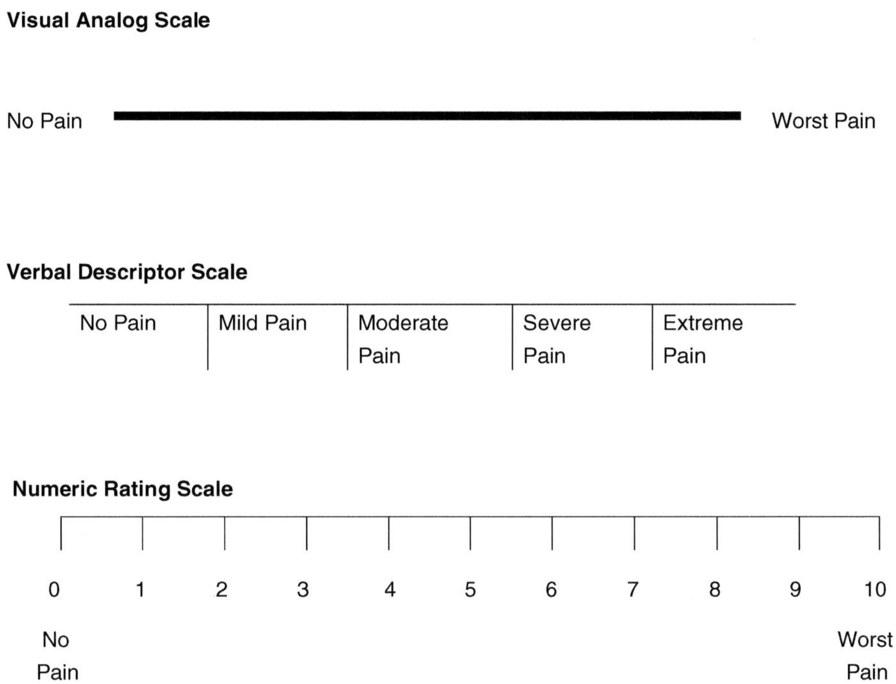

Fig. 2.5 Self-report scales

Table 2.3 Behavioral pain scale [29]

Item	Description	Score
Facial Expression	Relaxed	1
	Partially tightened (e.g., brow lowering)	2
	Fully tightened (e.g., eyelid closing)	3
	Grimacing	4
Upper Limbs	No movement	1
	Partially bent	2
	Fully bent with finger flexion	3
	Permanently retracted	4
Compliance with Ventilation	Tolerating movement	1
	Coughing but tolerating ventilation for most of the time	2
	Fighting ventilator	3
	Unable to control ventilation	4
Total		3–12

and assigns a score of 1–4 for each. The categories are facial expression, movement of upper limbs, and tolerance of mechanical ventilation (Table 2.3). The CPOT is another validated instrument that assesses behavioral pain according to four categories: facial expression, body movements, muscle tension, and tolerance of the ventilator (intubated patients) or vocalization (non-intubated patients) . The categories

Table 2.4 The critical-care pain observation tool (CPOT) [30]

Indicator	Description	Score
Facial expression	No muscular tension observed	Relaxed, neutral 0
	Presence of frowning, brow lowering, orbit tightening, and levator contraction	Tense 1
	All of the above facial movements plus eyelid tightly closed	Grimacing 2
Body movements	Does not move at all (does not necessarily mean absence of pain)	Absence of movements 0
	Slow, cautious movements, touching or rubbing the pain site, seeking attention through movements	Protection 1
	Pulling tube, attempting to sit up, moving limbs/thrashing, not following commands, striking at staff, trying to climb out of bed	Restlessness 2
Muscle tension evaluation by passive flexion and extension of upper extremities	No resistance to passive movements	Relaxed 0
	Resistance to passive movements	Tense, rigid 1
	Strong resistance to passive movements, inability to complete them	Very tense or rigid 2
Compliance with the ventilator (intubated patients) OR Vocalization (extubated patients)	Alarms not activated, easy ventilation	Tolerating ventilator or 0 movement
	Alarms stop spontaneously	Coughing but tolerating 1
	Asynchrony: blocking ventilation, alarms frequently activated	Fighting ventilator 2
	Talking in normal tone or no sound	Talking in normal tone or no sound 0
	Sighing, moaning	Sighing, moaning 1
	Crying out, sobbing	Crying out, sobbing 2
Total Range		0–8

are scored 0–2, with a range of possible sums from 0 (no pain) to 8 (extreme pain) [29, 30] (Table 2.4).

Despite the diversity of pain scales for the evaluation of patients with or without the capacity to communicate, there is a paucity of pain instruments which differentiate between the types of pain, that is, acute, neuropathic, chronic, and acute on chronic pain. This more granular degree of pain assessment has been used primarily in clinical research protocols, but it may be essential for the more precise delivery of targeted analgesics and the potential for opioid sparing analgesics.

Surrogate Indicators of Pain

In addition to the habitual pain assessment in individual ICU patients, surrogate assessments by proxy from family members, degree of opioid consumption, or by extent of physiologic perturbations have also been proposed [31, 32].

Proxy pain assessment by family members has been the subject of considerable investigation without any conclusive validation. Family members are considered inconsistent in their reporting and tend to over-estimate the degree of pain. In response, The Society for Critical Care Medicine does not endorse the substitution of family involvement for the ICU team's utilization of pain assessment tools [17, 31].

Degree of opioid consumption has been proposed as a measure of pain. Proponents of this approach argue that only the patient is aware of his or her analgesic requirements and, therefore, clinicians can measure cumulative opioid consumption as a marker for pain. Critics argue that considerable individual variability exists with respect to pain thresholds and opioid tolerance and that inference based on opioid consumption introduces a greater potential for Type I error [33]. Regardless, the use of a patient's opioid consumption as a real-time indicator of pain requires advanced statistical modeling and has also not been convincingly demonstrated.

Physiological perturbations such as tachycardia, heart rate variability, tachypnea, hypertension, diaphoresis, and mydriasis individually or in combination all serve as indicators of pain, but thus far they have not proven accurate or reliable in precisely measuring or identifying pain [17]. Nevertheless, the recent introduction of pupillometry to clinical practice has created an opportunity to study this technology as a potential marker for pain. According to one estimate, a 19% or greater change in pupillary size correlates with a Behavioral Pain Score of greater than 3 with 100% sensitivity and 77% specificity [34]. While the availability of pupillometry is not yet mainstream and not applicable to all critically ill patients in various physiologic states, the technology is at least promising for now.

At no time has the need for an alternative to verbal and behavioral pain assessment been more evident than during the COVID-19 pandemic. Since the administration of paralytics has been common practice in the management of patients with severe ARDS, clinicians have lost the ability to assess pain or the depth of sedation objectively. Concurrently, a growing consensus has emerged that critically ill patients with COVID-19 often require higher doses of analgesics and sedatives than non-COVID-19-infected patients. According to one estimate, patients with COVID-19 consume three times the amount of opioids compared to a non-COVID cohort in the ICU, albeit without any objective endpoints for titration [35]. Heart rate variability monitoring and processed EEG hold potential utility in quantifying pain and sedation in these patients, but the investigation of these modalities is just beginning to emerge [36].

Importance of Accurate Pain Phenotyping and Precision Analgesia

The end of the last century brought about an increased awareness of pain and the declaration by the Joint Commission that pain was to be measured as the fifth vital sign and treated in every patient [37]. This initiative was buttressed by the World Health Organization's (WHO) endorsement of the "pain ladder," a concept that emphasized the diligent management of pain, particularly in patients with cancer. These ambitious campaigns to increase awareness and management of pain have since been criticized as contributing to the opioid epidemic seen in the first decades of this century. As a result, many organizations including the Joint Commission and the WHO have issued revised recommendations that place greater emphasis on the risks of opioid overmedication and the risk of addiction and fatal overdose [38, 39].

Rightful concerns over the adverse effects of opioids should not however deter ICU providers from the goal of alleviating suffering at the most critical moments of patients' lives. Rather, a more precise measurement of pain and focused delivery of analgesics should be pursued within a deliberate opioid sparing strategy. The first step in this pursuit remains the meticulous evaluation of pain. However, available numerical, visual, and behavioral pain scales lack accuracy. Research is needed to discover and validate biomarkers which will expand the discriminative power of existing pain assessment tools and differentiate which patients are responsive to the analgesic effects of available treatments, as well as which patients are overly susceptible to the side effects of the same medications. This might be achieved via genotyping, serologic specimens, electrophysiologic, and imaging data that capture with higher accuracy the type and degree of pain experienced by critically ill patients, with the goal of achieving precision in analgesia.

References

1. Lummaa V, Vuorisalo T, Barr RG, Lehtonen L. Why cry? Adaptive significance of intensive crying in human infants. Evol Hum Behav. 1998;19:193–202.
2. Oertel B, Lotsch J. Genetic mutations that prevent pain: implications for future pain medication. Pharmacogenomics. 2008;9(2):179–94.
3. Carr DB, Goudas LC. Acute pain. Lancet. 1999;353(9169):2051–8.
4. Federation of State Medical Boards. Guidelines for the chronic use of opioid analgesics. 2017. Available at: https://www.fsmb.org/siteassets/advocacy/policies/opioid_guidelines_as_adopted_april-2017_final.pdf. Accessed 2 Dec 2020.
5. Merskey H, Bogduk N. Classification of chronic pain: descriptions of chronic pain syndromes and definitions of pain terms task force on taxonomy of the International Association for the Study of Pain Seattle. Washington, DC: IASP Press; 1994.
6. Elliott TE, Renier CM, Palcher JA. Chronic pain, depression, and quality of life: correlations and predictive value of the SF-36. Pain Med. 2003;4(4):331–9.
7. Hina N, Fletcher D, Poindessous-Jazat F, Martinez V. Hyperalgesia induced by low-dose opioid treatment before orthopaedic surgery: an observational case-control study. Eur J Anaesthesiol. 2015;32(4):255–61.

8. McAnally H. Rationale for and approach to preoperative opioid weaning: a preoperative optimization protocol. Perioper Med (Lond). 2017;6:19-017-0079-y. eCollection 2017
9. Institute of Medicine . Committee on advancing pain research, care, and education. Relieving pain in America. 2011:364.
10. Chanques G, Sebbane M, Barbotte E, Viel E, Eledjam JJ, Jaber S. A prospective study of pain at rest: incidence and characteristics of an unrecognized symptom in surgical and trauma versus medical intensive care unit patients. Anesthesiology. 2007;107(5):858–60.
11. Puntillo KA, Max A, Timsit JF, Vignoud L, Chanques G, Robleda G, et al. Determinants of procedural pain intensity in the intensive care unit. The Europain(R) study. Am J Respir Crit Care Med. 2014;189(1):39–47.
12. Stoneham MD, Walters FJ. Post-operative analgesia for craniotomy patients: current attitudes among neuroanaesthetists. Eur J Anaesthesiol. 1995;12(6):571–5.
13. Gottschalk A, Berkow LC, Stevens RD, Mirski M, Thompson RE, White ED, et al. Prospective evaluation of pain and analgesic use following major elective intracranial surgery. J Neurosurg. 2007;106(2):210–6.
14. Morad AH, Winters BD, Yaster M, Stevens RD, White ED, Thompson RE, et al. Efficacy of intravenous patient-controlled analgesia after supratentorial intracranial surgery: a prospective randomized controlled trial. Clinical article. J Neurosurg. 2009;111(2):343–50.
15. Morad A, Winters B, Stevens R, White E, Weingart J, Yaster M, et al. The efficacy of intravenous patient-controlled analgesia after intracranial surgery of the posterior fossa: a prospective, randomized controlled trial. Anesth Analg. 2012;114(2):416–23.
16. Lentschener C, Tostivint P, White PF, Gentili ME, Ozier Y. Opioid-induced sedation in the postanesthesia care unit does not insure adequate pain relief: a case-control study. Anesth Analg. 2007;105(4):1143–7. table of contents
17. Devlin JW, Skrobik Y, Gelinas C, Needham DM, Slooter AJC, Pandharipande PP, et al. Clinical practice guidelines for the prevention and management of pain, agitation/sedation, delirium, immobility, and sleep disruption in adult patients in the ICU. Crit Care Med. 2018;46(9):e825–73.
18. American Psychiatric Association, American Psychiatric Association. DSM-5 task force. Diagnostic and statistical manual of mental disorders: DSM-5. 5th ed. Washington, DC: American Psychiatric Association; 2013.
19. Chanques G, Ely EW, Garnier O, Perrigault F, Eloi A, Carr J, et al. The 2014 updated version of the confusion assessment method for the intensive care unit compared to the 5th version of the diagnostic and statistical manual of mental disorders and other current methods used by intensivists. Ann Intensive Care. 2018;8(1):33-018-0377-7.
20. McCartney JR, Boland RJ. Anxiety and delirium in the intensive care unit. Crit Care Clin. 1994;10(4):673–80.
21. Rossi V, Pourtois G. Transient state dependent fluctuations in anxiety measured using STAI, POMS, PANAS or VAS: a comparative review. Anxiety Stress Coping. 2012;25(6):603–45.
22. Chlan L, Savik K. Patterns of anxiety in critically ill patients receiving mechanical ventilatory support. Nurs Res. 2011;60(3 Suppl):S50–7.
23. Parker AM, Sricharoenchai T, Raparla S, Schneck KW, Bienvenu OJ, Needham DM. Posttraumatic stress disorder in critical illness survivors: a metaanalysis. Crit Care Med. 2015;43(5):1121–9.
24. Sessler CN, Gosnell MS, Grap MJ, Brophy GM, O'Neal PV, Keane KA, et al. The Richmond agitation-sedation scale: validity and reliability in adult intensive care unit patients. Am J Respir Crit Care Med. 2002;166(10):1338–44.
25. Noble B, Clark D, Meldrum M, ten Have H, Seymour J, Winslow M, et al. The measurement of pain, 1945-2000. J Pain Symptom Manag. 2005;29(1):14–21.
26. Skrobik Y, Ahern S, Leblanc M, Marquis F, Awissi DK, Kavanagh BP. Protocolized intensive care unit management of analgesia, sedation, and delirium improves analgesia and subsyndromal delirium rates. Anesth Analg. 2010;111(2):451–63.

27. Hamill-Ruth RJ, Marohn ML. Evaluation of pain in the critically ill patient. Crit Care Clin. 1999;15(1):35–54. v-vi
28. Kim TK. Practical statistics in pain research. Korean J Pain. 2017;30(4):243–9.
29. Payen JF, Bru O, Bosson JL, Lagrasta A, Novel E, Deschaux I, et al. Assessing pain in critically ill sedated patients by using a behavioral pain scale. Crit Care Med. 2001;29(12):2258–63.
30. Gelinas C, Fillion L, Puntillo KA, Viens C, Fortier M. Validation of the critical-care pain observation tool in adult patients. Am J Crit Care. 2006;15(4):420–7.
31. Desbiens NA, Mueller-Rizner N. How well do surrogates assess the pain of seriously ill patients? Crit Care Med. 2000;28(5):1347–52.
32. Neice AE. Pupil size variation and pain-can the results be generalized? J Pain. 2018;19(5):569.
33. Dai F, Silverman DG, Chelly JE, Li J, Belfer I, Qin L. Integration of pain score and morphine consumption in analgesic clinical studies. J Pain. 2013;14(8):767–77.e8.
34. Lukaszewicz AC, Dereu D, Gayat E, Payen D. The relevance of pupillometry for evaluation of analgesia before noxious procedures in the intensive care unit. Anesth Analg. 2015;120(6):1297–300.
35. Kapp CM, Zaeh S, Niedermeyer S, Punjabi NM, Siddharthan T, Damarla M. The use of analgesia and sedation in mechanically ventilated patients with COVID-19 acute respiratory distress syndrome. Anesth Analg. 2020;131(4):e198–200.
36. Boselli E, Fatah A, Ledochowski S, Allaouchiche B. ANI and BIS variations in supine and prone position during closed-tracheal suction in sedated and myorelaxed ICU patients with severe COVID-19: a retrospective study. J Clin Monit Comput. 2020;6:1–7.
37. Phillips DM. JCAHO pain management standards are unveiled. Joint commission on accreditation of healthcare organizations. JAMA. 2000;284(4):428–9.
38. Baker DW. History of the joint commission's pain standards: lessons for today's prescription opioid epidemic. JAMA. 2017;317(11):1117–8.
39. World Health Organization Web statement on pain management guidance. 2019. Available at: https://www.who.int/medicines/areas/quality_safety/guide_on_pain/en/. Accessed 23 Jan 2020.
40. American Psychiatric Association, American Psychiatric Association. DSM-5 Task Force. Diagnostic and statistical manual of mental disorders: DSM-5. 5th ed. Washington, DC: American Psychiatric Association; 2013.
41. Ely, EW. Evaluation of delirium in critically ill patients: validation of the Confusion Assessment Method for the Intensive Care Unit (CAM-ICU). Crit Care Med. 2001;29(7):1370–9. https://doi.org/10.1097/00003246-200107000-00012.

Chapter 3
Pharmacology and Pharmacokinetics of Opioids in the ICU

Jessica R. Crow, Stephanie L. Davis, and Andrew S. Jarrell

Opioid Mechanism of Action

Opioids exhibit effects at the cellular level by binding to the opioid receptors μ (mu), δ, (delta), and κ (kappa). The International Union of Pharmacology refers to the μ, κ, and δ receptors as MOP, KOP, and DOP, respectively [1]. These receptors are present throughout the central nervous system (CNS) and the periphery. Binding of an opioid agonist to these G-protein coupled receptors results in inhibition of adenylyl cyclase with reduced intracellular cyclic adenosine monophosphate levels, inhibition of calcium channels, and potassium channel efflux. These changes result in hyperpolarization with reduced neurotransmitter release and cellular excitability to nociceptive stimuli [1, 2]. Clinical effects of opioid receptor stimulation include analgesia (μ, δ, κ), respiratory depression (μ, κ), gastrointestinal dysmotility (μ), sedation (μ, κ), dysphoria (κ, δ), and pruritus (μ). Opioids may also have effects on N-methyl-d-aspartate (NMDA) receptors, which can lead to tolerance and hyperalgesia [3].

Opioid agonists possess affinity and efficacy directed at opioid receptors, while partial agonists have affinity with partial efficacy, and antagonists have receptor affinity but no efficacy [4]. Partial agonist/antagonist opioids act as partial μ-receptor agonists but may also function as μ-receptor antagonists, as well as κ-receptor agonists. At higher doses the analgesic effects of partial agonist/antagonists will plateau and then exhibit antagonistic effects, including withdrawal symptoms. Affinity of opioids to the different opioid receptors is described in Table 3.1. Opioids can be

J. R. Crow (✉) · S. L. Davis
Department of Pharmacy, The Johns Hopkins Hospital, Baltimore, MD, USA
e-mail: jcrow3@jhmi.edu; sdavis87@jhmi.edu

A. S. Jarrell
Department of Pharmacy, Oregon Health & Science University, Portland, OR, USA
e-mail: jarrella@ohsu.edu

J. L. Pascual, T. G. Gaulton (eds.), *Opioid Use in Critical Care*,
https://doi.org/10.1007/978-3-030-77399-1_3

Table 3.1 Affinity of opioids at opioid receptors [2, 5, 6]

Opioid	μ (mu), MOP	κ (kappa), KOP	δ (delta), DOP
Buprenorphine	Partial agonist	Weak antagonist	
Butorphanol	Partial agonist	Agonist	
Codeine	Weak agonist		Weak agonist
Fentanyl	Agonist	Weak agonist	No affinity
Hydromorphone	Agonist		
Meperidine	Agonist		Agonist
Methadone	Agonist		
Morphine	Agonist	Weak agonist	Weak agonist
Nalbuphine	Partial antagonist	Agonist	
Naloxone	Antagonist	Antagonist	Weak antagonist
Naltrexone	Antagonist	Antagonist	Weak antagonist
Oxycodone	Weak agonist	Moderate agonist	
Pentazocine	Partial agonist	Agonist	
Tramadol	Weak agonist		

classified in several different ways, such as by synthetic process, chemical groupings of synthetic compounds, and effect at opioid receptors. Several different classification schemes of opioids are described in Table 3.2.

Adverse Drug Effects

Adverse drug effects (ADEs) are classified as either type A (pharmacologically mediated) or type B (hypersensitivity reactions) [7]. Development of type A ADEs can lead to reduction in opioid dosing or frequency, resulting in ineffective analgesia. These ADEs are well-characterized and mediated in a dose-dependent manner through opioid receptors, as well as through hormonal and neuronal pathways [2, 8]. Common adverse effects of opioids include gastrointestinal and urinary disturbances, CNS and respiratory depression, and nausea and vomiting [8, 9]. In addition to class effects, certain opioids or their metabolites may exhibit unique adverse effects, such as QT-prolongation (methadone), serotonin syndrome (fentanyl, tramadol), and seizures (meperidine, morphine, tramadol) that may be potentiated in critically ill patients with altered pharmacokinetics and pharmacodynamics [8].

Opioid tolerance may develop to analgesia and to certain ADEs such as nausea, vomiting, respiratory depression, and sedation; however, tolerance does not usually occur for constipation. Potential management of adverse effects for critically ill patients may involve prophylactic use of laxatives for constipation, as well as prokinetic agents and serotonin antagonists for nausea and vomiting [9]. Since a multimodal approach to treating adverse effects is most effective, the potential adverse effects of adjunctive medications must be considered as well. For adverse effects deemed intolerable, opioid rotation is recommended and is discussed later in the chapter [9, 10].

Table 3.2 Classification of opioids [1, 4, 6]

Classification scheme	Classes		
Traditional Classification	Natural compounds	Semi-synthetic compounds	Synthetic compounds
	Codeine Morphine Papaverine Thebaine	Buprenorphine Hydrocodone Hydromorphone Oxycodone Oxymorphone	Alfentanil Butorphanol Fentanyl Levorphanol Meperidine Methadone Methylnaltrexone Nalbuphine Naltrexone Propoxyphene Remifentanil Sufentanil Tramadol
Structural Classification	*Phenanthrenes* Codeine Morphine	*Phenanthrenes* Buprenorphine Hydrocodone Hydromorphone Oxycodone Oxymorphone	*Diphenylheptanes* Methadone Propoxyphene *Phenanthrenes* Butorphanol (morphinian) Levorphanol (morphinian) Methylnaltrexone Nalbuphine Naloxone Naltrexone *Phenylpiperidines* Meperidine Alfentanil Fentanyl Remifentanil Sufentanil *Anilidopiperidine* Alfentanil Fentanyl Remifentanil Sufentanil *Phenylpropylamines* Tramadol

(continued)

Table 3.2 (continued)

Classification scheme	Classes		
Functional Classification	Agonists	Partial agonists	Antagonists
	Alfentanil Codeine Fentanyl Hydrocodone Hydromorphone Meperidine Methadone Morphine Oxycodone Oxymorphone Propoxyphene Remifentanil Sufentanil	Buprenorphine Butorphanol Nalbuphine Pentazocine Tramadol	*Centrally acting antagonists* Naloxone Naltrexone *Peripherally acting antagonists* Alvimopan Methylnaltrexone Naldemedine Naloxegol

Opioid Hypersensitivity

True hypersensitivity reactions (i.e., allergies) to medications involve an immune system response and are considered to be dose-independent [7]. Many opioids cause histamine release, resulting in a non-immune mediated reaction via direct degranulation of mast cells. Histamine release can present with an array of symptoms that vary widely and can mimic anaphylaxis (e.g., wheal and flare, rash, pruritus, hypotension, or bronchospasm) [11, 12]. For opioids, histamine release is not dependent on opioid receptors and generally not precipitated by opioid-induced IgE antibody release; therefore, true hypersensitivity reactions to opioids are thought to be very rare [13].

The incidence of true opioid hypersensitivity has been reported to be up to 2% in the perioperative setting; however, this is likely overestimated due to lack of validated tests [12, 14]. There are currently no studies reporting hypersensitivity rates in a chronic pain population. Opioid allergies reported by patients may be confused with common adverse effects, such as gastrointestinal upset, fatigue, or pruritis. In one study, up to 50% of documented opioid allergies were attributed to patient intolerance of adverse effects [15].

Low-potency natural opioids (e.g., codeine, morphine) have the strongest likelihood to induce mast cell degranulation as they preferentially activate receptors on cutaneous mast cells in a concentration-dependent manner [12]. High-potency and synthetic opioids (e.g., fentanyl, remifentanil) do not appear to trigger histamine release from mast cells as their concentrations are low [13]. Additionally, morphine has direct vasodilatory effects on systemic vasculature, which may result in further hypotension and flushing. This effect may be exacerbated in critically ill patients, especially those with impaired cardiovascular function or shock.

For patients experiencing histamine release with opioid use, pre-treatment with both histamine-1 and −2 antagonists may be sufficient [13, 14]. For patients with suspected true hypersensitivity reaction, another opioid may be trialed after potential for cross-reactivity is assessed, as discussed in the next section.

Opioid Cross-Reactivity

Cross-reactivity between classes of opioids may theoretically occur due to structural similarity (i.e., natural, semi-synthetic, synthetic), but this is poorly studied. See Table 3.2 for a description of opioid classifications. No significant difference in the development of IgE-mediated reactions (IMR) was found when patients with a documented opioid allergy were challenged with a different class of opioid [15]. Additionally, rates of IMR were low when rechallenged with an opioid of the same class (natural or semi synthetic) and no patients challenged or rechallenged with a synthetic opioid experienced IMR.

As natural opioids may be more likely to cause a hypersensitivity reaction, synthetic opioids are the preferred alternative in patients suspected of having an allergy. However, if a synthetic opioid is the causative agent, then a natural or semi-synthetic opioid should be trialed. Addition of non-opioid, multimodal analgesic agents should also be considered.

Dosing Strategies

Suggestions for initial dosing strategies in opioid naïve, critically ill patients are described in Table 3.3. Doses should be titrated carefully based on patient response, pharmacokinetic properties, and expected alterations in opioid pharmacokinetics and pharmacodynamics. Pharmacokinetic properties of opioids and expected alterations in critically ill patients are discussed later in the chapter.

Table 3.3 Initial doses of commonly used opioids for critically ill, opioid-naive patients [6, 16]

Opioid	Route and formulation	Initial dose
Fentanyl	IV push	25–50 mcg every 30–60 min PRN
	IV continuous infusion	25–100 mcg/h
Hydromorphone	IV push	0.2–0.5 mg every 1–3 h PRN
	IV continuous infusion	0.5–2 mg/h
	PO immediate-release tablet, PO liquid	2–4 mg every 4–6 h PRN
Morphine	IV push	2–4 mg every 1–4 h PRN
	PO immediate-release tablet, PO liquid	10–30 mg every 4 h PRN
Oxycodone	PO immediate-release tablet, PO liquid	5–10 mg every 4–6 h PRN
Remifentanil	IV continuous infusion	0.01–0.05 mcg/kg/min
Tramadol	PO immediate-release tablet, PO liquid	50 mg every 4–6 h PRN

Table 3.4 Equianalgesic dosing of oral and intravenous opioids [6, 10]

To: **From:**	Morphine PO	Hydromorphone PO	Oxycodone PO
Morphine PO	–	5:1	1.5:1
Hydromorphone PO	1:3.7	–	1:4.1
Oxycodone PO	1:1.5	4.1:1	–
To: **From:**	Morphine IV	Hydromorphone IV	Fentanyl IV
Morphine IV	–	1:1.5	10:0.1
Hydromorphone IV	1.5:1	–	1.5:100
Fentanyl IV	0.1:10	100:1.5	–

Opioid rotation, the switching from one opioid to another for intolerance of adverse effects or for ineffective analgesia as tolerance develops, may also be indicated with changes in clinical status, such as renal or hepatic impairment or need for an alternate route of administration [10]. Calculating the appropriate equianalgesic dose is based on relative potency and can be challenging given the varied pharmacokinetic and pharmacodynamic properties of individual agents. Suggested equianalgesic doses may vary by several orders of magnitude and differ depending on route being interchanged and duration of therapy [17, 18]. This can lead to potentially fatal medication errors.

Table 3.4 provides a summary of equianalgesic ratios for oral and intravenous (IV) therapy, respectively, based on safety-focused guidelines [19]. Starting with these ratios, a dose of the new agent is calculated. An initial dose reduction of 25% to 50% should then be made with a larger percent dose reduction in patients with high opioid requirements or based on clinical context (e.g., sedation, age, frailty, new organ dysfunction). An assessment of prior pain control and adverse effects should then be performed and an increase or decrease of 15–30% in initial dosing should be considered based on these characteristics.

Methadone provides a unique challenge as the potency can often be underestimated and equianalgesic ratios vary widely depending on which opioid is being transitioned from. Several studies have found the conversion from morphine to methadone ranged from 3.71:1 to 16.8:1 depending on the amount of morphine exposure prior to the switch [17, 20]. Conversion to methadone should only be performed in opioid-experienced patients and under the supervision of a pain expert.

Successful conversion of one opioid to another requires effective communication between the patient and the provider to frequently assess pain control and adverse effects. Opioid rotation should be performed conservatively, favoring short-acting opioids and formulations to allow for effective titration until patients are stable.

Route of Opioid Administration in Critically Ill Patients

When selecting the optimal route of opioid administration in critically ill patients, pharmacokinetic and patient-specific factors must be considered. Table 3.5 describes opioid formulations and potential routes of administration. The onset,

Table 3.5 Formulations and route of administration of opioid agonists and antagonists [6]

Medication	Formulations and route of administration
Alfentanil	Injection: IV (IVP, PCA, CI, epidural)
Alvimopan	Capsule: PO
Buprenorphine	Injection: IVP, IM, SC Film: TM Tablet: SL Implant: SC Patch: TD
Buprenorphine/naloxone	Film: TM Tablet: SL
Butorphanol	Injection: IV, IM Spray: IN
Codeine	Tablet: PO
Fentanyl	Injection: IV (IVP, PCA, CI) IM, SC, epidural, IT Film: TM Lozenge: TM Tablet: TM, SL Spray: SL, IN Patch: TD Device: TD
Hydrocodone	ER capsule (12 h): PO ER tablet (24 h): PO Combination with acetaminophen as tablet, elixir, and solution: PO Combination with ibuprofen: PO
Hydromorphone	Injection: IV (IVP, PCA, CI), SC, IM (not recommended) Oral liquid: PO Tablet: PO ER tablet: PO Suppository: PR
Meperidine	Injection: IV (IVP, IM, SC) Solution: PO Tablet: PO
Methadone	Injection: IVP Tablet: PO Soluble tablet: PO Oral solution: PO
Methylnaltrexone	Solution: SC Tablet: PO
Morphine	Injection: IV (IVP, PCA, CI) IM, SC, epidural, IT IM device: IM IR tablet: PO ER tablet: PO Oral solution: PO Suppository: PR
Nalbuphine	Injection: IV, IM, SC
Naldemedine	Tablet: PO
Naloxegol	Tablet: PO

(continued)

Table 3.5 (continued)

Medication	Formulations and route of administration
Naloxone	Injection: IV (IVP, CI), SC, IM Nasal liquid: Inhalation, IN
Naltrexone	Injection: IM Tablet: PO
Oxycodone	Tablet: PO ER tablet: PO Oral solution: PO
Oxymorphone	Tablet: PO ER: PO
Pentazocine/naloxone	Tablet: PO
Remifentanil	Injection: IV (IVP, PCA, CI), epidural
Sufentanil	Injection: IV (IVP, CI, epidural) Tablet: SL

ER extended release, *GI* gastrointestinal, *IM* intramuscular, *IN* intranasal, *IR* immediate release, *IV* intravenous, *PO* oral, *SC* subcutaneous, *SL* sublingual, *TD* transdermal, *TM* transmucosal

bioavailability, duration, and risk of adverse effects of opioids differ based on the route of administration, and critically ill patients may experience conditions that further alter these parameters, which are described in detail later in the chapter. The novel coronavirus 2019 (COVID-19) pandemic has highlighted the importance of these concepts. With increased hospital admissions of critically ill patients with COVID-19 pneumonia and acute respiratory distress syndrome, many requiring high doses of opioids, all in the midst of national opioid shortages, clinicians have sometimes been required to employ nontraditional strategies for opioid utilization. This exemplifies the need to understand various opioid routes of administration, as well as dosing strategies, in critically ill patients.

Parenteral Administration

The 2013 SCCM guidelines for management of pain, agitation, and delirium in adult ICU patients consider IV opioids first-line for treatment of non-neuropathic pain [21]. They also state all IV opioids are equally effective when titrated appropriately, and the decision to administer intermittent or continuous IV opioids may depend on the pharmacokinetic properties of the selected opioid, the frequency and intensity of pain, and the patient's mental status.

Intravenous administration results in rapid medication delivery to the systemic circulation and 100% bioavailability, allowing for rapid onset of analgesia and ease of titration, but typically a shorter duration of action [22]. Compared to continuous administration, intermittent dosing may decrease the risk of opioid accumulation and adverse events in critically ill patients with decreased clearance, and may also reduce opioid tolerance. Intravenous bolus doses of opioids must be administered slowly over several minutes, as rapid administration may result in chest wall rigidity with impaired ventilation and potential for respiratory arrest [6].

Morphine and hydromorphone have a prolonged duration of approximately 3–5 h when administered as an intermittent IV bolus [6]. Fentanyl has a rapid onset and relatively short duration when given intermittently; however, when given as a continuous infusion for 9 days, the terminal half-life increased to 13 h due to its large volume of distribution [23]. A meta-analysis demonstrated critically ill patients had a longer sufentanil half-life and ten-fold decrease in morphine clearance compared to non-critically ill patients [24]. Anilidopiperidine opioids may be preferred for continuous infusion given the relatively short duration of action. Remifentanil is rapidly metabolized by blood and tissue esterases and therefore the duration of effect is not affected by the duration of continuous infusions; but pain can set in quickly when the infusion is stopped [6].

The 2016 American Pain Society (APS) guidelines for the management of postoperative pain recommend IV patient-controlled analgesia (PCA) for management of postoperative pain when the parenteral route is necessary for several hours and the patient has adequate cognitive function, but recommend against routine infusion of basal opioids in opioid-naïve patients due to the risk of respiratory depression [25]. The lockout interval, which is defined as the time that must elapse before a repeat bolus can be administered, should be guided by the onset and duration of the opioid [26].

Alternative parenteral routes of administration can be considered on a patient-specific basis, but the routine use in critically ill patients is discouraged due to erratic and potentially inadequate absorption [23]. Subcutaneous absorption of medications in critically ill patients may be altered by the presence of edema, hemodynamic instability, and the use of vasoactive infusions [27]. Intramuscular administration is generally avoided in critically ill and postoperative patients due to the potential for hematoma formation, variable absorption, painful injection, and lack of pharmacokinetic advantage compared to other routes of administration [25, 27, 28].

Neuraxial Administration

Neuraxial analgesia is an invasive method of administration but may provide superior analgesia with a lower incidence of adverse effects. Spinal administration targets opioid receptors in the dorsal horn and dorsal root ganglia of the spinal cord, but opioids may spread to receptors in the brain via the cerebrospinal fluid (CSF) and cause supraspinal effects including sedation and respiratory depression [29].

Pharmacokinetic factors affecting neuraxial opioid analgesia include spinal bioavailability and clearance from the CSF [29]. Spinal bioavailability is inversely proportional to lipid solubility, with higher bioavailability for hydrophilic opioids, such as morphine, compared to the lipophilic anilidopiperidines which have low to moderate intrathecal and epidural bioavailability. Lipophilicity also affects volume of distribution, as lipophilic opioids diffuse into epidural fat, resulting in decreased concentrations in the CSF and increased vascular reuptake with distribution to the blood [29, 30]. The volume of distribution of sufentanil is 40 times larger than morphine, and clearance of alfentanil into the plasma is ten-fold higher than morphine [29]. In general, lipophilic opioids have a rapid onset and short duration of action, whereas hydrophilic opioids have a slower onset and longer duration of action [31].

Direct opioid administration into the intrathecal space results in almost immediate peak CSF concentrations [31]. Since morphine is hydrophilic, it crosses the blood brain barrier slowly, binds to the hydrophilic gray matter in the dorsal horn, and has slow reuptake into the plasma and limited binding to epidural fat. Therefore, intrathecal morphine has a slow onset of action (60–120 min) compared to less than 10 min with fentanyl and sufentanil [32, 33]. The duration of intrathecal analgesia for morphine is prolonged at 18–24 h, compared to 1–4 h for fentanyl and 2–6 h for sufentanil [33]. The dose of intrathecal morphine is typically one-tenth the epidural dosage [6]. The onset of respiratory depression may be delayed up to 24 h in patients receiving intrathecal morphine but may occur early within 1 h for lipophilic opioids [6, 32, 34].

Epidural analgesia occurs proportionally with CNS absorption, as opioids must diffuse throughout the epidural space, meninges, CSF, and white matter to reach the hydrophilic gray matter of the dorsal horn [29]. Maximum morphine concentrations in the CSF occur 60–90 min after injection and approximately 4% of the epidural dose injected reaches the CSF. Morphine disposition in CSF exhibits a biphasic pattern with initial half-life of 1.5 h and late phase half-life of 6 h, with a duration up to 24 h [6, 32]. In an animal model of epidural opioids, the volume of distribution of fentanyl and sufentanil was significantly higher than morphine, and the dose-normalized area under the curve was significantly lower [35].

The onset, duration of action, and timing of potential respiratory depression of neuraxially administered opioids differ based on pharmacokinetic properties, and must be considered when selecting an appropriate agent. Preservative-free formulations must be used when administering intrathecal or epidural opioids [6]. The APS guidelines for management of postoperative pain recommend offering neuraxial analgesia (intrathecal opioid or local anesthetic epidural with or without opioids) to patients undergoing major thoracic, abdominal, cesarean section, or lower extremity surgery [25]. Epidural analgesia with opioids offers the advantage of administration as a continuous infusion or as patient-controlled analgesia compared to single dose intrathecal opioid spinal analgesia [25].

Enteral Administration

The APS guidelines for the management of postoperative pain state that oral opioids are generally preferred for management of postoperative pain in patients who can use the oral route; however, long-acting opioids are generally not recommended in the immediate postoperative period since acute pain management often requires dose titration [25]. Administration of enteral opioids in critically ill patients should be limited to patients with sufficient gastrointestinal absorption and motility [21].

Enteral opioids that are not available in a liquid form require crushing prior to administration via an enteral tube or in patients unable to swallow tablets, which may result in clogging of small-bore feeding tubes [27]. Extended-release or delayed-release tablets should not be crushed, as this can result in a rapid increase in opioid concentrations and the development of adverse effects, while also shortening the effective duration of action. See Table 3.5 for formulations of enteral opioid agonists and antagonists.

Transdermal Administration

Transdermal drug delivery offers a noninvasive route of administration via the skin surface; however, disadvantages for the use in critically ill patients are numerous [36]. Transdermal fentanyl is considered a high-alert medication by the Institute of Safe Medication Practices (ISMP) based on the number of errors and adverse events that have been reported [37]. Fentanyl patches are contraindicated for short-term management of acute, intermittent, mild, or postoperative pain, as well as in patients who are not opioid tolerant [6, 37].

Fentanyl is continuously released from transdermal patches and results in a depot as it accumulates in the outer layer of skin [6]. Alternative analgesia may be required as serum concentrations gradually increase in the first 12–24 h after administration and as concentrations gradually decrease with patch removal [6, 38]. Decreased peripheral blood flow can result in unreliable transdermal absorption in patients with shock, and absorption is decreased in cachectic patients due to decreased skin permeability [36, 39]. Exposure to heat (e.g., warming blankets, fever) can increase delivery of transdermal fentanyl by up to one-third and tight coverings or dressing should be avoided [36, 37, 40]. Patches should be applied to unbroken, non-irritated, and unshaven skin as the risk of overdose increases when applied to broken skin [6, 36].

Errors have also been reported in which multiple patches are inadvertently applied to hospitalized patients due to inadequate monitoring of patch removal and practitioners overlooking clear patches [41]. Patches also differ in whether it is safe to cut them based on their design, but such practices should generally be avoided [6, 42]. Lastly, fentanyl patches must be removed prior to magnetic resonance imaging, as they may contain metal that could result in burns and injury to the skin [6, 37]. Overall, the risks of transdermal patch systems for opioid administration in critically ill patients may outweigh any potential benefits and should likely be avoided.

Alterations of Pharmacokinetics in Critically Ill Patients

Opioids vary widely in their pharmacokinetic properties, including absorption, distribution, metabolism, and elimination. Tables 3.6 and 3.7 describe pharmacokinetic properties of opioid agonists and partial agonist/antagonists commonly used in the ICU. Critically ill patients may experience renal and hepatic dysfunction, as well as a number of other conditions that may affect absorption, distribution, protein binding, metabolism, and excretion of opioids. Alterations in pharmacokinetics of opioid agonists in critically ill patients are summarized in Table 3.8.

Renal Impairment

Renal impairment is common among critically ill patients and has important implications for opioid pharmacokinetics. Most directly, renal impairment increases the half-life of renally cleared medications. This can lead to toxicity due to the accumulation of the drug and active metabolites if unaddressed [49]. Opioid volume of distribution may also be affected by renal impairment secondary to an increase in total body fluid; this particularly affects hydrophilic opioids (e.g., morphine).

In patients with acute or chronic renal impairment, the creatinine clearance must be estimated in order to inform opioid selection and dosing. Most dosing guidance resources, including US Food and Drug Administration-approved prescribing information, utilize the Cockcroft-Gault estimate of creatinine clearance, which accounts for patient's age, ideal body weight, sex, and serum creatinine. However, this estimate has some limitations, as factors such as obesity, low muscle mass, and acutely changing renal function invalidate the estimate. Though not typically helpful in determining an estimate of creatinine clearance, urine output may indicate an acute change, serving as a cue for reassessment of medication selection and dosing in critically ill patients.

The Cockcroft-Gault estimate cannot be used in patients receiving renal replacement therapy. The two primary forms of renal replacement therapy, intermittent hemodialysis (IHD) and continuous renal replacement therapy (CRRT), eliminate medications differently. In IHD, all clearance of dialyzable medications occurs exclusively during the several hours that IHD is running, assuming minimal underlying renal function. Dosing of affected medications in IHD tends to lower and is less frequent than standard dosing. In comparison to dosing in IHD, dosing in CRRT is more aggressive, though typically still more conservative than standard dosing. Medication elimination is more stable in CRRT because it runs continuously, but if CRRT is interrupted (e.g., clot in filter, patient going for a procedure), re-evaluation of dialyzable medication doses must occur, as clearance will be reduced substantially.

The ideal opioid to use in a patient with renal impairment is one in which active drug and active metabolites are not renally eliminated. Remifentanil meets these

Table 3.6 Pharmacology and pharmacokinetics of opioid agonists and partial agonists/antagonists: part 1 [6, 43–48]

Opioid	Bioavailability and absorption	Lipophilicity and logP	Volume of distribution	Protein binding	Time to peak, plasma	Onset
Alfentanil	–	Lipophilic 2.16	0.4–1 L/kg	88–92% to AAG	N/A	Rapid within 5 min
Buprenorphine	IR IM: 70% TD patch: ~15%; heat may increase serum concentrations up to 55% TM film: 46–65%; ingestion of liquids decreases systemic exposure 23–37% SL tablet: 29%	Lipophilic 3.8	97–187 L/kg	~96% primarily to AAG	IR IM: ~1 h TM film: 2.5–3 h SL tablet: 0.5–1 h TD patch: steady state 3 days ER SC: 24 h (steady state 4–6 months) SD implant: 12 h after insertion (steady state 4 weeks)	IR IM: ≥ 15 min
Butorphanol	IN: 60–70%	N/A	305–901 L	~80%	IV: within minutes IM, nasal: ≤ 15 min	IV: 0.5–1 h IM, nasal: 1–2 h.
Codeine	Tablet: 53%	Hydrophilic 1.19	3–6 L/kg	7–25%	Tablet: 1 h	Tablet: 30–60 min

(continued)

Table 3.6 (continued)

Opioid	Bioavailability and absorption	Lipophilicity and logP	Volume of distribution	Protein binding	Time to peak, plasma	Onset
Fentanyl	TD patch: Serum concentrations increase over 24–24 h TD device: Serum concentrations increase over 15 min after activation TM film: 71%; absorption 50% mucosal and 50% GI TM lozenge: 50%; rapid absorption with 50% mucosal and 50% GI TM tablet: 65%; absorption 50% mucosal and 50% GI	Highly lipophilic 4.05	4–6 L/kg with 3-compartment distribution model	79–87% primarily to AAG, also to albumin and erythrocytes	SC: median 15 min TD patch: 20–72 h TM film: median 1 h TM lozenge: median 20–40 min TM tablet: median 47 min SL tablet: median 30–60 min SL spray: 90 min IN: median 15–21	IM: 7–8 min IV: Immediate but several min for maximal effects TD: 6 h after initial placement TM: 5–15 min
Hydrocodone	25%	Hydrophilic 1.2	1300 to 1400 L	19–45%	Capsule ER (12 h): 5 h Tablet ER (24 h): 6–30 h Combination with acetaminophen: 1 h Combination with ibuprofen: 1.7 h	10–20 min

Hydromorphone	IM: variable and delayed PO liquid: 24% Tablet: 24% Extended-release tablet: 24%, delayed Extensive first-pass effect with PO administration	Hydrophilic 0.9	4 L/kg	8–19%	Tablet: 30–60 min ER: 12–16 h	IV: 5 min PO liquid: 15–30 min Tablet: 15–30 min ER tablet: 6 h
Meperidine	IM, PO: highly variable	Lipophilic 2.6	3–4 L/kg	65–75% to AAG	IV: 5–7 min IM, SC: ~1 h PO: 2 h	IV: 5 min PO, IM, SC: 10–15 min
Methadone	Tablet: 36–100% Soluble tablet: 36–100% PO solution: 36–100%	Lipophilic 3.93	1–8 L/kg	85–90%	Tablet: 1–7.5 h Soluble tablet: 1–7.5 h PO solution: 1–7.5 h	IV: 10–20 min Tablet: 30–60 min Soluble tablet: 30–60 min PO solution: 30–60 min
Morphine	Tablet: 17–33% ER tablet: 20–40% PO solution: 17–33%	Hydrophilic 0.89	1–6 L/kg with distribution to skeletal muscle, liver, kidneys, lungs, intestines, spleen, brain	20–35%	IM: 30–60 min SC: 50–90 min Epidural: 1 h Tablet: 1 h ER tablet: 3–4 h PO solution: 1 h Suppository: 20–60 min.	IV: 5–10 min Tablet, PO solution: 30 min

(continued)

Table 3.6 (continued)

Opioid	Bioavailability and absorption	Lipophilicity and logP	Volume of distribution	Protein binding	Time to peak, plasma	Onset
Nalbuphine	IM/SC: N/A	Lipophilic 1.4	N/A	~50%	N/A	IV: 2–3 min IM, SC: <15 min.
Oxycodone	60–87%	Hydrophilic 0.3	2.6 L/kg	38–45%	30–60 min	IR tablet: 10–15 min
Oxymorphone	~10% Increased with high-fat meal	Hydrophilic 0.83	3 L/kg	10–12%	IR tablet: 30–60 min ER tablet: 1–2 h	IR tablet: 30–60 min ER tablet: 1–2 h
Pentazocine/ naloxone	Well-absorbed	Lipophilic 3.7	N/A	60%	N/A	1.7 h
Remifentanil	–	Lipophilic 1.4	Initial: 100 mL/kg Steady state: 350 mL/kg	70% primarily to AAG	3–5 min	1–3 min
Sufentanil	SL tablet: 53%	Lipophilic 2.8	1.7 ± 0.2 L/kg	91–93% primarily to AAG	SL tablet: 1 h	IV: 1–3 min Epidural: 10 min SL tablet: 30 min
Tramadol	IR tablet: ~75% ER tablet: ~85–95%	Lipophilic 2.4	Females: 2.9 L/kg Males: 2.6 L/kg.	~20%	IR tablet: 2–3 h	IR tablet: within 1 h

AAG α_1-acid glycoprotein, *ER* extended release, *GI* gastrointestinal, *IM* intramuscular, *IN* intranasal, *IR* immediate release, *IV* intravenous, *logP* log octanol/water partition coefficient, *N/A* information not available, *PO* oral, *SC* subcutaneous, *SD* subdermal, *SL* sublingual, *TD* transdermal, *TM* transmucosal

Table 3.7 Pharmacology and pharmacokinetics of opioid agonists and partial agonist/antagonists: part 2 [6, 44–48]

Opioid	Metabolism	Excretion	Half-life elimination	Duration
Alfentanil	Hepatic	Urine, only 1% excreted as unchanged	90–111 min	30–60 min, dose-dependent
Buprenorphine	Hepatic via N-dealkylation by CYP3A4 to norbuprenorphine (active) and glucuronidation of buprenorphine and norbuprenorphine	Urine 27–30% with 1% unchanged and 2.7% as norbuprenorphine Feces ~70% with 33% unchanged and 21% norbuprenorphine	IV 2.2–3 h TM film: 27–11 h SL tablet: ~37 h TD patch: ~26 h	IR IM: > 6 h ER SC: 28 days
Butorphanol	Hepatic to major metabolite hydroxybutorphanol	Urine 70–80% with ~5% unchanged Feces 15%	IV, IN: ~2–9 h	IV, IM: 3–4 h IN: 4–5 h
Codeine	Hepatic via UGT2B7 and UGT2B4 to codeine-6-glucuronide, via CYP2D6 to morphine (active), and via CYP3A4 to norcodeine. See morphine for additional information	Urine 90% primarily as metabolites and 10% as unchanged drug Feces 10%	Tablet: 3 h	Tablet: 4–6 h
Fentanyl	Hepatic via CYP3A4 by N-dealkylation to norfentanyl with hydroxylation to inactive metabolites	Urine 75% primarily as metabolites and <10% unchanged drug Feces ~9%	IV CI: 2–4 h but increases with prolonged infusions SC: 10 h TD device: 16 h TD patch: 20–27 h TM film: 14 h TM tablet: 3–12 h (dose-dependent). IN: 15–25 h	IM: 1–2 h IV: 0.5–1 h TD: concentrations decrease ~50% 20–27 h after removal but effects may last 72–96 h
Hydrocodone	Hepatic via CYP2D6 by O-demethylation to hydromorphone, CYP3A4 by N-demethylation to norhydrocodone, and non-CYP pathways (6-ketosteroid reduction)	Urine 26% with 12% as unchanged drug	ER capsule (12 h): 8 h ER tablet (24 h): 7–9 h Combination with acetaminophen: 4 h Combination with ibuprofen: 4.5 h	Combination with ibuprofen 4–8 h

(continued)

Table 3.7 (continued)

Hydromorphone	Hepatic via glucuronidation to inactive metabolites; >95% metabolized to hydromorphone-3-glucuronide; minor amounts as 6-hydroxy reduction metabolites	Urine 99% primarily as glucouronide conjugates; 7% as unchanged drug Feces 1%	IV: 2–3 h PO liquid: 2–3 h Tablet: 2–3 h ER tablet: 8–15 h	IV: 3–4 h PO liquid: 3–4 h Tablet: 3–4 h ER tablet: 6 h Suppository: may provide longer duration of effect than PO tablet
Meperidine	Hepatic via N-demethylation to normeperidine (active metabolite with analgesic effects and CNS effects that may precipitate seizures) and hydrolysis to inactive metabolite	Urine as metabolites and 5% as unchanged drug	2.5–4 h Normeperidine 8–16 h	IV 2–3 h IM, SC, PO 2–4 h
Methadone	Hepatic with N-demethylation primarily via CYP3A4, CYP2B6, CYP2C19, CYP2C9, CYP2D6 to inactive metabolites	Urine 100% with <10% as unchanged drug	Tablet: 8–59 h Soluble tablet: 8–59 h PO solution: 8–59 h	Tablet: 4–8 h with single doses; 22–48 h with repeated doses Soluble tablet, PO solution: 4–8 h with single doses; 22–48 h with repeated doses
Morphine	Hepatic via conjugation with glucuronic acid primarily to morphine-6-glucuronide (active analgesic) morphine-3-glucuronide (inactive as analgesic); minor metabolites include morphine-3-6-diglucuronide; other minor metabolites include normorphine (active) and morphine 3-ethereal sulfate	Urine ~90% with 2–12% as unchanged drug Feces 7–10%	IV: 2–4 h Tablet: 2–4 h ER tablet: 11–13 h PO solution: 2–4 h	IV: 3–5 h Epidural: < 24 h Intrathecal: < 24 h Tablet: 3–5 h ER tablet: 8–24 h PO solution: 3–5 h Suppository: 3–7 h

Nalbuphine	Hepatic with extensive first-pass metabolism	Urine ~7% unchanged drug and metabolites Feces	5 h	3–6 h
Oxycodone	Hepatic via CYP3A4 to noroxycodone (weak active metabolite) and CYP2D6 to oxymorphone (active metabolite)	Urine 19% unchanged, >64% metabolites	IR 3.2–4 h ER tablet 4.5 h ER capsule 5.6 h	IR 3–6 h ER < 12 h
Oxymorphone	Hepatic via glucuronidation to inactive metabolites	Urine <1% unchanged Feces	IR 7–9 h ER 9–11 h	IR 4–6 h ER 12 h
Pentazocine/ naloxone	Hepatic via oxidative pathways and glucuronidation with extensive first-pass effect	Urine with small amount unchanged	3.6 h	≥3 h
Remifentanil	Rapid by blood and tissue esterases	Urine	10–20 min	3–10 min
Sufentanil	Hepatic and small intestine via demethylation and dealkylation	Urine 2% unchanged and 80% metabolites	IV 164 min. SL 2.5 h	IV 5 min Epidural 1.7 h SL 3 h
Tramadol	Hepatic via demethylation (CYP3A4 and CYP2D6 with active metabolite O-desmethyl tramadol), glucuronidation, and sulfation	Urine ~30% unchanged and 60% metabolites	Within 1 h	6 h after single dose

CI continuous infusion, *CNS* central nervous system, *ER* extended release, *IM* intramuscular, *IN* intranasal, *IR* immediate release, *IV* intravenous, *N/A* information not available, *PO* oral, *SC* subcutaneous, *SL* sublingual, *TD* transdermal, *TM* transmucosal

Table 3.8 Alterations in pharmacokinetics of opioid agonists in critically ill patients [6]

Medication	Absorption	Distribution	Protein binding	Metabolism	Excretion
Alfentanil	No alteration with IV formulation	Hypervolemia/ resuscitation and inflammatory states may have less impact on volume of distribution based on lipophilicity	Increased α_1-acid glycoprotein in critical illness may decrease free drug concentrations	Hepatic impairment may reduce metabolism to inactive metabolites, prolonging analgesic and adverse effects	Renal impairment does not affect half-life
Codeine	Tablet: may be decreased in hemodynamically unstable patients	Hypervolemia/ resuscitation and inflammatory states increase volume of distribution	Minimal clinically significant impact	Hepatic impairment may reduce metabolism to active morphine, limiting analgesic effect	Renal impairment may reduce excretion of morphine and active metabolites, prolonging analgesic and adverse effects
Fentanyl	All formulations except IV: may be decreased in hemodynamically unstable patients	Hypervolemia/ resuscitation and inflammatory states may have less impact on volume of distribution based on lipophilicity	Increased α_1-acid glycoprotein in critical illness may decrease free drug concentrations; binds to albumin to less extent and free fraction may increase with hypoalbuminemia	Hepatic impairment may reduce metabolism to inactive metabolites, prolonging analgesic and adverse effects	Renal impairment has minor impact since <10% eliminated as unchanged drug and metabolites are inactive
Hydrocodone	Tablet: may be decreased in hemodynamically unstable patients	Hypervolemia/ resuscitation and inflammatory states increase volume of distribution	Free fraction may increase with hypoalbuminemia due to moderate protein binding	Hepatic impairment may reduce metabolism to active hydromorphone, limiting analgesic effect	Renal impairment may reduce excretion of parent drug and increase concentrations up to 50%, prolonging analgesic and adverse effects

Hydromorphone	All formulations except IV: may be decreased in hemodynamically unstable patients	Hypervolemia/ resuscitation and inflammatory states increase volume of distribution	Minimal clinically significant impact	Hepatic impairment may reduce metabolism to inactive metabolites, prolonging analgesic and adverse effects	Renal impairment may reduce excretion of parent drug, prolonging analgesic and adverse effects
Meperidine	All formulations except IV: may be decreased in hemodynamically unstable patients	Hypervolemia/ resuscitation and inflammatory states may have less impact on volume of distribution based on lipophilicity	Increased α_1-acid glycoprotein in critical illness may decrease free drug concentrations	Hepatic impairment may reduce metabolism to inactive metabolites, prolonging analgesic and adverse effects (half-life 1.3–2 times greater in cirrhosis)	Renal impairment may reduce excretion of parent drug and normeperidine, prolonging analgesic and adverse effects. Use should be avoided.
Methadone	All oral formulations: may be decreased in hemodynamically unstable patients	Hypervolemia/ resuscitation and inflammatory states increase volume of distribution	Free fraction increases with hypoalbuminemia	Hepatic impairment may reduce metabolism to inactive metabolites, prolonging analgesic effects	Renal impairment may reduce excretion of parent drug, prolonging analgesic effects
Morphine	All formulations except, IV, IT, epidural: may be decreased in hemodynamically unstable patients	Hypervolemia/ resuscitation and inflammatory states increase volume of distribution	Minimal clinically significant impact	Hepatic impairment may reduce metabolism, prolonging analgesic effects	Renal impairment may reduce excretion of parent drug and active metabolites, prolonging analgesic and adverse effects
Oxycodone	All oral formulations: may be decreased in hemodynamically unstable patients	Hypervolemia/ resuscitation and inflammatory states increase volume of distribution	Free fraction may increase with hypoalbuminemia due to moderate protein binding	Hepatic impairment may increase parent drug concentrations up to 50%, with decrease in active metabolite concentrations by 30%	Renal impairment may reduce excretion of parent drug and active metabolites with increase of peak concentrations by up to 50%, prolonging analgesic and adverse effects

Table 3.8 Alterations in pharmacokinetics of opioid agonists in critically ill patients [6]

Oxymorphone	All oral formulations: may be decreased in hemodynamically unstable patients. Bioavailability significantly increased in patients with renal and/or hepatic impairment	Hypervolemia/ resuscitation and inflammatory states increase volume of distribution	Minimal clinically significant impact	Hepatic impairment may reduce metabolism, prolonging analgesic effects	Renal impairment may reduce excretion of active metabolites
Remifentanil	No alteration with IV formulation	Hypervolemia/ resuscitation and inflammatory states may have less impact on volume of distribution based on lipophilicity	Increased α_1-acid glycoprotein in critical illness may decrease free drug concentrations	No impact on pharmacokinetics	No impact on pharmacokinetics
Sufentanil	No alteration with IV formulation	Hypervolemia/ resuscitation and inflammatory states may have less impact on volume of distribution based on lipophilicity	Increased α_1-acid glycoprotein in critical illness may decrease free drug concentrations	Minimal clinically significant impact	Minimal clinically significant impact
Tramadol	All oral formulations: may be decreased in hemodynamically unstable patients	Hypervolemia/ resuscitation and inflammatory states may have less impact on volume of distribution based on lipophilicity	Minimal clinically significant impact	Hepatic impairment may reduce metabolism, prolonging analgesic effects	Renal impairment may reduce excretion of parent drug and active metabolites with increase warranting reduction in dose and frequency

criteria because it is metabolized quickly by blood and tissue esterases to inactive metabolites that are renally eliminated; therefore, no dose adjustment is needed for renal impairment. However, remifentanil is typically costly and its short half-life may not always be desirable. Fentanyl, though not as pharmacokinetically optimal, is still a good option in patients with renal impairment [16]. Less than 10% of fentanyl parent drug is eliminated in the urine and its metabolites are inactive, so renal impairment has a minimal effect on clearance in most cases [50, 51]. Though morphine parent drug is minimally impacted by renal impairment, its active metabolites, especially morphine-6-glucuronide, are renally eliminated and play a significant role in the negative sequelae of accumulation in renal impairment [51]. These characteristics make morphine a non-ideal opioid in patients with renal impairment. Additional information about the metabolism and elimination of other opioids is shown in Table 3.7.

Drug information resources can guide dosing of opioids in renal impairment or renal replacement therapy. If an ideal opioid cannot be utilized, it is important to dose conservatively initially. Opioid efficacy and toxicity can be readily monitored, so doses can subsequently be titrated to response. If naloxone is administered for opioid reversal, it is not affected by renal impairment, so repeat dosing or a continuous naloxone infusion may be necessary to sustain opioid antagonism until the opioid is eliminated.

Hepatic Impairment

Alterations in hepatic function due to multi-organ system failure or pre-existing comorbid conditions can result in prolonged exposure to opioids resulting in increased adverse effects. Assessment of hepatic impairment generally involves monitoring serum liver enzymes, bilirubin, and protein markers. Each of these markers has limitations when assessing liver function and may reveal some impairment, but are not indicative of how opioid dosing may need to change. Package labeling dose guidance for hepatic impairment is vague and involves core principles of dose reduction and close monitoring based on the pharmacokinetic changes described below.

Effect of Hepatic Impairment on Opioid Absorption

Most oral/enteral opioids are absorbed in the small intestine and enter enterohepatic circulation to undergo first-pass metabolism in the liver [52]. Hepatic extraction ratio refers to the amount of drug removed from circulation during first-pass metabolism. Hepatic extraction ratio for opioids range from low (methadone, tramadol), intermediate (codeine, hydromorphone, meperidine, oxycodone), to high (buprenorphine, fentanyl, morphine) [53, 54]. First-pass metabolism can be diminished in patients with compromised hepatic function, resulting in decreased extraction ratio with increased bioavailability and drug exposure. Medications with a high or intermediate extraction ratio will be most affected by changes in first-pass metabolism. This effect is perhaps most prominent in patients with cirrhosis where collateral flow shunts blood away from the portal circulation and significantly decreases extraction ratio.

Other factors which may complicate absorption of opioids in hepatic impairment include hypertensive gastropathy, gastritis, ulcers, and delayed gastric emptying [55, 56]. Use of immediate release oral formulations over extended or delayed-release is recommended for these patients. If compromised oral/enteral absorption is suspected, intravenous administration is the preferred route.

Effect of Hepatic Impairment on Opioid Distribution

Volume of distribution refers to the extent a medication moves from systemic circulation to other tissues or fluids in the body and is dependent on characteristics such as molecular size, degree of lipophilicity, and protein binding. See Tables 3.6, 3.7, and 3.8 for properties of specific opioids. Patients with hepatic disease commonly experience body fluid accumulation and changes in fluid distribution. This "third-spacing" (e.g., ascites in cirrhosis) causes an increase in volume of distribution and results in lower serum concentrations and decreased efficacy of hydrophilic opioids as they are distributed into tissue and body fluid [57, 58]. As patients undergo therapeutic interventions or improved clinical status, there may be acute changes in drug concentration as fluid and drug redistribute into the intravascular space. These changes are complex and difficult to predict; therefore, it is recommended to utilize short-acting, immediate-release formulations and initiate the lowest effective dose.

The liver is also responsible for the production of plasma binding proteins albumin and α_1-acid glycoprotein. Only "free" drug unbound from plasma proteins is available to bind to receptors. When plasma protein production is diminished due to hepatic impairment, the free fraction of highly protein bound drugs is increased and therefore more drug is available to exert a therapeutic effect.

Effect of Hepatic Impairment on Opioid Metabolism

Hepatic metabolism of opioids is a three-step process. Initially, drug enters enterohepatic circulation and undergoes first-pass metabolism. Once absorbed, opioids undergo phase I and phase II metabolism by the liver which results in active, inactive, or toxic metabolites.

Phase I metabolism occurs via cytochrome (CYP) P-450 systems and results in oxidation or hydrolysis of the compound. Opioids are metabolized by a variety of CYP isoenzymes (Table 3.7) and therefore have potential interactions with medications that are metabolized via these same isoenzymes. Most frequently this manifests as increased drug exposure and toxicity when opioids are administered with CYP enzyme inhibitors (e.g., methadone with ketoconazole). However, CYP enzyme inducers also pose a concern for opioids metabolized to active or toxic metabolites. For example, concurrent administration of tramadol and carbamazepine results in increased seizure risk from tramadol exposure [59]. Hepatic impairment may diminish any or all of the CYP isoenzyme systems resulting in two scenarios: (1) for opioids with inactive metabolites, decreased metabolism occurs and more active drug is available; or (2) for opioids with active metabolites, decreased metabolism occurs and decreased efficacy may be seen due to fewer active metabolites [52].

Phase II hepatic metabolism conjugates the drug with a hydrophilic substrate to prepare for excretion, most notably via glucuronidation. Phase II metabolism is generally not affected until severe hepatic impairment occurs and there is minimal clinical significance for opioids primarily metabolized by this method [52, 60]. However, in patients with cirrhosis drug exposure may be prolonged as phase II metabolism is diminished.

Effect of Hepatic Impairment on Opioid Excretion

Alterations in phase II metabolism as discussed above may diminish excretion of some opioids resulting in prolonged exposure. However, hepatic impairment is commonly associated with renal impairment, which may further impede clearance. Alterations of pharmacokinetics in patients with renal impairment has been previously discussed in this chapter.

Heart Failure

Heart failure (HF) is a clinical syndrome resulting from structural or functional impairment of ventricular filling or forward ejection, and includes HF with reduced ejection fraction (HFrEF) and HF with preserved ejection fraction (HFpEF) [61]. The significance of pharmacokinetic changes associated with HF likely varies based on the degree of compensation. In well-compensated patients, minimal pharmacokinetic changes can be expected, as guideline-directed medical therapy can preserve blood flow to the kidneys and liver and minimize volume overload.

Heart failure can affect a number of pharmacokinetic parameters [62]. Reduction in renal blood flow and glomerular filtration rate may occur in patients with HF, and therefore clearance may be decreased for medications dependent on flow-dependent renal and hepatic clearance. The reduction in clearance may be proportional to the severity of hemodynamic compromise. In addition, hepatic function may be impaired in patients with HF due to hepatocellular damage caused by hepatic congestion or hypoxemia. Volume of distribution may be significantly increased by peripheral edema as highly protein bound drugs distribute extensively in extracellular fluid. Serum albumin concentrations typically remain stable in well-nourished HF patients without hepatic impairment or critical illness; however, α_1-acid glycoprotein concentrations may be increased in patients with tissue damage and inflammation such as myocardial infarction. These changes in protein concentrations may alter the free fraction of medications that are highly protein bound.

Data describing pharmacokinetic changes of opioids in HF patients are extremely limited. A prospective cohort study evaluating fentanyl concentrations in ICU patients with respiratory failure or shock determined HF reduced fentanyl clearance substantially and significantly increased predicted plasma concentrations [50]. A pediatric study of patients undergoing cardiac surgery for congenital heart defects demonstrated that patients requiring higher levels of postoperative inotropic support had significantly lower morphine clearance, with the authors recommending a 50% reduction in morphine dose [63].

Morphine has traditionally been used in the management of acute HF based on its anxiolytic effects and decreased filling pressures, which can reduce both preload and afterload [64]. However, morphine may have adverse effects such as respiratory and CNS depression as well as hypotension. A propensity-matched study demonstrated that patients with acute HF who received morphine had increased mortality at 3, 7, 14, and 30 days, with the greatest risk at 3 days [65]. The 2016 European Society of Cardiology guidelines for acute and chronic HF recommend against routine use of opioids in acute HF, with cautious consideration in patients with severe dyspnea due to the risk of hypotension, bradycardia, respiratory depression with potential risk for invasive ventilation, as well as a potential increased risk of mortality [66].

Limited data exist regarding pharmacokinetic alterations with the use of opioids in patients with HF. Dose adjustments may be required in patients with significant edema or hemodynamic compromise that leads to renal and hepatic impairment. The potential for opioid adverse effects such as respiratory depression and hemodynamic compromise must be considered in patients with acute decompensation of HF.

Sepsis and Septic Shock

Patients with sepsis or septic shock exhibit a number of important pharmacokinetic changes that may have implications for opioid use. Early sepsis is characterized by inflammation, capillary leak, and third-spacing requiring fluid resuscitation, all of which increase drug volume of distribution, especially for hydrophilic opioids. Additionally, a compensatory increase in cardiac output occurs, often leading to an initial increase in creatinine clearance [49]. At the same time, serum albumin levels fall significantly, which may greatly increase the amount of unbound active drug in circulation, particularly for medications with high protein binding.

As sepsis progresses beyond the early phase, increased volume of distribution and hypoalbuminemia persist. However, renal and/or hepatic impairment may also occur, resulting in the previously discussed pharmacokinetic changes with those conditions [49, 53]. Hypoperfusion of the gastrointestinal tract, skin, and muscles may decrease absorption of enteral, transdermal, subcutaneous, and intramuscular medications [22, 53]. As the timing and magnitude of these pharmacokinetic changes are difficult to predict and because they have opposing implications for medication dosing, it is reasonable to initiate opioids at conservative doses, and then adjust as necessary. Since renal impairment is common in sepsis, utilization of an opioid that is minimally affected by renal impairment (e.g., fentanyl) is advisable.

Trauma

Critically ill patients with severe trauma exhibit many of the same pharmacokinetic changes seen in the early phase of sepsis. Increased volume of distribution secondary to inflammation, along with significant fluid resuscitation, is again present [49]. A hyperdynamic state with increased creatinine clearance and increased metabolism is also typically present. Additionally, these patients typically experience more pain inherent to their condition than other critically ill patients. All of these factors can increase opioid requirements, so clinicians should anticipate that more aggressive dosing may be necessary to adequately control pain, especially early in the patient's course. Because pain may be expected to persist, opioids with longer duration of action (e.g., hydromorphone, oxycodone) are often useful in patients with severe trauma. Since renal impairment is less common, renally eliminated opioids (e.g., oxycodone, morphine) that might be avoided in other populations can be considered in these patients. Notably, studies comparing morphine, fentanyl, and hydromorphone have not demonstrated significant differences in efficacy or toxicity when used for acute pain related to trauma, despite the pharmacokinetic differences between the medications [67].

Burns

Patients with burns may experience severe pain, including hyperalgesia and allodynia [68]. Opioids combined with non-opioid analgesics are the preferred therapy for management of general and procedure-related pain in burn patients, but requirements may be unpredictable due to changes in volume of distribution, protein binding, and hemodynamic changes affecting clearance [69, 70]. Pharmacokinetics may also be affected by patient-specific factors such as severity of burn, time since the burn injury occurred, age, underlying comorbid conditions, fluid resuscitation, and sepsis [71].

In patients with major burns, two distinct phases occur that affect pharmacokinetic and pharmacodynamic parameters of medications. In the acute burn shock phase, volume of distribution is typically increased due to generalized edema formation, while clearance may be decreased due to reduced cardiac output [68, 71]. Medication concentrations can be affected by altered protein binding from loss of plasma proteins through burned skin and dilution of remaining proteins by fluid resuscitation [70]. The hyperdynamic phase of burn injury evolves over several days to weeks, and therefore pharmacokinetic alterations may vary depending on the time elapsed after initial injury [71]. Cardiac output is significantly increased during the hyperdynamic phase, which may increase hepatic and renal elimination. Burn injury may result in hepatic impairment with decreased oxidation, reduction, and hydroxylation, but typically no alteration in conjugation. Hypoalbuminemia occurs due to decreased synthesis in the liver, increased intravascular permeability, and exudate loss. Hepatic synthesis of acute-phase proteins such as α_1-acid glycoprotein is increased, and therefore protein binding of medications continues to be highly variable.

A study evaluated fentanyl pharmacokinetics 4.5 h after a single dose in patients with burns (49 ± 4% total BSA 17 ± 3 days after injury) compared to control patients without burns [72]. The volume of distribution of fentanyl was two times higher for patients with burns; therefore higher doses may be required.

Five adult patients with burns (30–58% total BSA) received long-term morphine continuous infusion with titration based on pain ratings with bolus doses for procedural pain [73]. The effective dose of morphine infusion ranged widely from 4 to 39.5 mg/h and steady state concentrations of morphine demonstrated linear association with the infusion rate. There was no significant difference in systemic clearance of morphine during the 3-week study period; however, renal clearance decreased after 3 weeks. Slight hepatic impairment did not alter morphine disposition. This study demonstrated wide variability in required rate of morphine infusion in burn patients which was not directly related to clearance, and therefore dose should be titrated to clinical effect.

Methadone pharmacokinetics were evaluated in 14 burn patients receiving methadone loading dose followed by continuous IV infusion for 24 h [74]. The mean body surface area burned was 50 ± 22% (range 26–72%) and the median time from burn injury was 1 day (range 0–8 days). Clearance was significantly higher than standard values reported in the literature, and the estimated half-life was 2.6 ± 1.1 h. Significant predictors of clearance were serum albumin, time from burn injury, and age.

Opioid requirements in patients with burn injuries may vary widely based on patient-specific factors affecting opioid pharmacokinetics and pharmacodynamics. To manage opioid tolerance and hyperalgesia, switching of opioids and use of multimodal analgesia can be considered [68]. General pain can be managed with the use of patient-controlled analgesia, continuous infusion opioids, or the use of oral agents. For the management of procedural-related pain, opioids with a rapid onset of action and short duration are preferred [69].

Extracorporeal Membrane Oxygenation (ECMO)

Drug concentrations during ECMO depend on a variety of factors such as lipophilicity and protein binding of the medication, type and age of circuit, and the patient's underlying renal and hepatic function [75]. Pharmacokinetic data are primarily limited to ex vivo analyses, with concentrations measured at 24 h or less. Limited studies regarding opioid use in adult ECMO patients have been published, and practitioners should be cautious when applying neonatal data to the adult population due to differences in volume of distribution and clearance.

Extracorporeal membrane oxygenation can significantly increase in volume of distribution based on hemodilution and medication sequestration. Hemodilution from the circuit may decrease drug concentrations. Lipophilic drugs may bind to organic materials in circuit components such as polyvinyl chloride (PVC) tubing and the membrane oxygenator, which provide a large surface area for drug sequestration [75, 76]. Lipophilicity is measured by the octanol/water partition coefficient and logP is the log of the partition coefficient. Negative values of logP indicate hydrophilic compounds and high positive values indicate lipophilic compounds [77]. Opioid lipophilicity is listed in Table 3.6. The anilidopiperidines and methadone are lipophilic, whereas morphine, hydromorphone, and oxycodone are more hydrophilic and may be more appropriate in patients receiving ECMO.

The use of ECMO may also have variable effects on highly protein-bound medications. Hemodilution may decrease serum protein concentrations, which can result in increased free fraction of highly protein-bound medications, and therefore increase both efficacy and the risk of adverse effects [75]. Alternatively, serum proteins may also bind to circuit tubing, and highly protein-bound drugs may have significant reductions in serum concentrations [75, 76]. Protein binding of opioid agonists is listed in Table 3.6. Similar to the trend in lipophilicity, the anilidopiperidines and methadone are highly protein bound, whereas morphine, hydromorphone, and oxycodone exhibit less protein binding and may be more appropriate for use in patients receiving ECMO.

An ex vivo study evaluated drug concentrations in ECMO circuits primed with crystalloid, albumin, and fresh whole blood compared to controls of jars filled with fresh whole blood [78]. At 24 h the mean percent of drug recovered compared to baseline for fentanyl was only 3% in the ECMO circuits, compared to 82% in the controls, whereas there was no difference in morphine concentrations at 24 h. While morphine is preferable to fentanyl in terms of decreased circuit sequestration, the use of morphine in critically ill patients is limited by the risk of adverse effects [76]. Hydromorphone sequestration was evaluated in five pediatric ECMO circuits primed with crystalloid and whole blood [79]. The percent reduction in concentration was 55% for fentanyl and 24% for hydromorphone at 12 h. Hydromorphone may be preferable based on decreased sequestration compared to fentanyl and less risk of hemodynamic adverse effects compared to morphine.

A reasonable approach for opioid therapy in patients receiving ECMO is to initiate continuous infusion fentanyl as part of a sedation strategy at higher than standard doses, or to initiate opioids with lower lipophilicity and protein binding at standard doses [75]. Careful monitoring and titration is required to optimize dosing and balance opioid efficacy with the risks of toxicity with prolonged therapy. Drug binding sites within the circuit may eventually become saturated and therefore dosing requirements could potentially decrease with time. However, it is unclear if and when this occurs based on variable study results [76, 80, 81]. If circuit components are changed, dosing requirements may acutely increase due to the lack of saturation. Patients are at risk of prolonged sedation even after opioid discontinuation, as sequestered opioids continue to be released from the circuit. As patients are liberated from ECMO, an empiric reduction in dosing is likely warranted based on the decreased volume of distribution and lack of circuit sequestration; however, careful monitoring and titration is required to balance the risk of withdrawal and toxicity [75, 82].

Obesity

As obesity impacts more than 30% of adults in the United States, clinicians must be familiar with the pharmacokinetic implications of obesity. Volume of distribution is increased by obesity, primarily for lipophilic opioids (e.g., fentanyl, methadone) [83]. Table 3.6 contains information regarding the lipophilicity of specific opioids. Clinicians should expect obese patients to require higher initial doses of lipophilic opioids, though the doses will not be in direct proportion to their weight [83–85]. Lipophilic opioids will accumulate in adipose tissue, so maintenance doses should be reduced to avoid excessive or prolonged analgosedation. This is particularly relevant to scheduled dosing and continuous IV infusions of opioids. Use of hydrophilic opioids may be advantageous to avoid the risk of significant drug accumulation.

Conclusions

Opioids are commonly used in the ICU but organ dysfunction and critical illness may significantly impact pharmacokinetic and pharmacodynamic parameters. Careful consideration of the properties of the selected opioid, dose, and route of administration in addition to patient-specific attributes can reduce the incidence of adverse effects associated with opioid therapy.

References

1. Pathan H, Williams J. Basic opioid pharmacology: an update. Br J Pain. 2012;6(1):11–6. https://doi.org/10.1177/2049463712438493.
2. Trivedi M, Shaikh S, Gwinnut G. Pharmacology of opioids. Update in Anaesthesia. 2008 [updated 2008 Feb 24; cited 2019 Nov 14]. Available from www.wfsahq.org.
3. Fraser GL, Gagnon DJ. Pain and analgesia. CCSAP. 2016 [cited 2019 Nov 14]. Available from www.accp.com.
4. Trescot AM, Datta S, Lee M, Hansen H. Opioid pharmacology. Pain Physician. 2008;11(2 Suppl):S133–53.
5. Drewes AM, Jensen RD, Nielsen LM, Droney J, Christrup LL, Arendt-Nielsen L, et al. Differences between opioids: pharmacological, experimental, clinical and economical perspectives. Br J Clin Pharmacol. 2013;75(1):60–78. https://doi.org/10.1111/j.1365-2125.2012.04317.x.

6. Lexicomp Online. Hudson. Ohio: Wolters Kluwer Clinical Drug Information, Inc; 2013. Accessed on November 13, 2019
7. Böhm R, Proksch E, Schwarz T, et al. Drug hypersensitivity. Dtsch Arztebl Int. 2018;115:501–12.
8. Benyamin R, Trescot AM, Datta S, et al. Opioid complications and side effects. Pain Physician. 2008;11:S105–20.
9. Swegle JM, Logemann C. Management of common opioid-induced adverse effects. Am Fam Physician. 2006;74:1347–54.
10. Treillet E, Laurent S, Hadjiat Y. Practical management of opioid rotation and equianalgesia. J Pain Res. 2018;11:2587–601.
11. Barke KE, Hough LB. Opiates, mast cells and histamine release. Life Sci. 1993;53:1391–9.
12. Kalangara J, Potru S, et al. Clinical manifestations and diagnostic evaluation of opioid allergy labels: a review. J Pain Palliat Care Pharmacother. 2019; https://doi.org/10.1080/15360288.2019.1666955. [Epub ahead of print]
13. Baldo BA, Pham NH. Histamine-releasing and allergenic properties of opioid analgesic drugs: resolving the two. Anaesth Intensive Care. 2012;40:216–35.
14. Li PH, Ue KL, et al. Opioid hypersensitivity: predictors of allergy and role of drug provocation testing. J Allergy Clin Immunol Pract. 2017;5:1601–6.
15. Powell MZ, Mueller SW, et al. Assessment of opioid cross-reactivity and provider perceptions in hospitalized patients with reported opioid allergies. Ann Pharmacother. 2019;53:1117–23.
16. Jacobi J, Fraser GL, Coursin DB, Riker RR, Fontaine D, Wittbrodt ET, et al. Clinical practice guidelines for the sustained use of sedatives and analgesics in the critically ill adult. Crit Care Med. 2002;30(1):119–41.
17. Bruera E, Belzile M, Pituskin E, et al. Opioid rotation in patients with cancer pain. Cancer. 1996;78:852–7.
18. Dunbar PJ, Chapman CR, Buckley FP, et al. Clinical analgesic equivalence for morphine and hydromorphone with prolonged PCA. Pain. 1996;68:165–70.
19. Fine PG, Portenoy RK. Establishing "best practices" for opioid rotation: conclusions of an expert panel. J Pain Symptom Manag. 2009;38:418–25.
20. Ripamonti C, De Conno F, Groff L, et al. Equi-analgesic dose ratio between methadone and other opioid agonists in cancer pain: comparison of two clinical experiences. Ann Oncol. 1998;9:79–83.
21. Barr J, Fraser GL, Puntillo K, Ely EW, Gélinas C, Dasta JF, et al. Clinical practice guidelines for the management of pain, agitation, and delirium in adult patients in the intensive care unit. Crit Care Med. 2013;41(1):263–306. https://doi.org/10.1097/CCM.0b013e3182783b72.
22. Devlin JW, Roberts RJ. Pharmacology of commonly used analgesics and sedatives in the ICU: benzodiazepines, propofol, and opioids. Crit Care Clin. 2009;25(3):431–49., vii. https://doi.org/10.1016/j.ccc.2009.03.003.
23. Erstad BL, Puntillo K, Gilbert HC, Grap MJ, Li D, Medina J, et al. Pain management principles in the critically ill. Chest. 2009;135(4):1075–86. https://doi.org/10.1378/chest.08-2264.
24. Tse AHW, Ling L, Lee A, Joynt GM. Altered pharmacokinetics in prolonged infusions of sedatives and analgesics among adult critically ill patients: a systematic review. Clin Ther. 2018;40(9):1598–1615.e2. https://doi.org/10.1016/j.clinthera.2018.07.021. Epub 2018 Aug 31
25. Chou R, Gordon DB, de Leon-Casasola OA, Rosenberg JM, Bickler S, Brennan T, et al. Management of Postoperative Pain: a clinical practice guideline from the American pain society, the American Society of Regional Anesthesia and Pain Medicine, and the American Society of Anesthesiologists' committee on regional Anesthesia, executive committee, and administrative council. J Pain. 2016;17(2):131–57. https://doi.org/10.1016/j.jpain.2015.12.008.
26. Stewart D. Pearls and pitfalls of patient-controlled analgesia. U.S. Pharmacists. 2017 [updated 2007 Mar 17; cited 2019 Nov 14]. Available from www.uspharmacist.com.
27. Kruer RM, Jarrell AS, Latif A. Reducing medication errors in critical care: a multimodal approach. Clin Pharmacol. 2014;6:117–26. https://doi.org/10.2147/CPAA.S48530. eCollection 2014

28. Kestenbaum MG, Vilches AO, Messersmith S, Connor SR, Fine PG, Murphy B, et al. Alternative routes to oral opioid administration in palliative care: a review and clinical summary. Pain Med. 2014;15(7):1129–53. https://doi.org/10.1111/pme.12464. Epub 2014 Jul 4.
29. Bujedo BM. Spinal opioid bioavailability in postoperative pain. Pain Pract. 2014;14(4):350–64. https://doi.org/10.1111/papr.12099. Epub 2013 Jul 8
30. Mugabure BB. A clinical approach to neuraxial morphine for the treatment of postoperative pain. Pain Res Treat. 2012;2012:612145. Epub 2012 Jul 2
31. Kumar K, Singh SI. Neuraxial opioid-induced pruritus: An update. J Anaesthesiol Clin Pharmacol. 2013;29(3):303–7. https://doi.org/10.4103/0970-9185.117045.
32. Duramorph package insert. Deerfield, IL: Baxter Healthcare Corporation; 2005 [cited 2019 Nov 14]. Available from: www.accessdata.gov.gov.
33. DeSousa KA, Chandran R. Intrathecal morphine for postoperative analgesia: current trends. World J Anaesth. 2014;3(3):191–202. https://doi.org/10.5313/wja.v3.i3.191.
34. Hindle A. Intrathecal opioids in the management of acute postoperative pain. Cont Educ Anaesth Crit Care Pain. 2008;8(3):81–5. https://doi.org/10.1093/bjaceaccp/mkn016.
35. Bernards CM, Shen DD, Sterling ES, Adkins JE, Risler L, Phillips B, et al. Epidural, cerebrospinal fluid, and plasma pharmacokinetics of epidural opioids (part 1): differences among opioids. Anesthesiology. 2003;99(2):455–65.
36. Bajaj S, Whiteman A, Brander B. Transdermal drug delivery in pain management. Cont Educ Anaesth Crit Care Pain. 2011;11:39–43. https://doi.org/10.1093/bjaceaccp/mkq054.
37. Institute of Safe Medication Practices (ISMP). Fentanyl patches. 2013 [cited 2019 Nov 14]. Available from: https://www.ismp.org/sites/default/files/attachments/2018-11/fentanyl1-13.pdf.
38. Margetts L, Sawyer R. Transdermal drug delivery: principles and opioid therapy. Cont Educ Anaesth Crit Care Pain. 2007;7:5:171–6. https://doi.org/10.1093/bjaceaccp/mkm033.
39. Heiskanen T, Mätzke S, Haakana S, Gergov M, Vuori E, Kalso E. Transdermal fentanyl in cachectic cancer patients. Pain. 2009;144(1–2):218–22. https://doi.org/10.1016/j.pain.2009.04.012. Epub 2009 May 12
40. Carter KA. Heat-associated increase in transdermal fentanyl absorption. Am J Health Syst Pharm. 2003;60(2):191–2.
41. Institute of Safe Medication Practices (ISMP). ISMP Calls for more action to safeguard pain patches. 2005 [cited 2019 Nov 14]. Available from: https://www.ismp.org/news/ismp-calls-more-action-safeguard-pain-patches.
42. American Pharmacists Association (APhA). The danger with cutting medication patches. 2013 [cited 2019 Nov 14]. Available at: https://www.pharmacist.com/danger-cutting-medication-patches.
43. Compound summary. National Institutes of Health U.S. National library of medicine national center for biotechnology information. Accessed November 14, 2019. Available from: https://pubchem.ncbi.nlm.nih.gov/.
44. Dayer P, Desmeules J, Collart L. Pharmacology of tramadol. Drugs. 1997;53(Suppl 2):18–24.
45. Opana package insert. Chadds Ford, PA: Endo Pharmaceuticals; 2011 Aug [cited 2019 Nov 14]. Available from: https://www.accessdata.fda.gov/drugsatfda_docs/label/2012/021611s007lbl.pdf.
46. Opana ER package insert. Chadds Ford, PA: Endo Pharmaceuticals; 2012 [cited 2019 Nov 14].
47. Sloan P. Review of oral oxymorphone in the management of pain. Ther Clin Risk Manag. 2008;4(4):777–87.
48. Talwin package insert. Bridgewater, NJ: Sanofi-Aventis; 2011 [cited 2019 Nov 14]. Available from: https://www.accessdata.fda.gov/drugsatfda_docs/label/2011/018733s015lbl.pdf.
49. Boucher BA, Wood GC, Swanson JM. Pharmacokinetic changes in critical illness. Crit Care Clin. 2006;22(2):255–71.
50. Choi L, Ferrell BA, Vasilevskis EE, Pandharipande PP, Heltsley R, Ely EW, et al. Population pharmacokinetics of fentanyl in the critically ill. Crit Care Med. 2016;44(1):64–72.
51. Mercadante S, Arcuri E. Opioids and renal function. J Pain. 2004;5(1):2–19.

52. Bosilkovska M, Walder B, Besson M, et al. Analgesics in patients with hepatic impairment. Drugs. 2012;72:1645–69.
53. De Paepe P, Belpaire FM, Buylaert WA. Pharmacokinetic and pharmacodynamic considerations when treating patients with sepsis and septic shock. Clin Pharmacokinet. 2002;41(14):1135–51.
54. Gelot S, Nakhla E. Opioid dosing in renal and hepatic impairment. US Pharm. 2014;39:34–8.
55. Ishizu H, Shioni S, Kawamura E, et al. Gastric emptying in patients with chronic liver diseases. Ann Nucl Med. 2002;16:177–82.
56. Delcò F, Tchambaz L, Schlienger R, et al. Dose adjustment in patients with liver disease. Drug Saf. 2005;28:529–45.
57. Lin S, Smith BS. Drug dosing considerations for the critically ill patient with liver disease. Crit Care Nurs Clin North Am. 2010;22:335–40.
58. Yogaratnam D, Ditch K, Medeiros K, et al. The impact of liver and renal dysfunction on the pharmacokinetics and pharmacodynamics of sedative and analgesic drugs in critically ill adult patients. Crit Care Nurs Clin North Am. 2016;28:183–4.
59. Beakley BD, Kaye AM, Kaye AD. Tramadol, pharmacology, side effects, and serotonin syndrome: a review. Pain Physician. 2015;18:395–400.
60. Smith HS. Opioid metabolism. Mayo Clin Proc. 2009;84:613–24.
61. Yancy CW, Jessup M, Bozkurt B, Butler J, Casey DE Jr, Drazner MH, et al. ACCF/AHA guideline for the management of heart failure: a report of the American College of Cardiology Foundation/American Heart Association task force on practice guidelines. J Am Coll Cardiol. 2013;62(16):e147–239. https://doi.org/10.1016/j.jacc.2013.05.019. Epub 2013 Jun 5
62. Ogawa R, Stachnik JM, Echizen H. Clinical pharmacokinetics of drugs in patients with heart failure: an update (part 1, drugs administered intravenously). Clin Pharmacokinet. 2013;52(3):169–85. https://doi.org/10.1007/s40262-012-0029-2.
63. Dagan O, Klein J, Bohn D, Barker G, Koren G. Morphine pharmacokinetics in children following cardiac surgery: effects of disease and inotropic support. J Cardiothorac Vasc Anesth. 1993;7(4):396–8.
64. Naito K, Kohno T, Fukuda K. Harmful impact of morphine use in acute heart failure. J Thorac Dis. 2017;9(7):1831–4. https://doi.org/10.21037/jtd.2017.06.78.
65. Miró Ò, Gil V, Martín-Sánchez FJ, Herrero-Puente P, Jacob J, Mebazaa A, et al. Morphine use in the ED and outcomes of patients with acute heart failure: a propensity score-matching analysis based on the EAHFE registry. Chest. 2017;152(4):821–32. https://doi.org/10.1016/j.chest.2017.03.037. Epub 2017 Apr 12
66. Ponikowski P, Voors AA, Anker SD, Bueno H, Cleland JGF, Coats AJS, et al. 2016 ESC guidelines for the diagnosis and treatment of acute and chronic heart failure: the task force for the diagnosis and treatment of acute and chronic heart failure of the European Society of Cardiology (ESC). Eur Heart J. 2016;37(27):2129–200. https://doi.org/10.1093/eurheartj/ehw128. Epub 2016 May 20
67. MacKenzie M, Zed PJ, Ensom MHH. Opioid pharmacokinetics-pharmacodynamics: clinical implications in acute pain management in trauma. Ann Pharmacother. 2016;50(3):209–1.
68. Bittner EA, Shank E, Woodson L, Martyn JA. Acute and perioperative care of the burn-injured patient. Anesthesiology. 2015;122(2):448–64. https://doi.org/10.1097/ALN.0000000000000559.
69. Gregoretti C, Decaroli D, Piacevoli Q, Mistretta A, Barzaghi N, Luxardo N, et al. Analgo-sedation of patients with burns outside the operating room. Drugs. 2008;68(17):2427–43. https://doi.org/10.2165/0003495-200868170-00003.
70. Griggs C, Goverman J, Bittner EA, Levi B. Sedation and pain management in burn patients. Clin Plast Surg. 2017;44(3):535–40. https://doi.org/10.1016/j.cps.2017.02.026. Epub 2017 Apr 18
71. Blanchet B, Jullien V, Vinsonneau C, Tod M. Influence of burns on pharmacokinetics and pharmacodynamics of drugs used in the care of burn patients. Clin Pharmacokinet. 2008;47(10):635–54.

72. Kaneda K, Han TH. Comparative population pharmacokinetics of fentanyl using non-linear mixed effect modeling: burns vs. non-burns. Burns. 2009;35(6):790–7. https://doi.org/10.1016/j.burns.2008.12.006. Epub 2009 Jun 6
73. Perreault S, Choinière M, du Souich PB, Bellavance F, Beauregard G. Pharmacokinetics of morphine and its glucuronidated metabolites in burn injuries. Ann Pharmacother. 2001;35(12):1588–92.
74. Denson DD, Concilus RR, Warden G, Raj PP. Pharmacokinetics of continuous intravenous infusion of methadone in the early post-burn period. J Clin Pharmacol. 1990;30(1):70–5.
75. Dzierba AL, Abrams D, Brodie D. Medicating patients during extracorporeal membrane oxygenation: the evidence is building. Crit Care. 2017;21(1):66. https://doi.org/10.1186/s13054-017-1644-y.
76. Satyapriya SV, Lyaker ML, Rozycki AJ. Sedation, analgesia, delirium in the ECMO patient. Extracorporeal membrane oxygenation. In: Firstenberg MS, editor. Extracorporeal membrane oxygenation; 2016. https://doi.org/10.5772/64249. Available from: https://www.intechopen.com/books/extracorporeal-membrane-oxygenation-advances-in-therapy/sedation-analgesia-delirium-in-the-ecmo-patient.
77. Ha MA, Sieg AC. Evaluation of altered drug pharmacokinetics in critically ill adults receiving extracorporeal membrane oxygenation. Pharmacotherapy. 2017;37(2):221–35. https://doi.org/10.1002/phar.1882. Epub 2017 Feb 3.
78. Shekar K, Roberts JA, Mcdonald CI, Ghassabian S, Anstey C, Wallis SC, et al. Protein-bound drugs are prone to sequestration in the extracorporeal membrane oxygenation circuit: results from an ex vivo study. Crit Care. 2015;19:164. https://doi.org/10.1186/s13054-015-0891-z.
79. Heith CS, Hansen LA, Bakken RM, Ritter SL, Long BR, Hume JR, et al. Effects of an ex vivo pediatric extracorporeal membrane oxygenation circuit on the sequestration of Mycophenolate Mofetil, Tacrolimus, Hydromorphone, and Fentanyl. J Pediatr Pharmacol Ther. 2019;24(4):290–5. https://doi.org/10.5863/1551-6776-24.4.290.
80. Shekar K, Roberts JA, Ghassabian S, Mullany DV, Ziegenfuss M, Smith MT, et al. Sedation during extracorporeal membrane oxygenation-why more is less. Anaesth Intensive Care. 2012;40(6):1067–9.
81. Shekar K, Roberts JA, McDonald CI, Fisquet S, Barnett AG, Mullany DV, et al. Sequestration of drugs in the circuit may lead to therapeutic failure during extracorporeal membrane oxygenation. Crit Care. 2012;16(5):R194. https://doi.org/10.1186/cc11679.
82. Cheng V, Abdul-Aziz MH, Roberts JA, Shekar K. Optimising drug dosing in patients receiving extracorporeal membrane oxygenation. J Thorac Dis. 2018;10(Suppl 5):S629–41. https://doi.org/10.21037/jtd.2017.09.154.
83. Astle S. Pain management in critically ill obese patients. Crit Care Nurs Clin North Am. 2009;21(3):323–39.
84. Shibutani K, Inchiosa MA, Sawada K, Bairamian M. Accuracy of pharmacokinetic models for predicting plasma fentanyl concentrations in lean and obese surgical patients: derivation of dosing weight ("pharmacokinetic mass"). Anesthesiology. 2004;101:603–13.
85. Cheymol G. Effects of obesity on pharmacokinetics: implications for drug therapy. Clin Pharmacokinet. 2000;39(3):215–31.

Chapter 4
Opioid Drug Interactions

Amy L. Dzierba, Teresa Poon, and Justin Muir

Introduction

Pain experienced by patients in the intensive care unit (ICU) can manifest as acute, chronic, or acute-on-chronic. The majority of ICU patients suffer from moderate to severe pain that typically requires pharmacological interventions with a multimodal approach that will often include opioid analgesics [1]. While effective in treating pain, opioids are associated with potential drug interactions resulting in toxicity, intolerance, or therapeutic failure. An understanding of the complex interplay between drug interactions and the pharmacogenetics of opioids may provide insight into the individual variability in therapeutic response.

A drug interaction occurs when one drug modifies the action of another drug through prior or concurrent administration. Drug interactions can largely be classified as pharmacokinetic or pharmacodynamic [2]. Pharmacokinetic drug interactions result in changes to a drug's absorption, distribution, metabolism, or elimination resulting in augmented or diminished systemic concentrations. Conversely, pharmacodynamic reactions refer to the relationship between the concentration of the drug at the intended site and resulting drug effect. Pharmacodynamic drug interactions are classified as additive, synergistic, or antagonistic effects of two drugs on the same clinical endpoint. Pharmacogenomics refers to how genes affect an individual's response to drugs, potentially leading to pharmacokinetic and pharmacodynamic variability. These genetic polymorphisms may be responsible for the heterogeneity of opioid responses and potential for drug interactions.

A. L. Dzierba (✉) · T. Poon · J. Muir
Department of Pharmacy, NewYork-Presbyterian Hospital, New York, NY, USA
e-mail: ald9012@nyp.org; tep9027@nyp.org; jum9018@nyp.org

J. L. Pascual, T. G. Gaulton (eds.), *Opioid Use in Critical Care*,
https://doi.org/10.1007/978-3-030-77399-1_4

Potential drug interactions may occur in over half of ICU patients, a rate twice as high as patients on general wards; though, not all of these drug interactions are clinically significant [3, 4]. Approximately 5% of patients in the ICU experience an adverse drug event from a drug interaction which have been associated with prolonged ICU length of stay [3, 5]. Critically ill patients are more likely to suffer from an increased number of potential drug interactions given the intensity of their drug regimens and number of medication exposures [4]. The precise frequency and severity of opioid drug interactions in ICU patients have not been described. Therefore, an understanding of potential clinically important opioid drug interactions is a crucial component in the management of the critically ill patient.

Common Mechanisms of Opioid Drug Interactions

Since opioids are extensively metabolized by the liver, resultant drug interactions may occur via phase I and II hepatic enzymatic pathways. Phase I opioid metabolism converts the parent drug to a more water-soluble or reactive product through oxidation by cytochrome P450 (CYP450), hydrolysis, or reduction [6]. Opioid metabolism is largely driven through CYP450 enzymatic pathways, specifically the CYP3A4/5, CYP2D6, and CYP2B6 isoenzymes (Table 4.1). Drugs metabolized by CYP450 can be classified as substrates, inhibitors, or inducers. Several different drug interaction scenarios may arise with the addition or deletion of inducers and inhibitors (Fig. 4.1). For example, when a CYP450 inhibitor is combined with an opioid that is metabolized through the same isoenzyme, greater opioid concentrations will result with consequent enhanced clinical effects and a potential for toxicity. However, in cases when an opioid is a prodrug (inactive drugs metabolized to an active metabolite), the opposite scenario will occur. Phase II opioid metabolism promotes elimination through drug conjugation (e.g. glucuronidation). The most common enzymes that metabolize opioids are uridine diphosphoglucuronosyltransferases (UGTs). Conjugation of buprenorphine, codeine, hydrocodone, hydromorphone, morphine, oxycodone, and oxymorphone by UGTs results in either active or inactive metabolites [7].

Energy-dependent transporters such as permeability-glycoprotein (P-gp) and organic anion-transporting polypeptides (OATPs) are located in the gut, kidneys, and blood-brain barrier [6]. These transporters act as a biological barrier by expelling drug molecules out of cells resulting in significant changes in drug absorption and disposition. Drug interactions occur as a result of inhibition and induction of P-gp. Of note, many drug interactions involve both the P-gp and CYP450 system since they share many substrates that are physiologically linked; therefore, it is often challenging to determine the specific mechanism of interaction. Several opioids such as fentanyl, methadone, meperidine, morphine, and oxycodone are substrates of P-gp. Like the CYP450 system, P-gp inhibition can increase drug exposure and the potential risk for adverse events. There are several other medications used in the critical care setting that are also P-gp inhibitors and inducers (Table 4.2).

Table 4.1 Common metabolic pathways of opioid analgesics

	Phase I pathway			Phase II pathway
Opioid	CYP2B6	CYP2D6	CYP3A4/5	UGT
Buprenorphine	–	–	Norbuprenorphine[a]	Buprenorphine-3-glucuronide[a] Norbuprenorphine-3-glucuronide[a]
Codeine[b]	–	Morphine[a]	Norcodeine	Morphine 6-glucuronide[a] Morphine 3-glucuronide
Fentanyl	–	–	Norfentanyl	–
Hydrocodone[b]	–	Hydromorphone[a]	Norhydrocodone	Hydromorphone 3-glucuronide
Hydromorphone	–	–	–	Hydromorphone 3-glucuronide
Methadone	Inactive metabolites	Inactive metabolites	Inactive metabolites	–
Meperidine	–	–	–	–
Morphine	–	–	–	Morphine 6-glucuronide[a] Morphine 3-glucuronide
Oxycodone	–	Oxymorphone[a]	Noroxycodone[a]	Inactive metabolites
Oxymorphone	–	–	–	Inactive metabolites
Remifentanil	–	–	–	–
Sufentanil	–	–	Inactive metabolites	–
Tramadol[b]	–	O-desmethyl tramadol (M1)	N-desmethyl tramadol (M2)	–

CYP cytochrome P450, *UGT* uridine diphospho-glucuronosyltransferase
[a]Active metabolite
[b]Prodrug activated by cytochrome P450 enzyme

Inhibition of CYP450 or P-gp occurs faster than drug induction, occurring over several days after introducing the inhibitor. Drug interactions mediated by enzyme induction are delayed since it takes time for the production of new enzymes. A similar delay is observed for the dissipation of the interaction when the offending drug is removed as the enzyme system gradually declines to baseline function. The area under the concentration versus time curve (AUC) can be used in the context of opioid drug interactions to represent the variation of a plasma drug concentration over time.

Pharmacodynamic drug interactions can produce desired effects or unwanted adverse effects. In general, pharmacodynamic interactions occur via various mechanisms by acting on the receptor or by interfering with the feedback mechanism of a process targeted by the other medication. Opioids result in several clinical effects other than analgesia, many of which are undesirable. Across the drug class, these

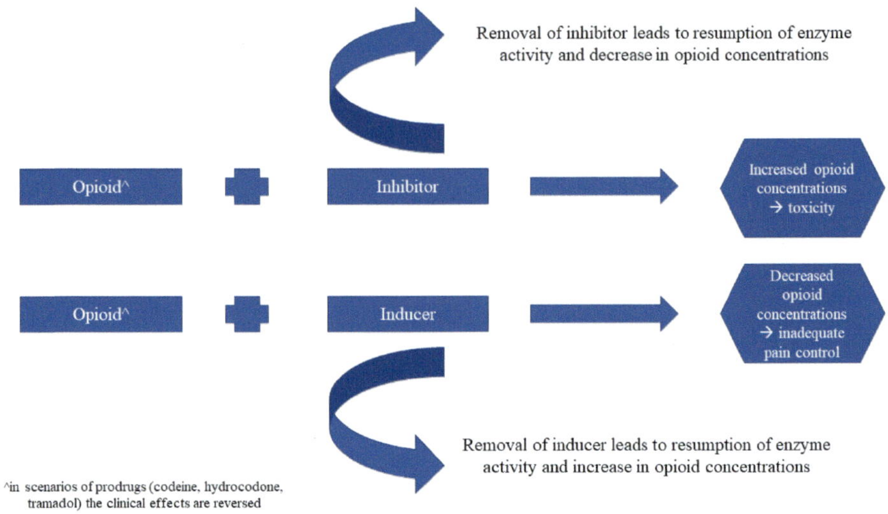

Fig. 4.1 Expected effects of opioid interactions with the addition of an inhibitor or inducer

Table 4.2 Common permeability-glycoprotein (P-gp) inhibitors and inducers

Inhibitors	Inducers
Amiodarone	Phenobarbital
Clarithromycin	Phenytoin
Cyclosporine	Rifampin
Diltiazem	
Erythromycin	
Itraconazole	
Ketoconazole	
Ritonavir	
Verapamil	

include central nervous system depression, respiratory depression, and constipation. Specific opioids harbor additional unique adverse effects related to central nervous system or cardiovascular toxicity.

Opioid Drug Interactions Commonly Encountered in the Critically Ill Patient

CYP450 Enzyme Modulation

Since many opioids are metabolized by the CYP450 system, they are susceptible to interactions with other drugs that inhibit or induce these enzymes. Many prescribed opioids in ICU patients, such as fentanyl, oxycodone, hydrocodone, tramadol, methadone, sufentanil, and buprenorphine, are metabolized predominantly by CYP3A4. A study of healthy volunteers found that inhibition of CYP3A4 with ketoconazole increased oxycodone's half-life from 4.1 to 5.5 hours and the AUC by 84% [8]. Conversely, the addition of a strong CYP2D6 inhibitor, quinidine, significantly increased oxycodone AUC by 42%, and the combination of the two inhibitors increased AUC by 209% as well as the peak concentration (Cmax) by 58% [8]. Induction of these enzymes may increase drug clearance and reduce analgesic effects for patients receiving opioids metabolized by the same pathway. Other opioids however, such as remifentanil and hydromorphone that are not metabolized through any CYP450 pathway, would not be subject to any CYP450 enzyme-mediated drug interactions.

Fentanyl is one of the most common opioids used in the ICU setting and is a major substrate of CYP3A4. However, because of its high hepatic extraction ratio, indicating that its clearance is primarily dependent on hepatic blood flow, enzyme interactions may be less apparent compared to that of other opioids. For example, a pharmacokinetic study in healthy volunteers found no difference in fentanyl concentrations with concomitant administration of itraconazole, a strong CYP3A4 inhibitor [9]. In contrast, voriconazole, an azole antifungal extensively metabolized by CYP450 isoenzymes, decreased fentanyl clearance by 23% and increased AUC by 39% [10]. Regarding enzyme induction, a study conducted in patients receiving chronic antiepileptic drugs reported substantial fentanyl dose escalations required to manage pain during craniotomy as the number of baseline antiepileptics increased [11]. Expected CYP-mediated drug interactions with fentanyl are displayed in Table 4.3.

CYP2D6 plays a role as a major pathway for codeine and a minor pathway for oxycodone, hydrocodone, tramadol, and methadone. Tramadol is additionally metabolized by CYP2B6 and methadone is metabolized by a number of additional enzymes including CYP2B6, CYP2C9, and CYP2C19. Notably, the true metabolic pathway for methadone has been scrutinized in recent years, with some investigations concluding that CYP3A4 is not a significant pathway for its clearance [12]. Certain opioids are prodrugs or are active drugs metabolized to active metabolites. In these examples, the effect of enzyme inhibition or interaction is more complex. For example, codeine is a prodrug that is predominantly metabolized to its active form morphine by CYP2D6, and a second pathway (CYP3A4) metabolizes codeine to norcodeine, an opioid with little activity. Inhibition of CYP2D6 will reduce the concentrations of morphine and therefore reduce the overall analgesic effect, while

Table 4.3 Effects of enzyme inhibition and induction on fentanyl

Enzyme effect of concomitant drug	Effects on substrate	Expected clinical effects
CYP3A4 inhibitor	↓ fentanyl metabolism ↑ fentanyl concentrations	↑ opioid effect
CYP3A4 inducer	↑ fentanyl metabolism ↓ fentanyl concentrations	↓ opioid effect

CYP cytochrome P450

Table 4.4 Effects of enzyme inhibition and induction on the effects of tramadol

Enzyme effect of concomitant drug	Effects on substrate and its metabolites	Expected clinical effects
CYP3A4 inhibitor	↑ tramadol ↑ M1 (active) ↓↓ M2 (inactive)	↑ serotoninergic effect ↑ opioid effect
CYP3A4 inducer	↓↓ tramadol ↓↓ M1 (active) ↑↑ M2 (inactive)	↓ serotonergic effect ↓↓ opioid effect
CYP2D6 inhibitor	↑ tramadol ↓↓ M1	↔/↑ serotonergic effect ↓↓ opioid effect
CYP2D6 inducer	N/A[a]	

CYP cytochrome P450, *M1* O-desmethyl tramadol, *M2* N-desmethyl tramadol
↑ and ↓ indicate a small increase/decrease; ↑↑ and ↓↓ indicate a large increase/decrease; ↔ indicates no change
[a]CYP2D6 generally considered not inducible

inhibition or induction of CYP3A4 will not have a significant impact on the drug's effect.

Another complex example is tramadol, which has weak opioid activity but inhibits reuptake of serotonin and norepinephrine. It is metabolized via CYP2D6 to a metabolite M1 (O-desmethyl tramadol) which has more potent opioid activity. CYP3A4 and, to a lesser extent, CYP2B6 also metabolize tramadol to inactive metabolites including M2 (N-desmethyltramadol). Although the opioid effects are mediated through CYP2D6, modulation of CYP3A4 can produce more or less parent drug available for conversion to M1. Concomitant administration of medications that induce or inhibit CYP3A4/2D6 thus increase the risk of substantial drug interactions with tramadol (Table 4.4).

Methadone has inconsistent and sometimes unpredictable interactions with different enzyme modulators. For example, administration with the CYP3A4/CYP2B6 inducer efavirenz decreases methadone Cmax and AUC by approximately 50%, necessitating a 22% increase in dose [13]. Similarly, other enzyme inducers like rifampin and antiepileptics will decrease methadone concentrations via CYP2B6 induction and may precipitate opioid withdrawal. However, antiretroviral regimens containing ritonavir, which predominantly acts as a CYP450 inhibitor of various enzymes, may have little effect or may actually decrease methadone concentrations (Table 4.5). The mechanism for this is unclear; despite the strong CYP3A4 inhibition from ritonavir there may be reduced methadone concentrations due to CYP2B6 induction or an atypical mechanism [12]. Case reports have described opioid toxicity and respiratory depression when ciprofloxacin was initiated in patients receiving chronic methadone, yet, considering that ciprofloxacin is a weak CYP3A4 and moderate CYP1A2 inhibitor, a significant interaction between the two would not generally be expected [14].

Several classes of drugs result in clinically important drug interactions with opioids. Various antimicrobials, antiepileptic drugs, cardiovascular drugs, and

Table 4.5 Expected drug interactions between antiretrovirals and opioids

Antiretroviral class[a]	Antiretroviral	Enzyme effects	Interactions with opioids
Protease Inhibitors	Atazanavir	3A4 inhibitor (strong)	All (except tipranavir) will ↑ opioid effects of oxycodone, fentanyl, hydrocodone, buprenorphine, and sufentanil
	Darunavir	3A4 inhibitor (strong), 2D6 inhibitor (moderate)	
	Fosamprenavir	3A4 inhibitor (moderate)	
	Indinavir	3A4 inhibitor (strong)	
	Nelfinavir	3A4 inhibitor (strong)	Darunavir and tipranavir may ↓ opioid effect of codeine and tramadol
	Ritonavir	3A4 inhibitor (strong), 2B6 inducer (moderate)	
	Saquinavir	3A4 inhibitor (strong)	
	Tipranavir	2D6 inhibitor (strong)	
Non-nucleoside Reverse Transcriptase Inhibitors	Delavirdine	3A4 inhibitor (weak)	Efavirenz and nevirapine will ↓ opioid effect of methadone
	Doravirine	None	Etravirine will ↓ opioid effects of oxycodone, fentanyl, hydrocodone, buprenorphine, and sufentanil
	Efavirenz	2B6 inducer (moderate), 3A4 inducer (moderate)	
	Etravirine	3A4 inducer (moderate)	
	Nevirapine	2B6 inducer (moderate)	
	Rilpivirine	None	
Others	Cobicistat	3A4 inhibitor (strong)	Cobicistat will ↑ opioid effects of oxycodone, fentanyl, hydrocodone, buprenorphine, and sufentanil
	Enfuvirtide	None	
	Maraviroc	None	

CYP cytochrome P450

[a]Nucleoside reverse transcriptase inhibitors and integrase inhibitors do not have any clinically relevant CYP450-mediated drug interactions

psychotherapeutics can affect CYP450 metabolism. Drugs that may be encountered in the ICU setting which modulate CYP3A4 or CYP2D6, the most prevalent enzymes responsible for opioid metabolism, are listed in Table 4.6. Careful dosage adjustments and monitoring are necessary in order to avoid adverse drug interactions.

Table 4.6 Drugs that inhibit or induce CYP3A4 and CYP2D6

CYP3A4 Inhibitors		CYP3A4 Inducers		CYP2D6 Inhibitors	
Moderate	Strong	Moderate	Strong	Moderate	Strong
Antiretrovirals Amprenavir Delavirdine Fosamprenavir	*Antiretrovirals* Atazanavir Cobicistat Darunavir Lopinavir Ritonavir Saquinavir	*Antiretrovirals* Efavirenz Etravirine	*Antiepileptics* Carbamazepine Phenobarbital Phenytoin	*Antiretroviral* Darunavir	*Antiretroviral* Tipranavir
Antibacterials Erythromycin		*Antitubercular* Rifabutin Rifapentine	*Antitubercular* Rifampin	*Antidepressant* Duloxetine	*Antidepressants* Bupropion Fluoxetine Paroxetine
Antifungals Fluconazole Isavuconazole	*Antibacterials* Clarithromycin	*Others* Bosentan Modafinil Nafcillin			
Cardiovascular Amiodarone Diltiazem Verapamil	*Antifungals* Itraconazole Ketoconazole Posaconazole Voriconazole				
Others Conivaptan	*Others* Nefazodone				

CYP cytochrome P450

P-glycoprotein Interactions

Induction of P-gp may lead to overexpression of P-gp and contribute to opioid tolerance specifically with morphine and fentanyl, but not meperidine [15]. When an opioid that is a P-gp substrate is introduced with a P-gp inducer, there will be a decreased concentration in the central nervous system, leading to a loss of analgesia. Carbamazepine, recommended by recent guidelines for the treatment of neuropathic pain in critically ill patients [1], acts as an inducer of both P-pg and CYP3A4. Chronic administration of carbamazepine can lead to tolerance of specific opioids through a dual interaction at the level of P-gp (decrease penetration into the brain due to the back-transport of the drug) and CPY3A4 (increased metabolism). On the contrary, an increase in sensitivity and duration of analgesia can occur with the acute administration of a P-gp inhibitor. Loperamide, an opioid used as an anti-diarrheal agent, does not exert sedative effects as a direct result of P-gp-mediated efflux at the blood-brain barrier. Combining loperamide with a P-gp inhibitor, such as quinidine, may result in moderate respiratory depression, not otherwise observed with loperamide [16]. Plasma morphine concentrations, but not its metabolites, were increased in the setting of P-gp inhibition with itraconazole in 12 healthy volunteers [17]. The authors concluded that P-gp inhibition of morphine may increase the concentration of the parent drug without affecting the downstream metabolism of the glucuronides. It was unclear whether this increase in morphine concentration in the plasma correlated to the concentration in the brain.

There are many in vitro P-gp studies looking at the possibility that P-gp substrates, including opioids, have inhibitory properties as well [18]. The few opioids studied include fentanyl, morphine, and sufentanil, with digoxin as the standard P-gp substrate used to test the opioids and determine if P-gp is inhibited. Morphine and its metabolites did not inhibit the transport of digoxin and therefore not considered a P-gp inhibitor. The other opioids inhibited P-gp activity at high concentrations. Nonetheless, it is difficult to translate this in vitro data into clinically meaningful conclusions.

While P-gp inhibition and induction can certainly cause significant drug interactions, it is important to recognize that it is often not possible to predict the magnitude of undesirable outcomes. Clinicians should monitor for opioid tolerance in patients who are receiving concomitant P-gp inducers and consider switching to agents that are not P-gp substrates. Of note, it may take up to a couple of weeks to see the maximum induction effect, exposing suboptimal pain management. For patients receiving P-gp inhibitors, it is prudent to monitor for enhanced analgesia and opioid-related adverse effects.

Synergistic Pharmacodynamic Interactions

Central Nervous System and Respiratory Depression

Central nervous system and respiratory depression are life-threatening effects that can arise from opioids, especially when used in combination with other medications with similar side-effect profiles. Aside from inappropriate dosing or enzyme-related drug interactions, synergistic effects with other sedating medications are thus a potential risk factor. This can be a significant problem in the ICU setting since multiple sedating medications are frequently used simultaneously to treat anxiety, agitation, and/or for procedural sedation.

A retrospective study of over 21 million hospitalized medical and surgical patients evaluated the risk of cardiac arrest associated with opioids and sedatives and patient-specific risk factors [19]. In addition to benzodiazepines, other sedating drugs including certain antidepressants, anticonvulsants, antiemetics, and sleep aids were included. Opioids and sedatives were both found to be significantly associated with cardiac arrest, though the risk was highest with both combined (adjusted odds ratio 3.83 for medical patients and 2.34 for surgical patients). Other risk factors common to both medical and surgical patients included Hispanic origin, mild liver disease, obesity, and chronic obstructive pulmonary disease. The Joint Commission has identified several other risk factors for oversedation and respiratory depression from opioids, including sleep apnea, older age, opioid naïve status, snoring, post-surgery, increased opioid dose requirement, longer length of time receiving general anesthesia, preexisting cardiac or other organ disease, thoracic or other surgical incisions, and smoking [20]. In 2016, the United States Food and Drug Administration (U.S. FDA) warned of the risks of the combination of opioid pain or cough medications with benzodiazepines and other sedating drugs [21]. They cited several studies, which link this combination with an increased risk of emergency department visits and fatal overdoses, and have since required opioid manufacturers to disclose these risks in boxed warnings. While these warnings are based on outpatient prescriptions, such drug combinations in inpatients should be approached cautiously, used only if alternatives are ineffective, and at the lowest effective doses.

Serotonin Syndrome

Opioids have been associated with serotonin syndrome at the neurotransmitter level in patients who are receiving serotonin reuptake inhibitors and other serotonergic medications. Serotonin syndrome is a potentially life-threatening syndrome caused by the excessive buildup of serotonin, leading to hyperactivity of the peripheral and central nervous systems. The proposed mechanisms for opioids' serotonergic effect include serotonin reuptake inhibition or an increase of serotonin release at presynaptic inhibitory serotonin neurons.

Pain and mental health disorders frequently coexist. For example, chronic pain can lead to depression, placing the patient at risk when opioids and antidepressants are prescribed together. In 2016, the FDA issued a safety announcement, warning of safety issues with opioid pain medications including the interaction with antidepressants and migraine medications increasing the risk of serotonin syndrome [22]. Although the FDA mandated label changes for all opioids to include these necessary warnings, not all opioids have been associated with serotonin syndrome. Individual case reports and animal studies have highlighted certain opioids such as tramadol, fentanyl, hydromorphone, oxycodone, meperidine, methadone, buprenorphine, and dextromethorphan, with tramadol and meperidine as the highest offenders [23–27]. Antidepressants at risk for interactions include selective serotonin reuptake inhibitors (SSRIs), serotonin-norepinephrine reuptake inhibitors (SNRIs), monoamine oxidase inhibitors (MAOIs), tricyclic antidepressants (TCAs), and atypical antidepressants which share unique or combined mechanisms (Table 4.7). Linezolid has also been rarely implicated as a precipitant for serotonin syndrome due to its effect as a weak MAOI [27].

Table 4.7 Expected drug interactions between antidepressants and opioids

Antidepressant class	Antidepressant	Enzyme inhibition	Interactions with opioids
Selective serotonin reuptake inhibitors	Citalopram	CYP2D6 (weak)	Serotonin syndrome[a]
	Escitalopram	CYP2D6 (weak)	
	Fluoxetine	CYP2D6 (strong)	Paroxetine and fluoxetine may ↓ opioid effect of codeine and tramadol
	Fluvoxamine	CYP2D6, CYP3A4 (weak)	
	Paroxetine	CYP2D6 (strong)	
	Sertraline	CYP2D6 (weak)	↑ seizure risk with tramadol, meperidine
	Vortioxetine	None	
	Vilazodone	None	
Serotonin-norepinephrine reuptake inhibitors	Desvenlafaxine	None	Serotonin syndrome[a]
	Duloxetine	CYP2D6 (moderate)	Duloxetine may ↓ opioid effect of codeine and tramadol
	Levomilnacipran	None	
	Milnacipran	None	
	Venlafaxine	CYP2D6 (weak)	Additive QT prolongation (especially citalopram, escitalopram) with methadone
			↑ seizure risk with tramadol, meperidine
Tricyclic antidepressants	Amitriptyline Amoxepine Clomipramine Desipramine Doxepin Imipramine Nortriptyline Protriptyline Trimipramine	None	Serotonin syndrome[a]
			Additive sedation (especially amitriptyline, doxepin, trimipramine)
			Additive QT prolongation (especially amitriptyline, doxepin, imipramine) with methadone
			↑ seizure risk with tramadol, meperidine
Serotonin reuptake inhibitor/antagonist	Trazodone	None	Additive sedation
	Nefazodone	CYP3A4 (strong)	Nefazodone will ↑ opioid effects of oxycodone, fentanyl, hydrocodone, buprenorphine, and sufentanil
			Serotonin syndrome[a]
			↑ seizure risk with tramadol, meperidine

(continued)

Table 4.7 (continued)

Antidepressant class	Antidepressant	Enzyme inhibition	Interactions with opioids
Monoamine oxidase inhibitors	Phenelzine Isocarboxazid Selegiline Trancylcypromine Meclobemide	None	Serotonin syndrome[a] ↑ seizure risk with tramadol, meperidine
Atypical antidepressants	Bupropion	CYP2D6 (strong)	Bupropion may ↓ opioid effect of codeine and tramadol
	Mirtazapine	None	↑ seizure risk with combination of bupropion with tramadol, meperidine

CYP cytochrome P450
[a]Especially meperidine and tramadol
[b]Meperidine contraindicated with monoamine oxidase inhibitors

Fentanyl is serotonergic through multiple potential mechanisms, including direct serotonin agonism and weak reuptake inhibitory properties. There are no reports of serotonin syndrome in patients on fentanyl monotherapy, despite the multiple mechanisms that increase serotonin levels. Most reports of fentanyl precipitating serotonin syndrome are in patients receiving a different serotonergic agent or on other opioids as well [24].

Tramadol is a central opioid receptor agonist and a serotonin and norepinephrine reuptake inhibitor. These characteristics make it an appealing agent for patients suffering from both pain and depression. At high doses, it may also induce the release of serotonin in addition to inhibiting reuptake, leading to reports of tramadol alone causing serotonin syndrome. There are also multiple cases of serotonin syndrome observed when tramadol is combined with antidepressants [25]. This combination has been specifically implicated as a frequent cause of fatal drug toxicity related to tramadol [28]. Additionally, certain antidepressants may alter the metabolism of tramadol and further increase its serotonergic effects. The timing of the onset of serotonin syndrome can vary from a few days to over a month after tramadol initiation in patients established on their antidepressant therapy.

Methadone is another agent frequently reported to be associated with serotonin syndrome. The mechanism of increased serotonin by methadone is through serotonin reuptake inhibition at a greater rate than other opioids. Serotonin syndrome has been reported when methadone is combined with serotonergic antidepressants and linezolid [26, 27].

Although a greater risk exists when combining opioids with other serotonergic medications, combining these agents is not an absolute contraindication. In general, the incidence of serotonin syndrome is very low and the number of cases involving opioids is even lower. The combination of drug classes can be prescribed safely with proper monitoring and patient counseling. In the event of serotonin syndrome development, clinicians should immediately remove offending agents and symptoms will likely subside quickly with a low likelihood of recurrence.

QT-Interval Prolongation and Torsades de Pointes

Several opioids have been associated with QT-interval prolongation and an increased risk of torsades de pointes (TdP). These drugs have the potential to inhibit the human ether a go-go related-gene (HERG) channel which prolongs the action potential and the QT interval. QT prolongation has been observed with oxycodone, buprenorphine, and methadone [29]. Numerous reports of TdP and sudden death have been linked to methadone, which appear to occur more frequently with high methadone doses and in individuals with long QT syndrome or hypokalemia. Similar reports are rare to nonexistent with oxycodone and buprenorphine [29].

A number of risk factors are associated with TdP, and several have implications for drug interactions. These include high drug concentration, administration of more than one drug that can prolong the QT interval, and electrolyte disturbances [30]. Therefore, QT-prolonging agents such as methadone are expected to have a higher risk of TdP when combined with other QT-prolonging drugs including azole antifungals, macrolide and fluoroquinolone antibiotics, some SSRIs and TCAs, calcium channel antagonists and amiodarone, and many antipsychotics. Additionally, drugs that increase methadone concentrations (e.g. CYP2B6 inhibitors) or promote hypokalemia (e.g. loop diuretics) may also increase the risk of TdP.

Seizures

Certain opioids have been associated with a rare incidence of seizures. Tramadol, at therapeutic doses and in overdoses, can precipitate seizures, and the prescribing information warns about concomitant use of tramadol with various antidepressant classes, other opioids, neuroleptics, and other drugs that reduce the seizure threshold. Other opioids that are potentially neuroexcitatory appear to be related to opioid metabolites including normeperidine, morphine-3-glucuronide, and hydromorphrone-3-glucuronide [31]. However, none of these metabolites are generated via CYP450 metabolism; therefore, drug interactions increasing this risk are unlikely, except theoretically the combination with drugs that decrease the seizure threshold.

Interaction at the Mu-Opioid Receptor

Medications that are opioid antagonists or partial agonists are expected to interact with pure opioid agonists. In certain scenarios, this is expected and desired, for example, administering naloxone (a pure opioid antagonist) to treat opioid toxicity or overdose or naltrexone (another pure opioid antagonist) for chronic opioid or alcohol dependence. However, partial agonists, including buprenorphine, nalbuphine, and butorphanol, may also reduce opioid effects and produce withdrawal symptoms when administered to patients on chronic opioid therapy [32]. The partial agonist can displace the opioid from the mu receptor but produce less agonism at the receptor.

Conversely, patients who are maintained chronically on a partial agonist, particularly important for buprenorphine used for opioid maintenance therapy, may experience reduced effects of pure opioid agonists and require increasing agonist doses for effect. This interaction may be particularly relevant for a patient on chronic buprenorphine who needs treatment for acute pain. There is no high-quality evidence to guide the appropriate management of patients maintained on buprenorphine who have acute pain, so recommendations differ regarding discontinuing or maintaining buprenorphine during acute illness. Naltrexone, on the other hand, should be held prior to a planned surgery (72 hours for oral naltrexone and 30 days for intramuscular) and can be resumed when opioid agonists are no longer required.

Project SHOUT (Support for Hospital Opioid Use Treatment) has recently provided guidelines on the treatment of acute pain in patients maintained on drugs for opioid use disorder [33]. Patients on buprenorphine who experience acute pain due to surgery, for example, can receive the same total daily dose split into three times daily dosing to maximize the analgesic effects of buprenorphine. Additional analgesia can be achieved with multimodal therapy depending on the type of pain or concomitant disease states. If opioids are required for severe pain, higher doses than usual may be required. In general, it is not recommended to discontinue buprenorphine, as higher opioid doses may be required, and patients may be at an increased risk for relapse of their opioid use disorder. It is important to confirm that the patient is currently taking buprenorphine if deciding to continuing therapy, and it is good practice to include the patient's outpatient provider in these decisions.

Pharmacogenomic-Related Interactions

It is important to consider pharmacogenomic factors in patients prescribed opioids metabolized by cytochrome P450 enzymes most notably, CYP2D6 and CYP3A4. Patients with CYP2D6 polymorphisms can be poor metabolizers and have a lower clearance of CYP2D6 substrates, leading to a buildup of the parent drug. On the other end of the spectrum, ultrarapid metabolizers, may lead to a rapid conversion of the parent drug to its metabolites. Both types of polymorphisms can increase the risk of drug interactions that may not carry any clinical relevance in another patient. Caucasians are the most common race associated with these polymorphisms, with the most common phenotype being the extensive metabolizer. Opioid analgesics metabolized by CYP2D6 include the prodrugs codeine, hydrocodone, and tramadol. Poor metabolizers can experience down to 14-fold lower concentrations of the active metabolite, leading to significant decrease in their analgesic effects [34]. Codeine is the most studied opioid analgesic as it relates to pharmacogenetics. It is inactive and is metabolized by CYP3A4 into norcodeine, which does not possess analgesic properties and by CYP2D6 into morphine, which is active and will undergo glucuronidation into additional active metabolites. Studies have shown higher concentrations of morphine in CYP2D6 rapid metabolizers compared to poor metabolizers, along with more frequent associated adverse events, such as constipation, sedation, and respiratory depression [35]. There have been reports of patient deaths associated with normal codeine administration in an ultra-rapid metabolizer due to respiratory depression [36].

Tramadol has minor serotonergic effects due to the (+) enantiomer. Various genetic polymorphisms of CYP2D6 may increase the concentration of the (+) enantiomer, leading to an increased risk of serotonin syndrome when combined with additional CYP2D6 inhibitors or serotonergic medications [28]. The variation in genetics can affect serotonin metabolism regardless of concomitant drug therapy because serotonin metabolism is also modulated by CYP2D6 and CYP3A4.

Hydrocodone is metabolized by CYP2D6 into a more active opioid, hydromorphone. Hydromorphone has up to a 33-fold greater affinity to the mu opioid receptor than hydrocodone. Although CYP2D6 polymorphisms alter the hydromorphone concentrations in patients taking hydrocodone, there are insufficient data to extrapolate to meaningful clinical effects [35].

Oxycodone is also an opioid partially metabolized by CYP2D6 into an even more active metabolite, oxymorphone. Due to pharmacogenomic differences, there may be a delayed analgesic effect in poor metabolizers, or the patient may experience a heightened response in rapid metabolizers. Similar to hydrocodone, patient reports on the effect of fluctuations in oxymorphone concentrations due to metabolizer status on oxycodone did not demonstrate significant clinical changes [35]. One study evaluated the variability of enzyme function in the metabolism of oxycodone due to genetic polymorphisms involving various types of CYP2D6 metabolizers and volunteers without genetic polymorphisms [8]. The enzyme inhibitors quinidine and ketoconazole were used to inhibit CYP2D6 and CYP3A4, respectively. The study found that when one enzyme was inhibited, there appeared to be a shunt of metabolism to the other enzymatic pathway. These findings were especially pronounced in those who had a different CYP2D6 genotypes.

Enzyme polymorphisms in patients taking opioid medications are well studied and reported to cause harm. However, routine pharmacogenetic testing is not routinely performed prior to prescribing them. Literature on the effect of drug interactions in patients with genetic polymorphisms is also scarce. It is important to recognize the need for pharmacogenetic screening in patients who experience inadequate analgesia, or exaggerated responses after taking opioids in normal doses. When genetic polymorphisms are suspected, alternative opioids not metabolized by CYP2D6, such as fentanyl, hydromorphone, morphine, and non-opioid agents are preferred.

Opioid Interactions with Drugs of Abuse

Increasing consumption of non-medical use (or misuse) of novel synthetic opioids (NSO) has risen over the last two decades in the United States and Canada [37]. To date little information is known about the exact metabolic pathway of NSOs; therefore, the frequency (predictability) and severity of drug interactions associated with these agents are largely unknown. Yet, given their increased potency, prolonged effects, and propensity to be used in combination with other substances, NSOs are particularly at risk for clinically relevant drug interactions and toxicity. Alcohol, barbiturates, benzodiazepines, or heroin combined with NROs may lead to increase in respiratory depression. Additionally, unexpected adverse effects may be observed when patients combine NSOs with stimulants such as cocaine or amphetamines. Furthermore, combining amphetamines with certain NSOs may lead to an increase in serotonin syndrome [38]. Co-ingestion of heroin and ethanol will lead to increases in morphine (heroin metabolite) as a result of ethanol induced inhibition of heroin metabolism [39]. In the setting of NSO misuse, clinicians should anticipate effects to be similar to fentanyl and morphine and anticipate untoward drug interactions with co-stimulant use.

Coronavirus Disease 2019 (COVID-19) and Opioid Interactions

Drugs used for the treatment of patients with COVID-19 such as remdesivir, dexamethasone, and tocilizumab do not have any known drug interactions with opioids. However, as patients with COVID-19 are enrolled in clinical trials using investigational drugs, clinicians should be vigilant in monitoring for potential drug interactions with opioids.

Critically ill patients with COVID-19 receiving mechanical ventilation may require continuous infusions of an opioid and sedative to treat pain and agitation. Shortages of intravenous fentanyl and hydromorphone during the pandemic have forced clinicians to use alternate intravenous or oral opioids with prolonged durations of action, active metabolites, and a potential for increased drug interactions.

Conclusion

Opioid analgesics are frequently administered in the ICU setting, and many of these drugs are metabolized or transported by enzymes prone to drug interactions, including CYP450 and P-gp. Opioids are also responsible for many undesired clinical effects which are often subject to several pharmacodynamic interactions discrete from the opioid receptor. Knowledge of these interactions of the most common opioids and non-opioids that are likely to interact can improve their appropriate use, facilitating effective patient analgesia while minimizing the risk of opioid toxicity and harm. As newer opioids are developed, it is important to study their metabolic pathway and potential for clinically relevant drug interactions.

References

1. Devlin JW, Skrobik Y, Gélinas C, Needham DM, Slooter AJC, Pandharipande PP, et al. Clinical practice guidelines for the prevention and management of pain, agitation/sedation, delirium, immobility, and sleep disruption in adult patients in the ICU. Crit Care Med. 2018;46(9):e825–e73.
2. Greenblatt DJ, von Moltke LL. Drug-drug interactions: clinical perspectives. In: Rodrigues AD, editor. Drug-drug interactions. 2nd ed. New York: Informa Healthcare; 2008. p. 643–64.
3. Uijtendaal EV, van Harssel LL, Hugenholtz GW, Kuck EM, Zwart-van Rijkom JE, Cremer OL, et al. Analysis of potential drug–drug interactions in medical intensive care unit patients. Pharmacotherapy. 2014;34(3):213–9.
4. Fitzmaurice MG, Wong A, Akerberg H, Avramovska S, Smithburger PL, Buckley MS, Kane-Gill SL. Evaluation of potential drug-drug interactions in adults in the intensive care unit: a systematic review and meta-analysis. Drug Saf. 2019;42(9):1035–44.
5. Moura C, Prado N, Acurcio F. Potential drug-drug interactions associated with prolonged stays in the intensive care unit: a retrospective cohort study. Clin Drug Investig. 2011;31(5):309–16.
6. Solhaug V, Molden E. Individual variability in clinical effect and tolerability of opioid analgesics - importance of drug interactions and pharmacogenetics. Scand J Pain. 2017;17:193–200.
7. Owusu Obeng A, Hamadeh I, Smith M. Review of opioid pharmacogenetics and considerations for pain management. Pharmacotherapy. 2017;37(9):1105–21.
8. Samer CF, Daali Y, Wagner M, Hopfgartner G, Eap CB, Rebsamen MC, et al. The effects of CYP2D6 and CYP3A activities on the pharmacokinetics of immediate release oxycodone. Br J Pharmacol. 2010;160(4):907–18.
9. Palkama VJ, Neuvonen PJ, Olkkola KT. The CYP 3A4 inhibitor itraconazole has no effect on the pharmacokinetics of i.v. fentanyl. Br J Anaesth. 1998;81(4):598–600.
10. Saari TI, Laine K, Neuvonen M, Neuvonen PJ, Olkkola KY. Effect of voriconazole and fluconazole on pharmacokinetics of intravenous fentanyl. Eur J Clin Pharmacol. 2008;64(1):25–30.
11. Tempelhoff R, Modica PA, Spitznagel EL. Anticonvulsant therapy increases fentanyl requirements during anaesthesia for craniotomy. Can J Anaesth. 1990;37(3):327–32.
12. Kharasch ED, Bedynek PS, Park S, Whittington D, Walker A, Hoffer C. Mechanism of ritonavir changes in methadone pharmacokinetics and pharmacodynamics I. Evidence against CYP3A mediation of methadone clearance. Clin Pharmacol Ther. 2008;84(4):497–505.
13. Clarke SM, Mulcahy FM, Tjia J, Reynolds HE, Gibbons SE, Barry MG, Back DJ. The pharmacokinetics of methadone in HIV-positive patients receiving the non-nucleoside reverse transcriptase inhibitor efavirenz. Br J Clin Pharmacol. 2008;51(3):213–7.
14. Samoy L. Interaction between methadone and ciprofloxacin. Can J Hosp Pharm. 2010;63(5):382–4.
15. Hamabe W, Maeda T, Fukazawa Y, Kumamoto K, Shang LQ, Yamamoto A, et al. P-glycoprotein ATPase activating effect of opioid analgesics and their P-glycoprotein-dependent antinociception in mice. Pharmacol Biochem Behav. 2006;85(3):629–36.
16. Sadeque AJ, Wandel C, He H, Shah S, Wood AJ. Increased drug delivery to the brain by P-glycoprotein inhibition. Clin Pharmacol Ther. 2000;68(3):231–7.
17. Heiskanen T, Backman JT, Neuvonen M, Kontinen VK, Neuvonen PJ, Kalso E. Itraconazole, a potent inhibitor of P-glycoprotein, moderately increases plasma concentrations of oral morphine. Acta Anaesthesiol Scand. 2008;52(10):1319–26.
18. Wandel C, Kim R, Wood M, Wood A. Interaction of morphine, fentanyl, sufentanil, alfentanil, and loperamide with the efflux drug transporter P-glycoprotein. Anesthesiology. 2002;96(4):913–90.
19. Izrailtyan I, Qiu J, Overdyk FJ, Erslon M, Gan TJ. Risk factors for cardiopulmonary and respiratory arrest in medical and surgical hospital patients on opioid analgesics and sedatives. PLoS One. 2018;13(3):e0194553.

20. Jarzyna D, Jungquist CR, Pasero C, et al. American Society for Pain Management nursing guidelines on monitoring for opioid-induced sedation and respiratory depression. Pain Manag Nurs. 2011;12(3):118–45.
21. FDA Drug Safety Communications. FDA warns about several safety issues with opioid pain medicines; requires label changes. 22 Mar 2016. https://www.fda.gov/downloads/Drugs/DrugSafety/UCM491302.pdf. Accessed 21 October 2019.
22. FDA Drug Safety Communications FDA warns about serious risks and death when combining opioid pain or cough medicines with benzodiazepines; requires its strongest warning. 31 August 2016. https://www.fda.gov/media/99761/download. Accessed 24 Oct 2019.
23. Baldo BA. Opioid analgesic drugs and serotonin toxicity (syndrome): mechanisms, animal models, and links to clinical effects. Arch Toxicol. 2018;92(8):2457–73.
24. Koury KM, Tsui B, Gulur P. Incidence of serotonin syndrome in patients treated with fentanyl on serotonergic agents. Pain Physician. 2015;18(1):E27–30.
25. Park SH, Wackernah RC, Stimmel GL. Serotonin syndrome: is it a reason to avoid the use of tramadol with antidepressants? J Pharm Pract. 2014;27(1):71–8.
26. Rastogi R, Swarm RA, Patel TA. Case scenario: opioid association with serotonin syndrome: implications to the practitioners. Anesthesiology. 2011;115(6):1291–8.
27. Gillman PK. Monoamine oxidase inhibitors, opioid analgesics and serotonin toxicity. Br J Anaesth. 2005;95:434–41.
28. Pilgrim JL, Gerostamoulos D, Drummer OH. Review: Pharmacogenetic aspects of the effect of cytochrome P450 polymorphisms on serotonergic drug metabolism, response, interactions, and adverse effects. Forensic Sci Med Pathol. 2011;7(2):162–84.
29. Wedam EF, Haigney MC. The impact of opioids on cardiac electrophysiology. Curr Cardiol Rev. 2016;12(1):27–36.
30. Nachimuthu S, Assar MD, Schussler JM. Drug-induced QT interval prolongation: mechanisms and clinical management. Ther Adv Drug Saf. 2012;3(5):241–53.
31. Lötsch J. Opioid metabolites. J Pain Symptom Manag. 2005;29(5 Suppl):S10–24.
32. Johnson RE, Strain EC, Amass L. Buprenorphine: how to use it right. Drug Alcohol Depend. 2003;70(2 Suppl):S59–77.
33. Project SHOUT. Acute pain and perioperative management in opioid use disorder: pain control in patients on buprenorphine, methadone, and naltrexone. https://www.projectshout.org/guidelines. Accessed 12 Nov 2019.
34. Nerenz RD, Tsongalis GJ. Pharmacogenetics of opioid use and implications for pain management. J Appl Lab Med. 2017;2(4):622–32.
35. Swen JJ, Nijenhuis M, de Boer A, Grandia L, Maitland-van der Zee AH, Mulder H, et al. Pharmacogenetics: from bench to byte–an update of guidelines. Clin Pharmacol Ther. 2011;89(5):662–73.
36. Ciszkowski C, Madadi P, Phillips MS, Lauwers AE, Koren G. Codeine, ultrarapid-metabolism genotype, and postoperative death. N Engl J Med. 2009;361(8):827–8.
37. Pérez-Mañá C, Papaseit E, Fonseca F, Farré A, Torrens M, Farré M. Drug interactions with new synthetic opioids. Front Pharmacol. 2018;9:1145.
38. Rickli A, Liakoni E, Hoener MC, Liechti ME. Opioid-induced inhibition of the human 5-HT and noradrenaline transporters in vitro: link to clinical reports of serotonin syndrome. Br J Pharmacol. 2018;175(3):532–43.
39. Thaulow CH, Høiseth G, Andersen JM, Handal M, Mørland J. Pharmacokinetic interactions between ethanol and heroin: a study on postmortem cases. Forensic Sci Int. 2014;242:127–34.

Chapter 5
Side Effects of Opioid Analgesic Therapy

Dane Scantling and Niels D. Martin

While this chapter will emphasize the acute side effects in the ICU, no discussion of the consequences of opioids is complete without reference to the crisis of opioid use disorder (OUD) in America and around the world. The first epidemic of OUD in the United States began perhaps as early as the 1840s with the huge influx of opium and morphine to the American continent. In the Civil War era, opioids were considered the panacea of pain relief but came to be banned in the early twentieth century. Later, they were redeployed again and legalized for well-moderated medical uses [3]. This period of medical redemption was short lived and OUD has skyrocketed since the arrival of OxyContin in 1996 and the advent of pain as the fifth vital sign; a concept that was endorsed by the Joint Commission in 2001 [3, 4]. From 1999 to 2018, opioid prescriptions increased by almost 400% [5], (Fig. 5.1). In recent years, their use has begun to decrease in the face of the increasing death toll and rising public awareness and concern [5]. Though a key tool instrument to alleviate suffering, opioids are certainly not without significant consequences and their many receptor targets involve nearly every physiologic system (Fig. 5.2). Regardless, about 80% of Americans using heroin began their opioid use with a legal narcotic prescription and, overall, 4–6% of those given a narcotic prescription will go on to use heroin [5, 3].

In the intensive care unit, as many as 80% of patients needing mechanical ventilation receive opioids. *Analgesia-first* sedation is associated with improved outcomes and fewer ventilator-dependent days, leading to very significant utilization of opioids like fentanyl in ICU settings [6, 7]. Moreover, anywhere from 33% to 73% of ICU survivors develop chronic pain syndromes [8]. It is logical to conclude a high rate of subsequent ongoing use and abuse, but study of the topic is lacking. Of overall ICU survivors, approximately 12% remain on opioids at

D. Scantling · N. D. Martin (✉)
Perelman School of Medicine at the University of Pennsylvania, Department of Surgery, Division of Traumatology, Surgical Critical Care & Emergency Surgery, Philadelphia, PA, USA
e-mail: Dane.Scantling@pennmedicine.upenn.edu; Niels.Martin@pennmedicine.upenn.edu

J. L. Pascual, T. G. Gaulton (eds.), *Opioid Use in Critical Care*,
https://doi.org/10.1007/978-3-030-77399-1_5

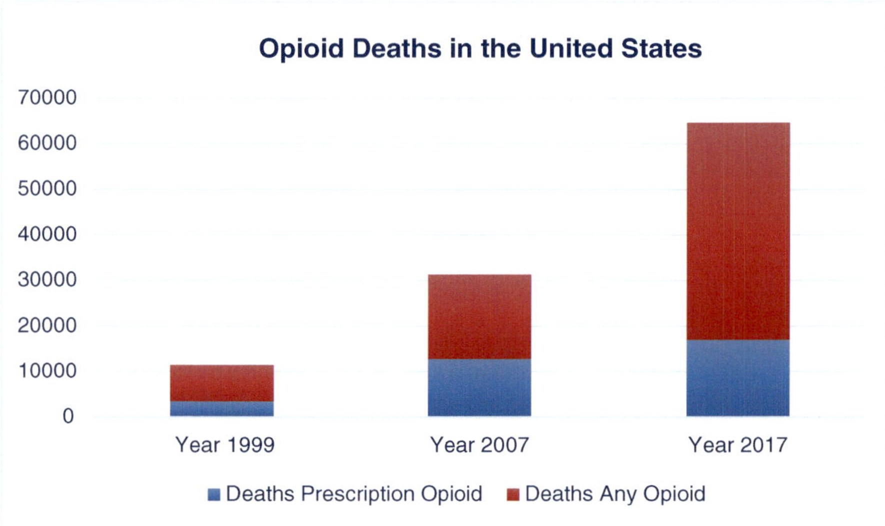

Fig. 5.1 Opioid deaths have increased exponentially in America. While prescription opioid control has conferred a lower percentage of overall opioid deaths, up to 6% of those given a script will develop an opioid use disorder (OUD). The vast majority of those using heroin began their OUD with a prescription. These individuals ultimately begin using heroin in response to a lack of access or affordability of prescription opioids. (Data from the Centers for Disease Control and Prevention)

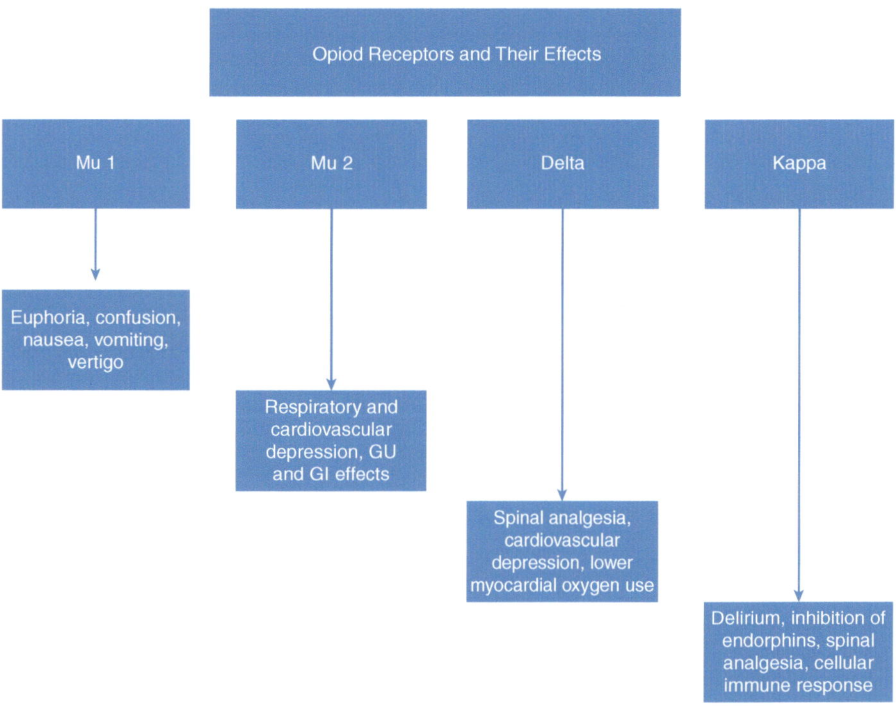

Fig. 5.2 A depiction of the various opioid receptors and their effects with activation. (Data from Molina et al. [1] and Plein et al. [2])

discharge from hospital and 4.4% are thought to still be obtaining prescriptions 4 years after discharge [8]. In a limited international study, length of hospitalization but not length of ICU stay was associated with increased chronic use [9]. Long-term post ICU OUD and the role that in-hospital opioid use plays in it is ultimately not well studied, but it is certainly worth being aware of given the potential societal toll. The topic of OUD will be covered more extensively elsewhere in this book. For the purposes of this chapter, we will now focus on a system-by-system discussion of the in-hospital consequences of opioid therapy.

Neurologic Side Effects

Physiologic Dependence

Description: Physiologic dependence is a state of altered physiology secondary to chronic opioid use which confers a risk of withdrawal when the medication is abruptly discontinued. It is related to increased somatic and autonomic activity [10, 11].

Incidence: Physiologic dependence is common in ICU patients [10, 11]. Opioid withdrawal in the ICU may be as frequent as 30% of mechanically ventilated patients who receive high-dose opioids for at least 1 week [11–13].

Diagnosis: Symptoms related to physiologic dependence may impact many body systems. This can include rhinorrhea, myalgias, nausea, vomiting, and autonomic hyperactivity including hypertension, tachycardia, hyperreflexia, and tachypnea. Validated clinical scores which aid in the diagnosis of opiate withdrawal exist and include the Clinical Opiate Withdrawal Scale (COWS), which assigns a diagnostic score based upon 11 clinical signs and symptoms [14].

Management: Dependence is best treated by prevention. Opioids should be utilized only as necessary and in the smallest possible doses. Multimodal pain management regimens avoiding opioids should be pursued whenever possible. Opioid withdrawal should be managed with therapy aimed at relieving symptoms (Fig. 5.3). The medication may also be given intermittently rather than in infusion form. If the sudden cessation of opioids was not intentional, the medication may be restarted and the doses tapered as tolerated.

Tolerance

Description: Tolerance is defined by a loss of analgesic potency for a given dose and may make dosing difficult, leading to uncontrolled pain [10]. Tolerance may be either innate or acquired. Innate tolerance is conferred by genetic factors, while acquired tolerance is derived from pharmacokinetic, pharmacodynamic, and learned factors [10]. Opioid tolerance is not related to drug clearance and is not well understood [6]. It is seen in all types of critically ill patients, but is most common in those

Withdrawal symptom	Treatment	Note
Insomnia	Sleep hygiene, melatonin, quetiapine or temazepam at bedtime	Use the lowest possible dose and consider simultaneous psychiatric diagnoses
Nausea/Vomiting	Metoclopramide, prochlorperazine, ondansetron	
Diarrhea	Loperamide, atropine/diphenoxylate	
Headaches/Joint Pains	Ibuprofen, acetaminophen	Use appropriate dosing in patients with HCV cirrhosis
Agitation/Anxiety	Diazepam	Avoid short acting benzodiazepines and do not use if concurrent benzodiazepine withdrawal
Hypertension and Hyperalgesia	Clonidine	In sedated patients, dexmedetomidine may be of use

Fig. 5.3 Potential treatment options for symptoms of opioid withdrawal

with major trauma and in children or patients who are mechanically ventilated or exposed to opioids for prolonged periods [6, 10].

Incidence: Opioid tolerance can readily occur in the acute ICU setting, there is no set time frame of administration or dose at which this predictably happens. It is not uncommon for patients to require drastically increasing opioid dosing for efficacious pain relief over weeks to months, but acute tolerance has been demonstrated in animal models in minutes to hours with unknown clinical significance [15]. Tolerance is worsened in the ICU setting as cytokine release can reduce blood-brain barrier penetration and reduce opioid efficacy [6].

Diagnosis: Tolerance is defined by a patient's efficacious opioid dose needing to be increased over time. Different opioids may also confer tolerance at different rates and cross tolerance may be incomplete between different drugs [10].

Management: As in physiologic dependence, the best treatment for tolerance is prevention. Opioids should be used in the minimum necessary dosing and a multimodal pain regimen employed whenever possible. Continuous infusions of opioids should be avoided as a means of sedation when possible. Intermittent opioids will produce less tolerance than continuous. When opioids cannot be avoided, they may be rotated to avoid-drug specific tolerance. This is specifically done between drugs that have active metabolites which may impair analgesia (morphine and hydromorphone) and those that do not (fentanyl) [6].

Hyperalgesia

Description: This condition is characterized by increased pain sensitivity, even in the face of increasing opioid use. It is believed to be related to the effect of opioid metabolites, such as morphine-3-glucuronide [10]. These metabolites are thought to induce GABA neuron apoptosis leading to changes in neurologic response and act as NMDA receptor agonists [10].

Incidence: Hyperalgesia may occur with opioid use and is associated with chronic pain in almost half of ICU survivors evaluated up to a year after discharge [16].

Diagnosis: This condition is characterized by increased pain sensitivity, even in the face of increasing opioid use. The diagnosis is a clinical one. Patients with chronic opioid therapy may exhibit pain out of proportion to that expected for a given stimulus, also demonstrating marked temperature intolerance in some cases.

Management: Treatment of hyperalgesia is geared toward appropriate analgesic therapy. Avoidance of certain opioids may be useful. Remifentanil in particular has been implicated in hyperalgesia in post-operative patients, though it is not commonly used in the ICU setting [16]. Clonidine and dexmedetomidine, alpha-2-adrenergic agonists, may be useful in symptomatic relief [6]. The use of calcium channel blockers such as amlodipine has been helpful and ketamine, methadone, and magnesium may also aid in therapy through NMDA receptor antagonism [10].

Delirium

Description: Delirium is an acute change in mental status characterized by disorientation or confusion. It may be hypoactive (somnolence) or hyperactive (agitation). It is characterized by its eb and flow with the symptoms appearing to come and go with time. Both benzodiazepines and opioids have been implicated in increasing the incidence of delirium in the critically ill and this is especially true in the elderly.

Incidence: Delirium is a common phenomenon in the intensive care unit, affecting 60–80% of patients who are mechanically ventilated and anywhere from 20% to 50% of those who are not [17, 18].

Diagnosis: The diagnosis of delirium is clinical and will, in this case, be related to the timing of administration of an opioid. Other causes of confusion and agitation should be considered, such as infection, stroke, or head trauma.

Management: Opioids should be avoided as possible and/or given at the lowest therapeutic dose. While their use can worsen delirium if the intent of their use is sedation, opioids used first confer lower delirium rates when utilized to address pain [13, 17–19]. This is ultimately related to the fact that untreated pain itself may cause delirium [6]. High-quality studies comparing specific opioids and their relation to delirium is currently lacking, although meperidine has been deemed causative in several studies and should be avoided [13, 20]. Standard approaches to delirium management outside of opioid titration include sleep hygiene optimization and frequent reorientation.

Seizures

Description: Seizures are classically defined by a sudden cerebral electrical disturbance. This may manifest itself as anything from an *absence* seizure to a generalized tonic-clonic seizure. Opioids are known to cause neuroinflammation and even direct neurotoxicity [6]. In many cases, it is the metabolites of opioids that cause these significant neurologic complications.

Incidence: Opioid-related seizures are uncommon unless an overdose has occurred. Specific rates are not well known. Normeperidine, a metabolite of meperidine, has a particularly long half-life and can accumulate in the body. It is not reversible and can lead to seizures and delirium [13]. Morphine-3-glucuronide, a neurotoxic metabolite of morphine, has also been implicated in seizure activity and its effects are most significant in the setting of renal failure when it cannot be adequately cleared [21]. Hydromorphone-3-glucuronide, a metabolite of hydromorphone, has theoretically similar complications but does not significantly accumulate in the setting of renal failure [16, 13, 21, 22]. Tramadol, in extreme doses, can also decrease seizure threshold. Fentanyl, which is quite commonly used in the ICU, has no active metabolites and has notably not been associated with seizures [16].

Diagnosis: Diagnosis is typically made based on a witness report of seizure activity alone. Additional diagnoses such as brain lesions or hemorrhagic strokes are typically ruled out utilizing brain imaging. If the diagnosis remains unclear, electroencephalogram (EEG) may be utilized.

Management: In the short term, seizures should be treated with intravenous benzodiazepine to stop the active seizing. Prevention of seizures involves appropriate opioid dosing and avoidance of extremely high opioid levels including tramadol, morphine, hydromorphone, and meperidine, which are not commonly administered in the ICU.

Sleep and Sedation

Description: Sleep and sedation are related in that both involve a diminished mental status. Sedation can be a goal of opioid use in the ICU, but it can also be an adverse effect. Opioid sedation is thought to be related to anticholinergic activity and is dose and tolerance dependent [10, 23].

Incidence: Sleep impairment and sedation from opioid use are thought to be nearly ubiquitous and have been demonstrated in randomized trials. Impacts are dose dependent. While many opioids, such as fentanyl, have a fairly short half-life with bolus administration and no metabolites, their use as a continuous infusion can lead to drug accumulation. Bolus dosing of fentanyl in particular has a short half-life, but this is due to its rapid re-distribution into different body compartments given its highly lipophilic nature rather than rapid clearance [24]. After discontinuation of an infusion, fentanyl deposited in peripheral adipose tissue is re-distributed into the plasma again and sedation may continue for quite some time [13, 24]. Ultimately, the "true" half-life of the drug is more related to its volume of distribution than its clearance and long-term infusions in the ICU can confer a longer than anticipated duration of action. This concept is known as a context-sensitive half time [13, 24].

While opioids may be sedating and induce sleep, they do not improve sleep quality. The caveat, of course, is that untreated pain can also be deleterious to sleep, but certainly a balance must be achieved. Opioids are associated with worsened sleep duration and quality, a reduction in REM and delta sleep, and an increased number of sleep-wake cycles [10, 25]. This finding has been replicated in healthy volunteers and is thought to be impactful in both acute and chronic opioid use settings [10, 25, 26].

Diagnosis: The diagnosis of these conditions is again a clinical one. Sedation from opioids can mimic hypoactive delirium but resolves with naloxone administration. Sleep disturbance and sedation can be best mitigated by using the lowest efficacious dose of the medications and avoiding opioids that lack active metabolites. Continuous fentanyl infusions should ideally be limited in favor of intermittent boluses.

Cardiovascular Side Effects

Description: Cardiac side effects range from bradycardia and hypotension to life-threatening arrhythmias. Methadone, which may be used to treat acute pain in the ICU, is a particular risk for cardiovascular complications, specifically *torsades de pointes* due to QT prolongation. Morphine is known to induce vasodilation and hypotension in response to histamine release at levels beyond other opioids, particularly as compared to fentanyl, which lacks any histaminic activity [16, 6, 10]. This can often be interpreted as an anaphylactic response although it is not. While given in myocardial ischemia to increase coronary perfusion through vasodilation and reduction in myocardial oxygen consumption, opioids do have deleterious cardiovascular effects [13]. Bradycardia and systemic hypotension may be caused by opioids through blunting of the stress response release of catecholamines [16, 27]. In particular, sympathetic nervous system control of the cardiovascular system is disrupted through opioid interactions with adrenergic receptors [1].

Incidence: The incidence of most cardiac complications related to opioids are not well chronicled, but they do exist. Methadone is the second most common drug-induced cause of ventricular arrhythmias [28]. It is associated with QT prolongation and may lead to *torsades de pointes*, conferring a mortality rate of almost 20% [16, 10]. Hypotension is thought to have an incidence of less than 5% [29].

Diagnosis: Identifying cardiovascular impacts of opioids often requires significant clinical suspicion and is largely based on the relation of the clinical change and drug administration. Electrocardiograms (ECGs) are useful in identifying a prolonged QT interval associated with methadone. When *torsades de pointes* occurs, the prior ECG pattern tends to be pathognomonic for a lengthened QT which is often drug related.

Management: Limit therapy to the lowest efficacious dose of medication. Some tolerance for a given dose may develop with time. For reversal of some cardiac effects, naloxone can be trialed and has been shown to increase peripheral vascular resistance and improve cardiac function in anesthetized swine and primate hemorrhage models [1]. Intravenous fluid administration or vasopressor support may be needed in extreme cases. With regard to *torsades de pointes*, ventricular tachycardia, and cardiac arrest, advanced cardiac life support (ACLS) measures should be undertaken immediately and prompt defibrillation is key. Serial ECGs should be done when using methadone to monitor for QTi elongation and the drug stopped if this develops. Other QT-altering drugs should be avoided as concurrent therapy and electrolytes should be routinely repleted, especially potassium and magnesium. A list of common drugs that may increase the QT interval is included in Fig. 5.4 [30]. There are many drugs not necessarily included here which may have similar effects. These drugs include some anti-emetics (ondansetron), antipsychotics (haloperidol and atypical antipsychotics), some antibiotics (fluoroquinolones and azole antifungals), and tricyclic antidepressants among numerous others [30].

Drug Types Causing QT Interval Elongation	Specific Medications
Anti-psychotics	Haloperidol, olanzapine, risperidone, thioridazine, ziprasidone
Antiarrhythmics	Amiodarone, dofetilide, flecainide, procainamide, quinidine, sotalol
Antibiotics	Macrolide and fluoroquinolone classes, azole antifungals, terbinafine
Antivirals	Atazanavir, darunavir, indinavir, fosamprenavir, nelfinavir, saquinavir, tiprinavir
Antidepressants	Amitriptyline, bupropion, citalopram, duloxetine, escitalopram, imipramine, paroxetine
Antiemetics	Droperidol, ondansetron, cisapride
Other	Cilostazol, donepezil, methadone, sumatriptan

Fig. 5.4 A list of common medications that may cause elongation of the QT interval and should be avoided with methadone use. (Data from Li et al. [21])

Pulmonary Side Effects

Description: Respiratory consequences of opioid use are among the most familiar to physicians and the public alike. Respiratory depression ranging from a decreased respiratory rate to total apnea leading to respiratory arrest and anoxic brain injury is a well-known consequence of opioid use in any setting, and this includes in the ICU [6, 10, 13]. Additional adverse pulmonary events include bronchospasm, though the incidence is not well defined [16, 6]. This is most associated with morphine administration. A reduction in functional residual capacity (FRC) and forced vital capacity (FVC) from opioid use may also impair clearance of secretions and contribute to pneumonia [13]. Conversely, inadequately controlled pain can cause abdominal muscle tensing and similarly decreased FRC and FVC with the same clinical outcome [13]. Additionally, there are reports of chest wall rigidity impairing mechanical ventilation with intravenous pushes of fentanyl [31].

Incidence: The incidence of respiratory depression with opioid analgesia is not well defined. This is primarily because of the varied end points that may be used to demonstrate hypoventilation. Studies may use variable definitions of hypoventilation: pulse oximetry of varying threshold levels, varying respiratory rates to define hypoventilation, levels for hypercapnia, or more vaguely any administration of naloxone. A meta-analysis of post-operative analgesia with differing administration techniques concluded that 0.3% of patients require naloxone, 1.1% have hypoventilation, 3.3% become hypercapneic, and 17% display some degree of oxygen desaturation [29]. Additional pulmonary effects are not well studied and their incidence is not well described.

Diagnosis: As described above, the definition of hypoventilation is not well circumscribed. A relative drop in pulse oximetry, an increase in end-tidal carbon dioxide, or a drop in respiratory rate may all be identified. In general, an attempt should be made to maintain end-tidal carbon dioxide within a normal range of 35–45 mmHg. Measurement of this is usually accomplished using a nasal prong and is often part of patient-controlled analgesia. Pulse oximetry can be an effective means of monitoring patients for oxygen desaturation and, in general, should be maintained above 92%.

Management: Quick recognition of hypoventilation is important. Pulse oximetry and end-tidal CO_2 monitoring are useful clinical adjuncts. Oxygen desaturation with otherwise adequate ventilation can be managed with supplemental oxygen administration in an otherwise arousable patient. Patients with hypercarbia or a diminished mental status from hypoventilation may require naloxone administration and those who are apneic or have significant respiratory compromise should receive immediate assistance with the use of a bag valve mask and intubation if the airway remains unsecured.

Gastrointestinal Side Effects

Description: Like the respiratory impacts of opioids, the gastrointestinal maladies are among the most common and well known. Constipation, ileus, Ogilvie's syndrome, nausea, and vomiting are the most common side effects of opioid therapy [6,

10]. Opioids are known to stimulate chemoreceptor trigger zones, acting to increase vestibular sensitivity and inducing nausea, vomiting, and decreased gastric motility [13]. Gastric emptying can be similarly impacted with slowed transit times and increased non-propulsing contractions [10]. Unlike many opioid side effects, constipation typically does not improve over time and can be a major source of morbidity and hospitalization length of stay [10].

Incidence: Constipation, mediated by mu receptor-controlled motility in the gastrointestinal tract, effects anywhere from 25 to 95% of opioid users [16, 6, 7, 10, 13]. Nausea and vomiting occur in about a quarter of patients using opioids [13]. Other side effects are not as well described.

Diagnosis: The diagnosis of gastrointestinal side effects is primarily a clinical one based upon the timing of symptoms and medication administration. Ileus and Ogilvie's may be diagnosed with abdominal X-rays or CT imaging if the X-ray is unclear.

Management: Gastric emptying can be improved with prokinetic agents for symptomatic relief and nausea and vomiting largely managed with anti-emetics. Both can be improved with dose reductions or multimodal pain regimens avoiding opioids as much as possible. Such multimodal therapy may include acetaminophen, non-steroidal anti-inflammatory drugs (NSAIDs), cyclooxygenase 2 (COX-2) inhibitors, local or regional anesthetics, and other adjunctive therapies. The same can be said for constipation and ileus, although it is especially hard to manage. Bowel regimens are often utilized. In patients who are opioid naïve and about to undergo major surgery that will necessitate opioid use, preoperative methylnaltrexone and alvimopan (mu receptor antagonists which inhibit peripheral but not central opioid activity) have shown some promise [10]. Patients with ileus may require gastric decompression until the ileus resolves, and patients with Ogilvie's may require neostigmine administration which can itself be life threatening.

Genitourinary Side Effects

Description: Genitourinary effects of opioids may include urinary retention and difficulty voiding. Opioids may impair detrusor contractility and block the urge to void. The feeling of bladder fullness and the urinary reflex are also inhibited [10]. This has specifically been demonstrated in study of morphine [10]. Regardless, the primary genitourinary impact of opioids may well be that existing renal dysfunction may decrease opioid clearance and enhance their other side effects [13, 21]. The extent of this is primarily related to metabolite accumulation and the level of renal failure [21].

Incidence: The genitourinary impacts of opioids are less common than their gastrointestinal counterparts, but may be clinically relevant as well. Anywhere from 3.8 to 18.1% of patients may get urinary retention believed to be related to opioids [6, 10]. Epidural morphine has a higher incidence of voiding dysfunction than other means of administration [10]. However, it is not always clear that this is due to the opioids themselves and this is not well delineated.

Diagnosis: The diagnosis of genitourinary effects is clinical and may be difficult to differentiate from other causes of voiding dysfunction.

Management: Genitourinary complications are best avoided through use of the minimum efficacious opioid dose. Naloxone is known to reverse opioid effects on the bladder, but will reverse many favorable effects of the opioids as well. Significant urinary retention should be treated with bladder catheterization until symptoms resolve.

Endocrine Side Effects

Description: Numerous endocrine impacts of opioids have been documented with varying clinical importance. Opioids are known to decrease serum levels of testosterone, estrogen, luteinizing hormone (LH), gonadotropin releasing hormone (GRH), corticotropin-releasing hormone (CRH), adrenocorticotropic hormone (ACTH), and dehydroepiandrosterone (DHEA) [10, 1]. Many of these effects act to mediate vascular and cardiac responses in stress [27]. Clinically, decreased testosterone and estrogen from opioid-induced hypogonadism is associated with decreased energy and increased depression, and these may be the most readily identifiable symptoms. While clinical symptoms may vary, some endocrine effects are evident in laboratory study within as little as 1 hour after administration and return to normal within 1 day after cessation [10]. In a rodent study, opioids increased catabolism and worsen hyperglycemia [1].

Incidence: Hormonal effects are thought to be frequent, but the incidence is not well characterized as most effects are clinically silent. Testosterone has been somewhat better studied and is known to acutely drop within four hours of opioid use. This effect is mitigated within a day of cessation of the drug [10].

Diagnosis: The diagnosis of endocrine dysfunction related to opioid use is typically clinical. It is often difficult to identify opioids as the specific cause. Hormonal levels can be assessed, but this is typically more relevant in the setting of chronic opioid use.

Management: Most hormonal effects are thought to be dose dependent. Dose reduction or cessation of use are the best treatment modalities for mitigating endocrine effects. However, acute untreated pain can cause much the same dysregulation and risks and benefits of therapy should be carefully considered [6].

Hematologic Side Effects

Description: Hematologic consequences of opioid therapy are poorly studied. It is known that drugs such as heroin impact levels of trace elements in the body, including iron [32]. The timing of this effect is largely unknown, however, as most studies utilized chronic opioid users [32]. Much data is extrapolated from populations of heroin and opium users, limiting clinical application. Chronic heroin users, when controlled to healthy individuals, have overall higher mean corpuscular volume, red cell distribution width, mean corpuscular hemoglobin, and iron-binding capacity [32, 33]. However, hemoglobin, hematocrit, platelet counts, and serum iron levels were significantly lower [32]. Increases in hemoglobin from their baseline during active heroin use were also found 1 month after withdrawal [33]. Most findings did relate to the route of administration of the drug with intravenous administration having the biggest effect. It is difficult to separate this from other lifestyle and dietary confounders in the studied populations.

Incidence: The incidence of hematologic changes from clinically used opioids is unknown.

Diagnosis: Any accomplished diagnosis would be difficult to pinpoint to opioid therapy and no certain conclusions could be made in a critically ill patient.

Management: As always, opioid therapy should be limited to the minimum efficacious dose and multimodal opioid-sparing techniques utilized whenever possible.

Immunologic Side Effects

Description: Opioids have been implicated in immunologic dysfunction and poor wound healing, beginning as early as the late 1800s [10, 21]. It was long ago discovered that the cellular immune response was impaired in an animal model treated with morphine [10]. Opioids may inhibit both innate and adaptive immune responses and specifically inhibit T-cells, B-cells, intestinal barrier integrity, natural killer cells, neutrophils, mast cells, cytokine expression, and phagocytosis [6, 10, 1, 2], (Fig. 5.5). Exposure to morphine may also result in TH-1 cell death but TH-2 cell differentiation [2]. Though immune cells do express opioid receptors, some immune

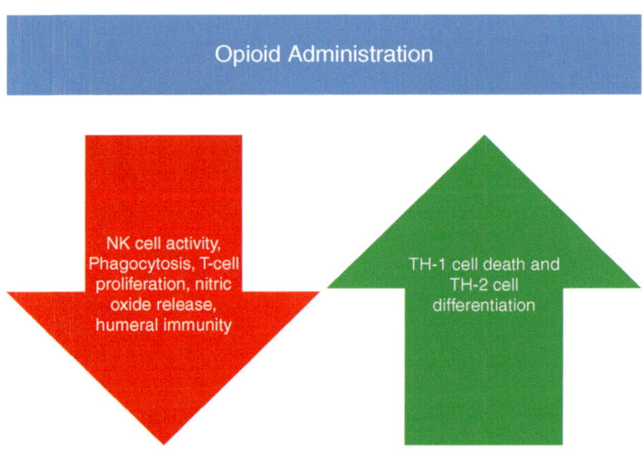

Fig. 5.5 Some of the wide ranging effects of morphine administration on the innate and adaptive immune systems. Most immunologic impacts have been catalogued in animal models; clinically significant effects on humans are not well studied. (Data from Benyamin et al. [10])

effects are actually mediated by opioid modulation of receptors in the central nervous system and hypothalamic-pituitary-adrenal (HPA) axis [1]. This pathway ultimately involves the cleavage of POMC to ACTH, alpha MSH, and beta endorphin, which specifically impacts immune cells [1]. The clinical importance of this is not well defined and much of the study is limited to animal models. Limited study in humans has also suggested immune modulation by opioids, including infection in ventilator-associated conditions [1, 34]. As in many of the impacts of opioids, untreated pain may have much the same immunologic impairment through stress response and similar interaction with the HPA [6].

Incidence: Effects on immune function are variable and the effect of opioids may be related to the underlying health of the host, the mode of drug administration, and the medication given [1]. Effects can be immediate and may last for up to a day after administration. Unpredictably, some study has actually shown an increase in cytotoxicity in NK cells of healthy hosts given fentanyl [1]. In short, clinical relevance is not well understood.

Diagnosis: As the clinical impacts of opioid therapy on the immune system are not well understood, a diagnosis is not easily achieved. Far more study is required to better understand which patients, if any, may clinically benefit from opioid reduction or cessation for immunomodulating purposes.

Management: There is no specific treatment related to immunomodulation due to opioids. Avoidance and discontinuation are the only known interventions, though again the clinical relevance is not well known.

Summary

The effects of opioids are wide ranging and impact almost every physiologic system. While some effects may be clinically silent or of unclear importance with contemporary research, others are well known and quickly lethal. Genitourinary, endocrine, immunologic, and hematologic effects in particular can be of unclear clinical relevance in the intensive care setting. A high level of caregiver vigilance and clinical suspicion is necessary to identify such outcomes, which may be mostly theoretical. Neurologic, respiratory, and cardiovascular effects are both rampant in clinical medicine and potentially life threatening. Opioid use disorder is a major source of morbidity and mortality in modern America and across the globe. Patients should always be monitored for physiologic dependence, tolerance, over-sedation, hypoventilation, and cardiovascular compromise from opioid therapy. Many, if not all, of the adverse effects of opioid therapy are best managed with avoidance. The minimum efficacious dose should always be pursued, continuous infusions avoided, and multimodal pain regimens that spare opioids initiated.

Conflicts of Interest No author has a relevant conflict of interest or financial disclosure necessary.

References

1. Molina PE. Opioids and opiates: analgesia with cardiovascular, haemodynamic and immune implications in critical illness. J Intern Med. 2006;259:138–54.
2. Plein LM, Rittner HL. Opioids and the immune system – friend or foe. Br J Pharmacol. 2018;175:2717–25.
3. Kolodny A, Courtwright DT, Hwang CS, Kreiner P, Eadie JL, Clark TW, Alexander GC. The prescription opioid and heroin crisis: a public health approach to an epidemic of addiction. Annu Rev Public Health. 2015;18(36):559–74.
4. Phillips DM. JCAHO pain management standards are unveiled. Joint commission on accreditation of healthcare organizations. JAMA. 2000;284(4):428–9.
5. Centers for Disease Control and Prevention. Understanding the Epidemic [Internet]. Centers for Disease Control and Prevention; 2018 [updated 2018, cited 2019 November] Available from: https://www.cdc.gov/drugoverdose/epidemic/index.html.
6. Martyn JA, Mao J, Bittner EA. Opioid tolerance in critical illness. N Engl J Med. 2019;380(4):365–78.
7. Erstad BL. Attempts to limit opioid prescribing in critically ill patients: not so easy. Not So Fast Ann Pharm. 2019;53(7):716–25.
8. Stamenkovic DM, Laycock H, Karanikolas M, Ladjevic NG, Neskovic V, Bantel C. Chronic pain and chronic opioid after intensive care discharge – is it time to change practice? Front Pharmacol. 2019;10(23)
9. Yaffe PB, Green RS, Butler MB, Witter T. Is admission to the intensive care unit associated with chronic opioid use? A 4-year follow-up of intensive care unit survivors. J Intensive Care Med. 2017;32(3):429–35.
10. Benyamin R, Trescot AM, Datta S, Buenaventura R, Adlaka R, Sehgal N, Glaser SE, Vallejo R. Opioid complications and side effects. Pain Physician. 2008;11:S105–20.
11. Cammarano WB, Pittet JF, Weitz S, Schlobohm RM, Marks JD. Acute withdrawal syndrome related to the administration of analgesic and sedative medications in adult intensive care unit patients. Crit Care Med. 1998;26(4):676–84.
12. Hall L, Oyen LS, Murray MJ. Analgesic agents: pharmacology and application in critical care. Crit Care Clin. 2001;17:899–925.
13. Go R, Cole BE, Broglio K. Managing pain in intensive care units. Pract Pain Manag. 2007; 7(7).
14. Wesson DR, Ling W. The clinical opiate withdrawal scale (COWS). J Psychoactive Drugs. 2003;35(2):253–9.
15. Ballantyne JC. Opioids for chronic pain: taking stock. Pain. 2006;125(1–2):3–4.
16. Fraser GL, Gagnon DJ. Pain and analgesia. In: Dasta JF, Carothers J, Bartel B, editors. CCSAP 2016 book 3: pain and sedation/support. Kansas: ACCP; 2016.
17. Brummel NE, Girard TD. Preventing delirium in the intensive care unit. Crit Care Clin. 2013;29(1):51–65.
18. Kamdar BB, Niessen T, Colantuoni E, King LM, Neufield KJ, Bienvenu J, Rowden AM, Collop NA, Needham DM. Delirium transitions in the medical ICU: exploring the role of sleep quality and other factors. Crit Care Med. 2015;43(1):135–41.
19. Agarwal V, O'Neill PJ, Cotton BA, Pun BT, Haney S, Thompson J, Kassebaum N, Shintani A, Guy J, Ely EW, Pandharipande P. Prevalence and risk factors for development of delirium in burn intensive care unit patients. J Burn Care Res. 2010;31(5):706–15.
20. Swart LM, van der Zanden V, Spies PE, de Rooj SE, van Munster BC. The comparative risk of delirium with different opioids: a systematic review. Drugs Aging. 2017;34(6):437–43.
21. Ehieli E, Yalamuri S, Brudney CS, Pyati S. Analgesia in the surgical intensive care unit. Postgrad Med J. 2017;93:38–45.
22. Gagnon DJ, Riker RR, Glisic EK, et al. Transition from dexmedetomidine to enteral clonidine for ICU sedation: an observational pilot study. Pharmacotherapy. 2015;35:251–9.

23. Wang HT, Hill AD, Gomes T, Wijesundera DN, Pinto R, Scales DC, Fowler R, Wunsch H. Opioid use after ICU admission among elderly chronic opioid users in Ontario: a population-based cohort study. Crit Care Med. 2018;46(12):1934–42.
24. Bailey JM. Context sensitive half times and other decrement times of inhaled anesthetics. Anesth Analg. 1997;85(3):681–6.
25. Tripathi R, Dhawan A, Rao R, Mishra AK, Jain R, Sinha S. Assessment of subjective sleep problems in men with opioid dependence maintained on buprenorphine. J Addict Med. 2020;14:132–8.
26. Dimsdale JE, Norman D, DeJardin D, Wallace MS. The effect of opioids on sleep architecture. J Clin Sleep Med. 2007;3:33–6.
27. Marino PL. Standard complications including bradycardia. Analgesia and sedation. In: Marino PL, Sutin KM, editors. The ICU book. 3rd ed. Philadelphia, PA: Lippincott Williams & Wilkins; 2007. p. 885–907.
28. Chou R, Cruciani RA, Fiellin DA, Compton P, Farrar JT, Haigney MC, et al. Methadone safety: a clinical practice guideline from the American pain society and college on problems of drug dependence, in collaboration with the heart rhythm society. J Pain. 2014;15:321–37.
29. Cashman JN, Dolin SJ. Respiratory and haemodynamic effects of acute postoperative pain management: evidence from published data. Br J Anaesth. 2004;93(2):212–23.
30. Li M, Ramos LG. Drug-induced QT prolongation and Torsades de pointes. PT. 2017; 42(7):473–7.
31. Klausner JM, Caspi J, Lelcuk S, Khazam A, Marin G, Hechtman HB, Rozin RR. Delayed muscular rigidity and respiratory depression following fentanyl anesthesia. Arch Surg. 1988;123(1):66–7.
32. Guzel D, Yazici AB, Yazici E, Erol A. Evaluation of Immunomodulatory and hematologic outcome in heroin/opioid addicts. J Addict. 2018:2036145.
33. Haghpanah T, Afarinesh M, Divsalar KA. Review on hematological factors in opioid-dependent people (opium and heroin) after the withdrawal period. Addict Health. 2010;2(1–2):9–16.
34. Lewis SC, Li L, Murphy MV, Klompas M. Risk factors for ventilator-associated events: a case-control multivariable analysis. Crit Care Med. 2014;42(8):1839–48.

Chapter 6
Rational Selection and Utilization of Opioid Analgesics in Critical Care

Christina Boncyk, Kyle Bruns, Christina J. Hayhurst, and Christopher G. Hughes

Introduction

An important part of patient care is facilitating comfort and reducing anxiety in order to improve interactions between the patients, staff, and caregivers. Pain is frequently present in critically ill patients regardless of whether they are admitted to medical or surgical units [1]. Although pain is often attributed to invasive procedures, monitoring devices, or wounds, a significant number of patients report pain *at rest* while in the intensive care unit (ICU) [1]. Recognition of pain is important, not only to be able to relieve the discomfort and suffering of the patient but also to mitigate downstream physiologic effects including increased stress hormone production, hemodynamic instability, vasoconstriction, increased catabolism, impaired tissue perfusion, immunosuppression, and impaired wound healing. Other long-term effects including chronic pain and post-traumatic stress symptoms (PTSS) are highly prevalent among ICU survivors [2]. The first step in treating discomfort or pain, however, is recognizing it. Critically ill patients are frequently intubated, sedated, or otherwise unable to communicate their symptoms to healthcare providers. Unless regularly screened for and treated with targeted interventions, pain can be mismanaged and lead to worsened psychological and physical outcomes.

Pain management has emerged as a major focus in critical illness as sedation practices have shifted and providers target lighter sedation with the goal of having more interactive patients. These changes are driven by emerging research demonstrating benefits of decreased sedation, increased patient interactions, and more frequent mobilization [3, 4]. Along with improved patient awareness is the increased recognition and need to keep patients comfortable and calm. The management of

C. Boncyk (✉) · K. Bruns · C. J. Hayhurst · C. G. Hughes
Department of Anesthesiology, Division of Anesthesia Critical Care Medicine, Vanderbilt University Medical Center, Nashville, TN, USA
e-mail: christina.s.boncyk@vumc.org; Kyle.bruns@vumc.org; christina.j.hayhurst@vumc.org; christopher.hughes@vumc.org

J. L. Pascual, T. G. Gaulton (eds.), *Opioid Use in Critical Care*,
https://doi.org/10.1007/978-3-030-77399-1_6

pain with opioids to assist in these practices has become a major goal of ICU practitioners that has led to the practice of analgesia-based sedation, or "analgosedation." Within this practice, analgesia is prioritized over sedation or hypnosis to encourage a more interactive, lucid, and comfortable patient [2]. Unless contraindicated, current guidelines recommend for the use of targeted analgesia-based sedation with limited use of additional sedative or hypnotic medications [3]. Once initiated, targeted pain management with assessment-driven clinical practices can improve the quality of care provided to patients as well as their outcomes following ICU survival. The evidence behind a targeted analgesia-based approach has proven to be associated with a reduction in hypnotic agents use, duration of mechanical ventilation, and ICU length of stay [3].

This chapter aims to describe pain in the critically ill patient, identify tools to aid in diagnosis and quantification of pain, provide guidance when choosing opioids in patients with various pathophysiologic derangements, and define clinical targets for titration of medications.

Origins of Pain in Critical Illness

Pain is the unpleasant sensory or emotional experience associated with actual or potential tissue damage [5]. This definition allows for the broad interpretation of the diagnosis and experience of pain in patients owing to the multiple physiologic and psychologic pathways that interplay to contribute to this condition. The experience of pain is not limited to those patients who are conscious enough to describe it—pain is frequently reported as a significant memory among critical illness survivors despite appearing unaware or unconscious [6]. For both the psychiatric and physiologic benefits of patients, it is particularly important to assess and treat pain in critically ill populations unable to articulate their experiences. Additionally, there is an increasing prevalence of chronic pain within the community, affecting approximately 1 in 10 adults at baseline [7]. Such patients present with baseline pain levels and can have hyperalgesic (pain out of proportion to stimulus) or allodynic (pain cause by non-painful stimulus) [8] responses to stimuli while in the ICU. For these reasons, it is important to have a systematic and consistent approach to the assessment and management of pain across all patients.

Pain in the ICU can be most simply broken down into rest pain and procedural pain. Rest pain is pain or discomfort that exists while the patient is inactive. This includes baseline chronic pain, musculoskeletal pain from immobility or pressure, wound, fracture, or surgical site pain, gastrointestinal discomfort, or pain related to indwelling lines or tubes [2]. Procedural pain involves regular activities including patient turning, bathing, oral care, or invasive procedures (monitor placement, drain insertion, suture laceration, etc.) that elicit discomfort for the patient while the finite activity is ongoing. Distinction between these types of pain is noteworthy as they carry different sets of risk factors. Recognition by bedside providers of these

Table 6.1 Risk factors for rest and procedural pain [3, 9–15]

Rest pain risk factors	Procedural pain risk factors
Younger age	Younger age
Anxiety	Female sex
Depression	Non-white ethnicity
Comorbidities	Patient positioning
Baseline disability	Type of procedure
History of surgery	Pre-procedural pain intensity
Delay in analgesic initiation	Peri-procedural opioid use[a]
Disproportionate to expectations	Underlying surgery or trauma
Increased ICU length of stay	
Expectation of future poor quality of life	

[a]Conflicting evidence [16, 17]

different types of pain allows identification of patients at increased risk of unrelieved pain—allowing earlier implementation of pain management strategies to mitigate discomfort. A summary of risk factors for resting and procedural pain is listed in Table 6.1.

As shown, this list includes both non-modifiable and potentially modifiable risk factors for active pain. Potentially modifiable risk facts should be addressed as soon as possible to mitigate downstream pain and discomfort for patients as well as stress and anxiety of family members.

In the broader realm of acute pain management, pain is classified by origin of insult as either nociceptive or neuropathic since treatment approaches and efficacy of strategies for pain management differ between these types of pain. Nociceptive pain represents ongoing tissue injury and can be further broken down into somatic pain (affecting superficial and/or peripheral tissues, i.e., skin, tissue, muscle, or bone pain) or visceral pain (affecting the abdomen or organ-related injury, i.e., internal organ pain) [18]. Neuropathic pain is often the result of abnormal nervous system function or dysregulation [18]. It is frequently associated with hyperalgesia and/or allodynia—additional consequences of a dysregulated nervous system. Patients are not limited to one classification, however, and frequently experience a combination of these types of pain. It is helpful to distinguish the origin of pain as treatment options will vary in efficacy depending on pain type (Table 6.2).

In addition to identifying the type of pain to better assign effective treatment therapies, it is also important to identify pain that can signal further risk to the patient. Pain is a basic protective mechanism teleologically. History and physical exam is the most important factor in classifying pain. For example, pain from a fractured leg can be an appropriate cause of somatic rest pain in a critically ill patient. But failing to perform a physical exam when the pain is worsening can delay the identification of neuropathic pain caused by acute compartment syndrome, which carries different albeit as acute of a condition if this change in pain is unrecognized or inappropriately classified.

Table 6.2 Classification, origin, and management strategies for acute pain [18–20]

Classification of pain	Origin of pain	Examples	Pain management strategies
Nociceptive	Ongoing tissue damage		Treat underlying cause, non-steroidal anti-inflammatory drugs, acetaminophen, ketamine, dexmedetomidine, anticonvulsants (e.g., gabapentin, carbamazepine), neuraxial analgesia or peripheral nerve blocks, music therapy
	Somatic	Burns, fractures, invasive lines	
	Visceral	Angina, pancreatitis, bowel distension	
Neuropathic	Damaged nerves or dysregulated nervous system	Spinal cord injury pain, phantom limb pain, multiple sclerosis, neuropathy (diabetic, alcoholic, chemotherapy-related)	Antidepressants (e.g., serotonin-norepinephrine reuptake inhibitors, bupropion), anticonvulsants (e.g., gabapentin, pregabalin), ketamine, topical anesthetics (e.g., lidocaine), opioids, peripheral nerve blocks, physical therapy and complementary therapies (transcutaneous electrical nerve stimulation [TENS], relaxation or massage therapy, music therapy)

Diagnosing and Quantifying Pain in the ICU Patient

Acute pain is highly individual and patients have different experiences, expectations, and tolerance for pain. For these reasons, critical care providers should not assume a linear relationship between injury severity and pain experienced. Validated tools to objectively quantify and qualify pain are available and should be routinely employed to optimize recognition of pain and delivery and titration of analgesic medications. Traditionally, pain has been assessed by a self-reported pain scale such as the numerical rating scale (NRS) or the numerical rating scale with a visual format (NRS-V), see Chap. 7 [21, 22]. Such pain scales are frequently administered along with verbal and/or the visual pain scales, such as the Wong-Baker FACES Pain Rating Scale [23] discussed in Chap. 7. Most ICU patients, however, are unable to participate reliably with the NRS-V, verbal, or facial scales due to mental status derangements from illness, sedation, presenting pathology, or a combination thereof and alternative assessment methods must be utilized. In the scenario where the patient is unable to verbalize due to intubation or other causes, the Behavior Pain Scale (BPS) [24] or the Critical-Care Pain Observation Tool (CPOT) [25] may be used to quantify pain. Both of these scales are well validated within the critically ill population and recommended by current guidelines (see Chap. 7) [26, 27].

As shown in Table 6.3, the CPOT is divided into four main behavioral domains: facial expression, body movements, ventilator compliance (when applicable), and muscle tension. This assessment can be performed quickly by a bedside nurse or

Table 6.3 Critical-care pain observation tool scoring table [25]

Indicator	Description	Score	
Facial expression	No muscular tension observed	Relaxed, neutral	0
	Presence of frowning, brow lowering, orbit tightening, and levator contraction	Tense	1
	All of the above facial movements plus eyelid tightly closed	Grimacing	2
Body movements	Does not move at all (does not necessarily mean absence of pain)	Absence of movements	0
	Slow, cautious movements, touching or rubbing the pain site, seeking attention through movements	Protection	1
	Pulling tube, attempting to sit up, moving limbs/thrashing, not following commands, striking at staff, trying to climb out of bed	Restlessness	2
Muscle tension Evaluated by passive flexion and extension of upper extremities	No resistance to passive movements	Relaxed	0
	Resistance to passive movements	Tense, rigid	1
	Strong resistance to passive movements, inability to complete them	Very tense or rigid	2
Compliance with the ventilator (intubated patients)	Alarms no activated, easy ventilation	Tolerating ventilator or movement	0
	Alarms stop spontaneously	Coughing but tolerating	1
	Asynchrony: Blocking ventilation, alarms frequently activated	Fighting ventilator	2
OR			
Vocalization (extubated patients)	Talking in normal tone or no sound	Talking in normal tone or no sound	0
	Signing, moaning	Signing, moaning	1
	Crying out, sobbing	Crying out, sobbing	2
Total, range			0–8

other clinical care providers. Each domain is scored between 0 and 2, with total possible scores ranging from 0 to 8. A score of 3 or greater indicates pain. Importantly, this tool assesses for the presence of pain and is not a linear scale. It also does not correlate to the same number score on the self-reported scales.

Another common tool used to assess pain in the ICU is the Behavior Pain Scale (BPS) [24]. The BPS is broken down into three main behavioral domains: facial expression, upper limb movements, and compliance with mechanical ventilation. These are scored from 1 to 4, as shown in Table 6.4. A score of ≤ 3 indicates no pain, 4–5 indicates mild pain, 6–11 unacceptable amount of pain, and ≥ 12 indicates maximum pain. This scale is similar to the CPOT in that it

Table 6.4 Behavior pain scale scoring table

Indicator	Description	Score
Facial expression	Relaxed	1
	Partially tightened (e.g., brow lowering)	2
	Fully tightened (e.g., eyelid closing)	3
	Grimacing	4
Upper limb movements	No movement	1
	Partially bent	2
	Fully bent with finger flexion	3
	Permanently retracted	4
Compliance with mechanical ventilation	Tolerating movement	1
	Coughing but tolerating ventilation for most of the time	2
	Fighting ventilator	3
	Unable to control ventilation	4
Total		
	No pain	0–3
	Mild pain	4–5
	Unacceptable amount of pain	6–11
	Maximum pain	12

can also be done quickly and effectively at the bedside with good reliability and validity [28]. One major difference is that the BPS scale additionally quantifies the degree of pain, whereas CPOT is designed primarily for identification of the presence of pain [29].

While both of these scoring methods have been validated and shown effective at identifying pain in conscious and unconscious critically ill patients, neither has been shown to be superior in sensitivity or specificity [30]. As such, the routine use of any of these validated pain tools is the most important aspect of assessment. Hemodynamic changes and intermittent non-validated qualitative assessments by bedside providers are not a reliable method for assessing pain in critical care and result in the failure to recognize pain—particularly in unconscious patients. Although recognition of these changes are important aspects of bedside care and should not be ignored, they also cannot be depended on for routine pain assessments in critically ill patients. Protocol-based analgesia and sedation approaches are not only important from a humane perspective in that they improve patient pain scores [31], but they offer additional proven clinical benefits as well. Institution of protocol-guided analgesia and sedation administration have been shown to reduce total sedation received [32], days of mechanical ventilation, and ICU length of stay [33, 34]. It is therefore imperative that validated screening methods be implemented and routinely performed throughout the ICU stay for all patients.

Pathophysiology and Opioid Selection

There are several factors that should be included when making the decision of which opioid medication to administer. These include medication availability, underlying pathophysiology, patient-specific factors, as well as staff familiarity, and local practice. Per current guidelines, pain should be treated first in a targeted-practice strategy with sedation used to augment patient comfort, per analgesia-based sedation or "analgosedation." Pain management strategies, however, are not limited to opioid medications. Pain management should involve multimodal components including patient positioning, non-pharmacologic strategies, regional analgesia as indicated, and non-opioid medications (i.e., muscle relaxants, intravenous lidocaine/ketamine, gabapentinoids, non-steroidal anti-inflammatory drugs, or NSAIDs) as indicated for optimal results. These adjunct medications, however, are not benign and accumulation of either medication or active metabolites secondary to impaired metabolism can cause significant, even life-threatening, complications. Additionally, although they may help accomplish other clinical goals, adjunct medications may not be reliably associated with reduction in opioid use [35, 36]. It is recommended that doses be adjusted for metabolic clearance or avoided entirely if patients have evident decreased renal or hepatic metabolism. Table 6.5 lists non-opioid analgesics recommended for use by current guidelines for pain, along with their primary route of clearance and relative contraindications [3].

Non-pharmacologic strategies to be considered include music therapy, relaxation techniques, massage, or transcutaneous electrical nerve stimulator (TENS) therapy. Where these opioid sparing and non-pharmacologic strategies fail, opioids should be considered for additional acute pain management. The optimal opioid medication is cost-effective, quick acting, has a short context-sensitive half-life, is rapidly titratable, and does not interact with other medications or hemodynamic parameters. While no opioid medication on the market fully meets all of these criteria, we will discuss their relative indications and contraindications.

Opioids recommended for pain management in the ICU include remifentanil, fentanyl, hydromorphone, and morphine [3]. All will have dose-dependent side effects, with higher doses associated with greater respiratory depression and

Table 6.5 Non-opioid analgesics, primary metabolic clearance, and relative contraindications

Medication	Metabolic clearance	Contraindication
Acetaminophen	Hepatic	Cirrhosis (> 2 g/24 h)
Gabapentinoids	Renal	Renal failure
Ketamine	Hepatic	PTSD/psychiatric disorders
NSAIDs[a]	Renal	Food and Drug Administration warning after coronary artery bypass graft surgery, renal impairment

[a]recommended for discrete use in infrequent procedures as an alternative to opioids

Table 6.6 Pharmacokinetics of commonly utilized opioid medications [37]

Medication	Onset (IV)	Elimination half-life	Context-sensitive half-life	Active metabolites	Metabolic pathway
Remifentanil	1–3 min	3–10 min	3–4 min	No	Hydrolysis by plasma esterases
Fentanyl	1–2 min	2–4 hrs	200 min (6 hr. infusion); 300 min (12 hr. infusion)	No	Demethylation CYP3A4 substrate
Hydromorphone	5–15 min	2–3 hrs	N/A	No	Glucuronidation
Morphine	5–10 min	3–4 hrs	N/A	6- and 3-glucuronide metabolite	Demethylation, Glucuronidation

hypotension. When deciding which agent to use, one should factor in time of onset, planned duration of use, alterations in renal or hepatic metabolism, respiratory status, and external factors such as utilization of extra-corporeal membrane oxygenation (ECMO). Table 6.6 describes pharmacokinetic properties of commonly utilized opioid medications in the ICU that should factor in to opioid choice. In addition to these, individual medication factors must also be considered.

For example, fentanyl is a quick-acting opioid medication owing in large part to its relative lipophilicity. This same property, however, will allow it to absorb within ECMO cannula tubing [38]. While not necessarily a contraindication, higher doses may be required for these patients to achieve target concentration. Alternatively, one could transition to a less lipophilic alternative such as morphine or hydromorphone. Additionally, several opioid medications have been shown to cause clinically significant histamine release impacting patient hemodynamics. Morphine is the most frequently implicated in this adverse event and patients should be monitored closely, especially if presenting with a history of immunologic sensitivity [39]. Finally, remifentanil is often used for short procedures given the cost of prolonged infusions as well as its association with increased hyperalgesia following discontinuation [40]. In patients with impaired renal function, prolonged infusions have been associated with glycine toxicity and should be used with caution in ICU patients with impairments in renal metabolism [41]. In general, because fentanyl causes less histamine release than morphine and does not undergo renal elimination, it is the preferred opioid analgesic in hemodynamically unstable patients or those with renal insufficiency.

Few comparative trials between opioid regimens have been performed in the ICU. Remifentanil appears to provide better outcomes than morphine with regard to time at sedation target, use of supplemental sedation, and duration of mechanical ventilation in one randomized double-blind study [42, 43]. Meanwhile, remifentanil and fentanyl have displayed equal efficacy in achieving time at target sedation with no difference in extubation times [43]. Patients receiving fentanyl required more frequent administration of additional sedatives but experienced less pain after extubation compared to those receiving remifentanil [43].

Regardless of the opioid medication used, patients should be continually assessed using validated scoring systems following medication administration for titration of medication and early identification of adverse events.

Targeted Opioid Medication Utilization

The Saturday Review in 1895 published an article by George Bernard Shaw in which he used the phrase "a shot in the dark." In present day medicine, we are fortunate to have guidelines and validated scales to shed light on our target. Intensivists are challenged with the task of providing sedation that is analgesia-based and assessment-driven [3]. Several studies have produced results demonstrating improved outcomes when analgesia is managed primarily [37, 39–42]. We will describe this strategy below.

Analgosedation protocols begin using the same tools presented earlier in this chapter. Multimodal pain management strategies are initiated for patients guided by validated CPOT or BPS scales. When indicated, providers should choose opioids with the previously mentioned considerations as a guide. They should then titrate these medications to achieve adequate pain relief as determined using either CPOT, BPS, or other validated scoring systems. An earlier review of appropriate opioid selection should guide the critical care team in devising a protocol appropriate for each unique institution while considering the clinical condition and cost. A step-wise approach in concordance with current recommendations guiding opioid utilization for managing acute pain is presented in Table 6.7.

In the case that the patient remains agitated, sedation should then be initiated (i.e., propofol, dexmedetomidine) and guided by validated sedation scare targets. There are several validated scales that can be utilized to describe patient sedation or agitation—the most common being the Ramsay Scale [44] and the Richmond Agitation-Sedation Scale (RASS) [45], described in Tables 6.8 and 6.9. Following these scales, clinicians should target sedation to achieve a Ramsay score of 1–2 or a RASS score of −1 to +1.

Table 6.7 General approach to treating acute pain in critical illness

Situation	Preferred intervention
Acute pain	Intermittent (IV or enteral) opioid administration
Acute pain that persists/recurs	Opioid infusion +/− IV boluses for breakthrough pain
Acute pain in chronic opioid user	Account for previous opioid use when using IV opioid; may consider ketamine or other multimodal adjunct
Planned transition out of ICU and patient on IV opioid infusion	Initiate scheduled enteral opioid therapy

Table 6.8 Ramsay scale

Ramsay scale	
Scale	Description
1	Anxious, agitates, or restless
2	Cooperative, oriented
3	Response to commands only
4	Brisk response to light touch or loud auditory commands
5	Sluggish response to light touch or loud auditory commands
6	No response to light touch or loud auditory commands

Table 6.9 Richmond agitation-sedation scale (RASS)

Richmond agitation-sedation scale (RASS)		
Score	Term	Description
+4	Combative	Overtly combative or violent; immediate danger to staff
+3	Very agitated	Pulls on or removes tube(s) or catheter(s) or has aggressive behavior toward staff
+2	Agitated	Frequent non-purposeful movement or patient-ventilator dyssynchrony
+1	Restless	Anxious or apprehensive but movements not aggressive or vigorous
0	Alert and calm	
-1	Drowsy	Not fully alert, but has sustained (more than 10 s) awakening, with eye contact, to voice
-2	Light sedation	Briefly (less than 10 s) awakens with eye contact to voice
−3	Moderate sedation	Any movement (but no eye contact) to voice
−4	Deep sedation	No response to voice, but any movement to physical stimulation
−5	Unarousable	No response to voice or physical stimulation

Once the targeted sedation level is achieved, clinicians should continue to re-assess and adjust sedative medications for continued maintenance of light sedation in addition to continued concurrent pain assessments and control. These re-assessments and interventions are critical to maintaining a safe and alert patient with optimized pain control. Importantly, for all patients intubated and maintained on sedation, daily pauses in sedation should be performed along with daily spontaneous breathing trials, unless otherwise contraindicated. When performed together, this practice is associated with a decrease in ventilator days, ICU days, and improved survival up to 1 year following hospital discharge [46].

Further, the use of analgesic-based sedative regimens targeting light sedation have shown clinical benefits across study centers and in diverse populations. Patients maintained on primary analgesia-driven sedation with protocolized assessments and minimal, as-needed, sedation have also been shown to have decreased length of stay in the ICU, more days alive without mechanical ventilation, and improved sedation scores [31, 47, 48]. These analgesia-based protocols serve as a tool for providers to both target and titrate analgesic and sedative regimens in critically ill patients. Although specific medications and doses can vary among protocols, the primary basis remains administration of short-acting, readily titratable medications driven by frequent patient assessments.

While opioids have been discussed here as the primary tool for analgosedation and acute pain, the clinician must not minimize the current opioid crisis. The previously stated adverse effects should remind providers to employ a multimodal approach to analgesia that incorporates both pharmacologic and non-pharmacologic agents. Utilizing the whole spectrum of the critical care team (clinical psychologists, physical and occupational therapists, nursing staff, physicians) is further recommended to achieve success in this realm.

Summary

Inappropriate sedation and pain management contribute to worse patient outcomes [47, 48]. The shift away from deep sedation in mechanically ventilated patients to more awake and interactive patients has directed the focus toward analgesia-based strategies in critical illness. Recognizing the cause and type of pain present in patients is the first step toward treatment. A foundational knowledge of opioids and non-opioid adjuncts is essential for implementation and targeted pain relief therapy. Clinicians should employ opioid adjuncts to pain management with individual derangements in pathophysiology and institutional constraints and familiarity in mind. Most importantly, ICUs should employ and perform validated assessments of pain and modify analgesia and sedation using targeted goal-directed protocols. Adherence with these goal-directed analgesia and pain management strategies has been shown to improve outcomes for critically ill patients.

References

1. Chanques G, Sebbane M, Barbotte E, Viel E, Eledjam JJ, Jaber S. A prospective study of pain at rest: incidence and characteristics of an unrecognized symptom in surgical and trauma versus medical intensive care unit patients. Anesthesiology. 2007;107(5):858–60.
2. McGovern C, Cowan R, Appleton R, Miles B. Pain, agitation and delirium in the intensive care unit. Anaesthe Intens Care Med. 2018;19(12):634–40.
3. Devlin JW, Skrobik Y, Gelinas C, et al. Clinical practice guidelines for the prevention and management of pain, agitation/sedation, delirium, immobility, and sleep disruption in adult patients in the ICU. Crit Care Med. 2018;46(9):e825–73.
4. Treggiari MM, Romand JA, Yanez ND, et al. Randomized trial of light versus deep sedation on mental health after critical illness. Crit Care Med. 2009;37(9):2527–34.
5. Bonica JJ. The need of a taxonomy. Pain. 1979;6(3):247–8.
6. van de Leur JP, van der Schans CP, Loef BG, Deelman BG, Geertzen JH, Zwaveling JH. Discomfort and factual recollection in intensive care unit patients. Crit Care. 2004;8(6):R467–73.

7. Mansfield KE, Sim J, Jordan JL, Jordan KP. A systematic review and meta-analysis of the prevalence of chronic widespread pain in the general population. Pain. 2016;157(1):55–64.
8. Jensen TS, Finnerup NB. Allodynia and hyperalgesia in neuropathic pain: clinical manifestations and mechanisms. Lancet Neurol. 2014;13(9):924–35.
9. Carroll KC, Atkins PJ, Herold GR, et al. Pain assessment and management in critically ill postoperative and trauma patients: a multisite study. Am J Crit Care Off Publ Am Assoc Crit Care Nurs. 1999;8(2):105–17.
10. Al Sutari MM, Abdalrahim MS, Hamdan-Mansour AM, Ayasrah SM. Pain among mechanically ventilated patients in critical care units. J Res Med Sci. 2014;19(8):726–32.
11. Navarro-Garcia MA, Marin-Fernandez B, de Carlos-Alegre V, et al. Preoperative mood disorders in patients undergoing cardiac surgery: risk factors and postoperative morbidity in the intensive care unit. Rev Esp Cardiol. 2011;64(11):1005–10.
12. Desbiens NA, Wu AW, Broste SK, et al. Pain and satisfaction with pain control in seriously ill hospitalized adults: findings from the SUPPORT research investigations. For the SUPPORT investigators. Study to understand prognoses and preferences for outcomes and risks of treatment. Crit Care Med. 1996;24(12):1953–61.
13. Puntillo KA, Morris AB, Thompson CL, Stanik-Hutt J, White CA, Wild LR. Pain behaviors observed during six common procedures: results from thunder project II. Crit Care Med. 2004;32(2):421–7.
14. Arroyo-Novoa CM, Figueroa-Ramos MI, Puntillo KA, et al. Pain related to tracheal suctioning in awake acutely and critically ill adults: a descriptive study. Intensive Crit Care Nurs. 2008;24(1):20–7.
15. Faigeles B, Howie-Esquivel J, Miaskowski C, et al. Predictors and use of nonpharmacologic interventions for procedural pain associated with turning among hospitalized adults. Pain Manag Nurs. 2013;14(2):85–93.
16. Puntillo KA, Max A, Timsit JF, et al. Determinants of procedural pain intensity in the intensive care unit. The Europain(R) study. Am J Respir Crit Care Med. 2014;189(1):39–47.
17. Puntillo K, Weiss SJ. Pain: its mediators and associated morbidity in critically ill cardiovascular surgical patients. Nurs Res. 1994;43(1):31–6.
18. Pandharipande PP, et al. Effect of sedation with dexmedetomidine vs lorazepam on acute brain dysfunction in mechanically ventilated patients: the MENDS randomized controlled trial. J JAMA. 298(22):2644–53.
19. Treede RD, Jensen TS, Campbell JN, et al. Neuropathic pain: redefinition and a grading system for clinical and research purposes. Neurology. 2008;70(18):1630–5.
20. Kerstman E, Ahn S, Battu S, Tariq S, Grabois M. Neuropathic pain. Handb Clin Neurol. 2013;110:175–87.
21. Chanques G, Viel E, Constantin JM, et al. The measurement of pain in intensive care unit: comparison of 5 self-report intensity scales. Pain. 2010;151(3):711–21.
22. Rahu MA, Grap MJ, Ferguson P, Joseph P, Sherman S, Elswick RK Jr. Validity and sensitivity of 6 pain scales in critically ill, intubated adults. Am J Crit Care Off Public Am Assoc Crit Care Nurs. 2015;24(6):514–23.
23. Chambers CT, Hardial J, Craig KD, Court C, Montgomery C. Faces scales for the measurement of postoperative pain intensity in children following minor surgery. Clin J Pain. 2005;21(3):277–85.
24. Payen JF, Bru O, Bosson JL, et al. Assessing pain in critically ill sedated patients by using a behavioral pain scale. Crit Care Med. 2001;29(12):2258–63.
25. Gelinas C, Fillion L, Puntillo KA, Viens C, Fortier M. Validation of the critical-care pain observation tool in adult patients. Am J Crit Care Off Public Am Assoc Crit Care Nurs. 2006;15(4):420–7.
26. Dehghani H, Tavangar H, Ghandehari A. Validity and reliability of behavioral pain scale in patients with low level of consciousness due to head trauma hospitalized in intensive care unit. Arch Trauma Res. 2014;3(1):e18608.

27. Joffe AM, McNulty B, Boitor M, Marsh R, Gelinas C. Validation of the critical-care pain observation tool in brain-injured critically ill adults. J Crit Care. 2016;36:76–80.
28. Rijkenberg S, Stilma W, Bosman RJ, van der Meer NJ, van der Voort PHJ. Pain measurement in mechanically ventilated patients after cardiac surgery: comparison of the Behavioral pain scale (BPS) and the critical-care pain observation tool (CPOT). J Cardiothorac Vasc Anesth. 2017;31(4):1227–34.
29. Ahlers SJ, van der Veen AM, van Dijk M, Tibboel D, Knibbe CA. The use of the Behavioral pain scale to assess pain in conscious sedated patients. Anesth Analg. 2010;110(1):127–33.
30. Severgnini P, Pelosi P, Contino E, Serafinelli E, Novario R, Chiaranda M. Accuracy of critical care pain observation tool and Behavioral pain scale to assess pain in critically ill conscious and unconscious patients: prospective, observational study. J Intensive Care. 2016;4:68.
31. Faust AC, Rajan P, Sheperd LA, Alvarez CA, McCorstin P, Doebele RL. Impact of an analgesia-based sedation protocol on mechanically ventilated patients in a medical intensive care unit. Anesth Analg. 2016;123(4):903–9.
32. Georgiou E, Hadjibalassi M, Lambrinou E, Andreou P, Papathanassoglou ED. The impact of pain assessment on critically ill patients' outcomes: a systematic review. Bio Med Res Int. 2015;2015:503830.
33. Payen JF, Bosson JL, Chanques G, Mantz J, Labarere J. Pain assessment is associated with decreased duration of mechanical ventilation in the intensive care unit: a post hoc analysis of the DOLOREA study. Anesthesiology. 2009;111(6):1308–16.
34. Mehta S, Burry L, Cook D, et al. Daily sedation interruption in mechanically ventilated critically ill patients cared for with a sedation protocol: a randomized controlled trial. JAMA. 2012;308(19):1985–92.
35. Perbet S, Verdonk F, Godet T, et al. Low doses of ketamine reduce delirium but not opiate consumption in mechanically ventilated and sedated ICU patients: a randomised double-blind control trial. Anaesth Crit Care Pain Med. 2018;37(6):589–95.
36. Fabritius ML, Geisler A, Petersen PL, et al. Gabapentin for post-operative pain management - a systematic review with meta-analyses and trial sequential analyses. Acta Anaesthesiol Scand. 2016;60(9):1188–208.
37. Barr J, Pandharipande PP. The pain, agitation, and delirium care bundle: synergistic benefits of implementing the 2013 pain, agitation, and delirium guidelines in an integrated and interdisciplinary fashion. Crit Care Med. 2013;41(9 Suppl 1):S99–115.
38. Wildschut ED, Ahsman MJ, Allegaert K, Mathot RA, Tibboel D. Determinants of drug absorption in different ECMO circuits. Intensive Care Med. 2010;36(12):2109–16.
39. Flacke JW, Flacke WE, Bloor BC, Van Etten AP, Kripke BJ. Histamine release by four narcotics: a double-blind study in humans. Anesth Analg. 1987;66(8):723–30.
40. Yu EH, Tran DH, Lam SW, Irwin MG. Remifentanil tolerance and hyperalgesia: short-term gain, long-term pain? Anaesthesia. 2016;71(11):1347–62.
41. Bonnet MP, Minville V, Asehnoune K, et al. Glycine and ammonia plasma concentrations during sedation with remifentanil in critically ill patients. Intensive Care Med. 2007;33(7):1179–82.
42. Dahaba AA, Grabner T, Rehak PH, List WF, Metzler H. Remifentanil versus morphine analgesia and sedation for mechanically ventilated critically ill patients: a randomized double blind study. Anesthesiology. 2004;101(3):640–6.
43. Muellejans B, Lopez A, Cross MH, Bonome C, Morrison L, Kirkham AJ. Remifentanil versus fentanyl for analgesia based sedation to provide patient comfort in the intensive care unit: a randomized, double-blind controlled trial [ISRCTN43755713]. Crit Care. 2004;8(1):R1–R11.
44. Ramsay MA, Savege TM, Simpson BR, Goodwin R. Controlled sedation with alphaxalone-alphadolone. Br Med J. 1974;2(5920):656–9.
45. Sessler CN, Gosnell MS, Grap MJ, et al. The Richmond agitation-sedation scale: validity and reliability in adult intensive care unit patients. Am J Respir Crit Care Med. 2002;166(10):1338–44.

46. Girard TD, Kress JP, Fuchs BD, et al. Efficacy and safety of a paired sedation and ventilator weaning protocol for mechanically ventilated patients in intensive care (awakening and breathing controlled trial): a randomised controlled trial. Lancet. 2008;371(9607):126–34.
47. Breen D, Karabinis A, Malbrain M, et al. Decreased duration of mechanical ventilation when comparing analgesia-based sedation using remifentanil with standard hypnotic-based sedation for up to 10 days in intensive care unit patients: a randomised trial [ISRCTN47583497]. Crit Care. 2005;9(3):R200–10.
48. Rozendaal FW, Spronk PE, Snellen FF, et al. Remifentanil-propofol analgo-sedation shortens duration of ventilation and length of ICU stay compared to a conventional regimen: a Centre randomised, cross-over, open-label study in the Netherlands. Intensive Care Med. 2009;35(2):291–8.

Chapter 7
Monitoring of Opioid Analgesic Use and Its Effects in Acute Care

Akhil Patel, Kunal Karamchandani, and Ashish K. Khanna

Introduction

Due to the complex nature of issues plaguing the critically ill patient, it is vital to employ adequate and appropriate pain management strategies. While treating acute pain and preventing the short- and long-term effects of inadequate pain control are a priority, it is also important that pain management is tailored to individual patient needs in order to avoid detrimental effects of excessive analgesia. Opioids remain the mainstay of treating pain in the acute care setting and are also used to provide analgo-sedation in this patient population. They may cause a myriad of side effects which can cause deleterious effects acutely as well as contribute to the post-ICU syndrome. Depression of the respiratory and neurological systems is the most feared complication of overdosing, along with the negative impact on the cardiovascular system. On the other hand, patients' pain in the acute care setting may be undertreated, thus leading to worse outcomes [1, 2]. This is of concern since many procedures performed in the ICU are extremely painful and must be treated appropriately [3]. The SCCM

A. Patel
Department of Anesthesiology, Cooper University Hospital, Cooper Medical School of Rowan University, Camden, NJ, USA

K. Karamchandani
Department of Anesthesiology and Pain Management, UT Southwestern Medical Center, Dallas, TX, USA
e-mail: kunal.karamchandani@utsouthwestern.edu

A. K. Khanna (✉)
Department of Anesthesiology, Section on Critical Care Medicine, Wake Forest School of Medicine, Wake Forest Baptist Medical Center, Winston-Salem, NC, USA

Outcomes Research Consortium, Cleveland, OH, USA
e-mail: akhanna@wakehealth.edu

J. L. Pascual, T. G. Gaulton (eds.), *Opioid Use in Critical Care*,
https://doi.org/10.1007/978-3-030-77399-1_7

(Society of Critical Care Medicine) ABCDEF bundle and the PADIS (Pain, Agitation, Delirium, Immobility and Sleep) guidelines emphasize appropriate choices of analgesia and sedation [3]. To help assist providers in assessing and managing pain, several grading systems and algorithms have been developed [4, 5]. However, assessment or quantification of pain can be challenging, as patients may have barriers to communication such as agitation, encephalopathy, or mechanical ventilation. Although monitoring techniques and scales that objectively assess pain have been developed, implementation and use is not universal. Similarly, monitoring and provision of sedation in acute care setting is challenging. The American Society of Anesthesiology (ASA) has defined sedation as mild, moderate, and deep based on patients' response to various degree of stimuli and have mandated provider certification to deliver the different levels of sedation [6–10]. The ASA has also developed recommendations for opioid monitoring in the perioperative setting to reduce the incidence of adverse respiratory events, and these recommendations can also be applied in the acute care setting.

Pain Assessment and Treatment

Routine assessment of pain in the acute care setting can prevent overmedication and hence the harmful side effects of opioids. Treatment plans should follow a basic gradation of severity of pain, and there should be an escalation plan for pain management based on severity. Multimodal analgesia including use of non-opioid medications such as NSAIDs, acetaminophen, gabapentin, and carbamazepine as well as regional analgesia should be implemented to avoid excessive use of narcotics. Enteral administration of medications should be encouraged whenever feasible restricting breakthrough pain to be treated with intravenous opioids. Intravenous Patient-Controlled Analgesia (IVPCA) is an option in appropriate patients immediately after surgery that cannot tolerate enteral medications [1, 2].

Assessment of a patient's pain in the acute care setting can be challenging and can be impacted by residual anesthesia, encephalopathy, and postoperative delirium among other factors. Numerous scales are available to assist providers with assessment of pain. The Numerical Rating Scale (NRS) and Visual Analog Scale (VAS) are two scoring systems commonly used to measure the severity of the pain in patients who are able to communicate [11]. The NRS scale is a scale from 0 to 10 and patients are asked to rate their pain on this scale with 0 being no pain and 10 being the worst pain they have or can imagine to ever experience. The VAS is a visual depiction of faces with varying expressions from smiling to crying. These pictures correlate with the NRS scale of 0–10 with a smiling face representing 0 and a crying face presenting a 10 (Fig. 7.1).

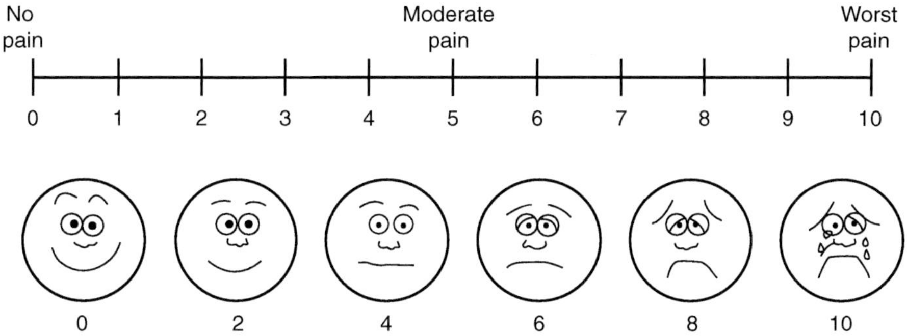

Fig. 7.1 Numerical rating scale (NRS) on top with the visual analog scale (VAS) to match on bottom. Scale ranging from 0 to 10 with 0 representing no pain and 10 representing the worst pain. (Adapted with permission from Yale University [Internet]. Visual Analogue Scale | Yale Assessment Module Training. [cited 2019Nov10]. Available from: https://assessment-module.yale.edu/im-palliative/visual-analogue-scale)

Table 7.1 Behavioral pain scale used for intubated and non-intubated patients. Higher score relates to increased pain

Facial expression	Relaxed	1
	Partial tighten	2
	Fully tighten	3
	Grimace	4
Upper limbs	No movement	1
	Partial flexion	2
	Full flexion	3
	Permanent retraction	4
Vent compliance	Tolerate movement	1
	Coughing	2
	Fighting	3
	Desynchrony	4

Adapted with permission from Severgnini et al. [14] Creative Commons Public Domain Dedication Waiver: https://creativecommons.org/publicdomain/zero/1.0/. Changes made to the wording

In patients who are unable to self-report pain but have intact motor function and observable behaviors, pain scales such as the Behavioral pain scale (BPS) and Critical Care Pain Observation Tool (CPOT) have been found to be moderately effective [12, 13]. These scales (Tables 7.1 and 7.2) take physical exam findings into consideration to produce a numerical value which categorizes pain severity [4, 14, 15]. However, currently available pain assessment methods are inadequate, and there remains a need for better tools, particularly for the objective assessment of pain in nonverbal individuals [14, 16, 17].

Table 7.2 CPOT: Can be used for either intubated or non-intubated patients. When using scale for non-intubated patients, disregard vent compliance section. For intubated patient, disregard speech section. Higher scores are related to increased pain sensed by the patient

Facial expression	Relaxed	0
	Tense	1
	Grimace	2
Movement	None	0
	Guarded	1
	Restless	2
Muscle tension	Relaxed	0
	Partially tense	1
	Fully tense	2
Speech	Normal tone	0
	Moaning	1
	Crying	2
Vent compliance	Tolerating vent	0
	Coughing	1
	Fighting	2

Adapted with permission from Severgnini et al. [14] Creative Commons Public Domain Dedication Waiver: https://creativecommons.org/publicdomain/zero/1.0/. Changes made to the wording

Respiratory Monitoring Techniques

There is always a risk of overdose when utilizing opioids for pain management. Patients in extreme pain may be unwilling to wait the required amount of time for opioids to take effect and reach maximal effectiveness or may manipulate providers into giving additional doses or other medications. Objective data from the aforementioned scales are helpful for spot assessments but often insufficient for continuous monitoring and treatment. National organizations have now studied and developed guidelines and practice advisories to advise continuous monitoring in patients receiving opioid therapy to prevent respiratory compromise [2]. In 2014, the Centers for Medicare and Medicaid Services (CMS) recommended "serial assessments of vital signs," including blood pressure, temperature, respiratory rate, pain level, respiratory status, and sedation level measurements to avoid opioid-induced respiratory depression (OIRD) [4]. They recommend frequent assessments, every 2.5 h for the first 24 h and 4.5 h thereafter during ongoing treatment including bolus administration and patient-controlled analgesic infusions. In 2016, the ASA provided guidelines for neuraxial administration of opioids which categorize a respiratory rate less than 10/minute, arterial saturation less than 90%, or arterial carbon dioxide greater than 6.66 kPa as signs of respiratory depression requiring urgent intervention [18]. Respiratory rate can be measured at the bedside by frequent clinical assessments or by continuous monitoring techniques. Repeated and frequent ventilation assessments can be completed at the bedside and can help identify early respiratory compromise;

however, this is labor intensive and expensive. This is also limited by the provider skill and expertise in diagnosing respiratory compromise.

Various non-invasive continuous monitoring techniques have been proposed to help overcome the limitations listed above. Pulse oximetry is the most commonly used method of non-invasive, continuous respiratory monitoring. A pulse oximeter comprises a light-emitting diode that emits light rays at a wavelength of 660 nm (red light) and 940 nm (infrared light), and the ratio of the amount of red light and infrared light absorbed by the red blood cells within the vasculature is recorded. This ratio is then converted to a percentage using the Beer-Lambert law. It provides a measure of blood oxygenation, with no information regarding the patient's ventilation. Since hypoxemia is a late sign of hypoventilation, especially in an oxygen-enriched environment, the ability of oximetry to detect respiratory depression before it becomes clinically important is limited. Thus, pulse oximetry may indicate high oxygen saturation regardless of the presence of hypoventilation and significant hypercapnia in patients receiving supplemental oxygen. Moreover, it is not a very reliable early indicator of hypoxemia since there is often a delay in recorded measurements. Finally, the waveform of pulse oximetry can be affected by low perfusion states, pigmented skin, nail polish, and patient movement [12, 18–20].

Inductance plethysmography allows continuous monitoring of a patient's respiratory status by measuring the change of impendence of two electrodes on the chest and producing a waveform to count cycles. These cycles represent breaths which can then be counted to calculate a respiratory rate [2]. While this modality is promising, the waveform is very sensitive, and hence, any movement can overestimate the respiratory rate. Body habitus can also limit the accuracy as cardiac oscillations can be mistaken for breaths in patients with very small habitudes. Plethysmography also does not measure oxygenation or ventilation and therefore unable to detect hypoxemia or hypoventilation [12, 19]. If a patient is to suffer airway obstruction, the respiratory rate may remain normal, due to persistent chest wall movement. Plethysmography is also unable to measure airflow and, hence, will not alert the provider in conditions where airflow is impaired.

Bioimpedance is similar to plethysmography, utilizing surface electrodes; however, it goes a step further in analyzing the electrical conductance to estimate respiratory rate, tidal volume, and minute ventilation. Although motion artifact can still affect the readings, there is data suggesting that bioimpedance-guided monitoring may be able to detect impending respiratory failure prior to a decrease in saturation [2, 12, 18].

Capnography provides non-invasive, continuous, and immediate assessment of the respiratory mechanics. Capnography has been recommended for opioid-treated patients receiving supplemental oxygen after surgery [21]. Since capnography measures ventilation as opposed to oxygenation, it has the ability to detect hypoventilation and OIRD earlier and more reliably. The waveform can help calculate the end tidal carbon dioxide values ($ETCO_2$) and can also be used to measure the respiratory rate. An increase in $ETCO_2$ values along with somnolence and a decrease in respiratory rate usually indicate impending respiratory failure. Respiratory depression can thus be quickly identified even if patients are given supplement oxygenation.

Limitations of capnography include the requirement to place nasal cannula and the difficulty in correlating the relationship between end tidal carbon dioxide and arterial CO_2. The accuracy of $ETCO_2$ measurement is only correlated with alveolar CO_2 when patients take a full vital capacity breath, which is uncommon in the immediate postoperative period [22]. Improper placement of nasal cannula, occlusion of cannula with secretions, altered nasal anatomy, nasal obstruction, and oxygen administration by mask and mouth breathing may all provide inaccurate readings which can raise false alarms and result in unnecessary interventions. Disease processes may change the gas exchange at the level of the alveoli, and thus, a normal $ETCO_2$ value may not equate to a normal arterial carbon dioxide and so reassessment and physical examination must be considered [12, 18, 19].

Mechanical ventilation via an invasive airway device allows for monitoring of patient's respiratory rate and also incorporates various safety features to prevent hypoventilation. Ventilators have the ability to set alarms for minimum respiratory rate and tidal volumes, thus allowing for early detection of hypoventilation. Most ventilators have a backup mode of ventilation that is triggered when a defined threshold for respiratory rate and/or minute ventilation is reached [12, 19]. It is safe to say, that at present, there is no proven single monitoring system or set of alarm thresholds that can detect all respiratory patterns associated with unexpected death events. Overall sensitivity to detecting impending events may be increased by using multiple monitoring modalities to detect patterns of change. Combining respiratory rate with oximetry and capnography may help with early detection of OIRD as well as other disease processes.

Newer Monitoring Technologies and Assessment Scales

As discussed above, limitations often exist for achieving consistent monitoring that is accurate in capturing adverse events from narcotic administration in a timely manner. Research is ongoing to develop and validate newer monitors with smarter alert systems. Algorithms combining multiple individual physiologic parameters to produce a single threshold level may increase the sensitivity of threshold systems and avoid false alarms making safe monitoring easier for providers. One such example is the Modified Early Warning Score (MEWS). The MEWS system is a simple additive threshold alarm that combines multiple monitors into one score for documentation and alerts. It takes into consideration the respiratory rate, heart rate, blood pressure, urine output, temperature, and neurological status. In the future, development of new systems that will analyze changing patterns among several combined vital signs is likely to become more widespread. Systems are being developed to set a single score based on multiple vital signs and exam findings to identify patients at risk for respiratory depression, similar to MEWS [19]. These systems may allow for timely intervention, and perhaps reduction of untoward events and in overall patient morbidity and mortality.

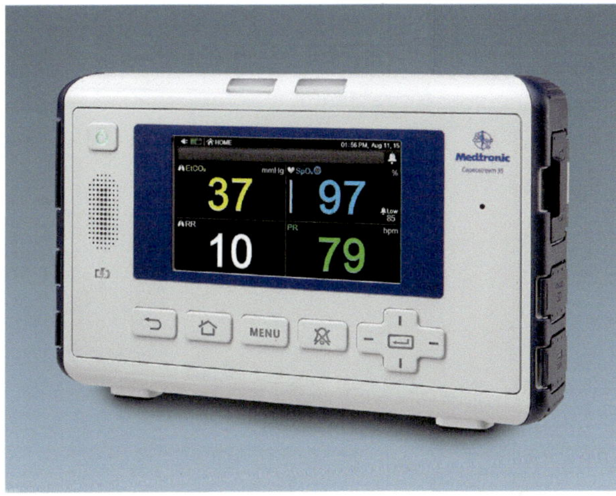

Fig. 7.2 Medtronic Capnostream 35p respiratory monitor showing $EtCO_2$, SpO_2, RR, and HR. The device has the capability to measure and display the Integrated Pulmonary Index (IPI) as well. (With permission from Medtronic)

One such system is the Integrated Pulmonary Index, or IPI, which takes into consideration $ETCO_2$, respiratory rate (RR), pulse rate (PR), and arterial oxygenation [23]. The IPI algorithm is a mathematical model combining SpO_2, RR, PR, and $ETCO_2$ into a single value between 1 and 10 that reflects the adequacy of ventilation and oxygenation at a given point in time. Figure 7.2 shows the Medtronic 35p capnostream monitor that has the ability to measure IPI. The algorithm was designed using a fuzzy logic inference model to incorporate expert clinical opinions. The validity of the index was tested on 523 patients and correlated well with expert interpretation of the continuous respiratory data (R1/40.83; $P < 0.01$), with an agreement of -0.5 ± 1.4 [24]. Integrated systems that monitor respiratory status (e.g., pulse oximetry and capnography) and medication-delivery systems (e.g., IV PCA pumps) provided an added advantage of concurrent assessment of, and intervention for, emerging signs of respiratory depression. A monitor using such smart algorithms can identify early signs of respiratory depression, discontinue further opioid administration, and also alert the medical staff [25]. Another variation to integrated monitoring is smaller, more portable "all-in-one" monitoring devices such as FDA-cleared ViSi mobile. This offers wearable, continuous multi-parameter monitoring that also includes continuous blood pressure and posture detection, in addition to SpO_2, RR, HR, and atrial fibrillation detection. Figure 7.3 shows the portable wrist-mounted ViSi mobile monitor.

While respiratory rate can currently be measured with capnography via a sampling line, it has significant limitations as described above. Acoustic monitoring is a newer, attractive option to measure respiratory rate based on generation of sound waves and has an advantage of not requiring direct patient contact. They have been used extensively in pediatric patients and studies have shown it to have similar sensitivity to manual breath counting with the added benefit of continuous monitoring [26]. Radar is yet another system available for respiratory rate monitoring. It utilizes

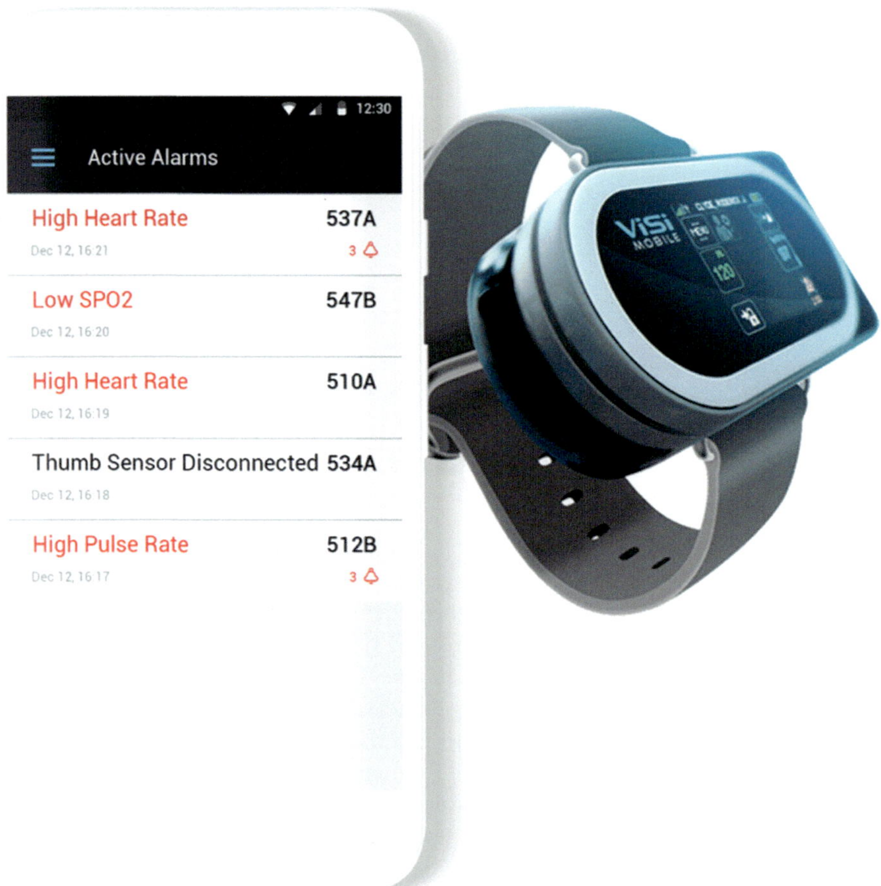

Fig. 7.3 The portable wrist-mounted ViSi mobile (Sotera wireless, San Diego, CA) monitor which has the capability for continuous blood pressure and hemodynamic monitoring in addition to standard respiratory vital signs. (With permission from Sotera wireless)

frequency modulated continuous wave radar to provide a contactless, non-invasive, and continuous way of monitoring respiratory rate. Preliminary studies assessing its utility in postoperative patients suggest that it may be accurate for measuring respiratory rate in mechanically ventilated patients but less accurate in spontaneously breathing patients [27]. Limitations also include artifacts from patient movements. Table 7.3 gives a summary of the prevalent and available monitoring technology for OIRD. There is emerging data on the use of a combination of continuous respiratory monitoring and clinical data to identify at-risk patients that can help plan early interventions and avoid the morbidity and mortality associated with OIRD. The PRediction of OpioiD-Induced respiratory depression in patients monitored by capnoGraphY (PRODIGY) trial used continuous respiratory monitoring (capnography

Table 7.3 A detailed comparison of new non-invasive respiratory monitoring techniques

Monitors	Parameters	Advantages	Disadvantages
Integrated pulmonary index	SpO_2, $EtCO_2$, RR, and HR	Easy clinical interpretation integrating all parameters into single numerical output	Not validated for all patients
Integrated delivery and monitoring devices	SpO_2, $EtCO_2$, and RR	Monitoring system is connected to drug delivery system System is disabled prior to notifying practitioners	Expensive Not widely available Require oximeter and carbon dioxide sampling line
Acoustic monitor	RR	Tolerated by children Detects and VF Detects apnea	Prone to artifacts High false positives Alarm fatigue
Radar monitor	RR	No patient contact Tolerated by children Detects and VF Detects apnea	Prone to artifacts High false positives Alarm fatigue
Bioimpedance	RR, TV, and MV	Sensitivity to ventilation Detects apnea Detects ventilation prior to SpO_2	Expensive Cumbersome equipment Prone to artifacts High false positives False negatives for obstructive apnea
Inductance plethysmography and audiometry	RR, SpO_2, and airway patency	Sensitivity to ventilation Detects apnea Detects OSA Detects ventilation prior to SpO_2 Detects isolated SpO_2	Expensive Cumbersome equipment Prone to artifacts High false positives Alarm fatigue

Adapted with permission from "Ayad et al. [3]"
SpO_2 pulse oximetry, *$EtCO_2$* end tidal carbon dioxide, *RR* respiratory rate, *HR* heart rate, *OSA* obstructive sleep apnea

and oximetry) and clinical data to develop an assessment score for patients at risk of developing OIRD on the general care ward [28]. The results of the trial would help fill this very important void.

At-Risk Population

Respiratory depression is common and often unpredictable in the post-surgical inpatient population [29]. OIRD has catastrophic consequences, including but not limited to anoxic brain injury and mortality. A closed claims analysis identified that half of all such events occur about 2 h after the last nursing check and almost all were preventable with better education and monitoring [30]. Knowing that patients with obstructive sleep apnea and those receiving long acting opioids may be at a highest risk, attempts have been made to use screening tools such as the STOP-BANG (snoring, tiredness, observed apnea, blood pressure, body mass index, age, neck circumference, and gender) as surrogates for postoperative hypoxemia; however, a consistent relationship between obstructive sleep apnea and postoperative hypoxemia could not be established [22, 31, 32]. It is Important to understand that hypoventilatory events may be more common than hypoxemic events in OIRD [16] and that the combination of sedatives and narcotics may have more damaging effects that either of them being used individually [33, 34]. Further, patients at the extremes of age are more sensitive to opioids and dosing should be adjusted accordingly [35]. It is reasonable to start with smaller doses and up titrate based on individual patient response and dosing intervals should be based on the pharmacokinetics of the individual drugs. Patients with a history of obstructive sleep apnea or obesity-related hypoventilation syndrome (OHS, Pickwickian syndrome) are at a significantly high risk of OIRD, and hence, judicious use of narcotics in these patients is warranted. Elderly, female sex, chronic obstructive pulmonary disease, cardiac disease, diabetes mellitus, hypertension, neurologic disease, renal disease, obesity, two or more comorbidities, and opioid dependence are other significant patient-related risk factors for postoperative OIRD [36]. The use of a combination of narcotic medications and routes (i.e., oral, IV, intrathecal) can potentially lead to a higher systemic concentrations and greater risk of respiratory depression. Safety checks should thus be in place to avoid accidental administration of different drugs via multiple routes for the same indication. Patients with kidney or liver dysfunction should also have dose modifications. As certain opioid are metabolized and excreted through hepatic or renal routes, there may be an increase in active metabolites which can result in longer duration of action. High-risk patients should be closely monitored and frequently assessed with any combination of the tools listed above [36]. The PRODIGY risk score which identifies increasing age, male sex, chronic heart failure, opioid naivety, and sleep disordered breathing, in various combinations, can be helpful in predicting the risk of OIRD. This score is novel since the risk index was developed using continuous monitoring of capnography and oximetry in patients receiving opioids on hospital wards. This is in contrast to the traditional risk factors that are a result of associative models mostly based on retrospective datasets and OIRD defined from diagnostic codes or as a surrogate from the use of reversal medications such as naloxone [33].

It is important to determine an appropriate level of care specific to individual patient's needs to adequately monitor for respiratory decompensation. The level of care determines the patient to nurse ratio and the frequency of "spot" checks per patient. In general, most hospital floors function with 4–6 hourly checks on any given patient [29]. However, most acute cardiorespiratory events leading to sudden respiratory or cardiac arrest often start with a series of abnormal vital signs well before the actual event and an increasing frequency of such events portend a poor prognosis [37]. With this in mind, patients who have been identified to have a higher risk of respiratory depression should be maintained at a level of care and monitoring that benefits from an adequate patient to nurse ratio with more frequent "spot checks" continuous monitoring to allow for early bedside intervention [38, 39]. In essence, appropriate monitoring systems on general wards can prevent acute respiratory compromise and consequent rapid responses, codes, and unplanned ICU admissions, thus preventing strain on critical care resources within a hospital [39]. While continuous portable monitoring seems promising, the use of these monitors must balance the risk of alarm fatigue and needs validation of monitor data using stringent criteria, prior to embarking on larger operations or intervention trials [40].

More recently, we have experienced the challenges associated with critically ill patients with COVID-19 disease. This group poses significant challenges with sedation management. Appropriate sedation is essential in those who require mechanical ventilation to allow for paralytic use, preventing unintentional extubation, and to promote ventilator synchrony. These patients require unusually high doses of sedatives and often need administration of multiple agents, thus increasing the potential risks of side effects. The duration of mechanical ventilation is also longer in these patients, thus the need for prolonged duration of sedation. With high doses of opioids often required in addition to other sedatives, it is imperative that sedation is appropriately monitored. However, the logistical challenges associated with reducing frequent entry of providers in the room and preserving personal protective equipment limit monitoring options.

Continuum of Sedation

In 2013, the American Society of Anesthesiologist (ASA) published guidelines defining the continuum of sedation [6]. This was later updated in 2014 and has now been used to define mild, moderate, and deep sedation in contradistinction to general anesthesia. The level of sedation is directly related to the patient's responsiveness, airway assessment, spontaneous ventilation, and cardiovascular function (Table 7.4). As the depth of sedation increases, there should be a corresponding increase in the ventilatory and cardiovascular assistance required [7–10]. As such, providers working in acute care settings should be aware of the sedation continuum and receive adequate training to distinguish the depths of sedation. Certifications are now required for providers to administer medications to achieve different levels of sedation and proficiency is mandatory when managing cardiorespiratory function with deeper levels of sedation [9, 10].

Table 7.4 Depth of sedation as defined by the ASA

	Mild	Moderate	Deep	GA
Responsiveness	Normal	Purposeful	To noxious stimuli	Unarousable
Airway	Normal	Normal	May require assistance	Requires assistance
Ventilation	Normal	Adequate	May require assistance	Requires assistance
CV	Normal	Normal	Normal	Potentially depressed

Based on Continuum of depth of sedation: definition of general anesthesia and levels of sedation/analgesia. Approved by ASA House of Delegates on October 13, 1999, and last amended on October 15, 2014, by the American Society of Anesthesiologists. A copy of the full text can be obtained from ASA, 1061 American Lane Schaumburg, IL 60173–4973, or online at www.asahq.org [6]

Mild sedation is defined as a state in which the patient can respond normally to commands without any changes in their responsiveness, airway status, spontaneous breath, or cardiovascular function. As the patient is further sedated to moderate sedation, there will be a change in the responsiveness to a purposeful response to verbal or tactile stimulation. In deep sedation, responsiveness will decrease with the requirement of repeated or painful stimulus and airway manipulation may be necessary. Airway manipulation may warrant the use of nasal trumpets, oropharyngeal airways, chin lift, or jaw thrust maneuvers. General anesthesia encompasses unconsciousness, and the patient will require mechanical ventilation via a laryngeal mark airway or endotracheal tube. The provider must be capable of recognizing and treating cardiovascular compromise at this level of sedation [6].

Practice guidelines by the ASA for sedation by the non-anesthesiologists strongly recommend that practitioners providing mild to moderate sedation must have pharmacological education and the ability to react to OIRD if the patient is progressing to deep sedation [7]. The same is necessary for those providing deep sedation with transition to general anesthesia. There is also a strong recommendation for at least one Base Life Support qualified individual to be present in the room at all times and at least one individual qualified in Advanced Cardiovascular Life Support skills (intubation, defibrillation, ability to recognize cardiac waveforms, and delivery rescue medications) reachable within 1–5 min for all patients receiving moderate to deep sedation [7–10].

According to the 2018 practice guidelines by the ASA, benzodiazepines, dexmedetomidine, and opioids are accepted medications for moderate sedation. Induction agents such as propofol and etomidate are intended for general anesthesia and must therefore adhere to requirements as such. However, ketamine may be titrated to reach the desired level of sedation and can be managed accordingly [7].

Sedation Certification

In 2016 and 2017, the ASA created statements regarding the credentials required by non-anesthesiologists to administer moderate and deep sedation. As per the guidelines for moderate sedation, "The non-anesthesiologist sedation practitioner who is to supervise or personally administer medications for moderate sedation should have satisfactorily completed a formal training program in: [1] the safe administration of sedative and analgesic drugs used to establish a level of moderate sedation, and [2] rescue of patients who exhibit adverse physiologic consequences of a deeper-than-intended level of sedation. This training may be a part of a recently completed residency or fellowship training (e.g., within 2 years), or may be a separate educational program"[1] [9]. Subject areas to be included in training include reviewing ASA practice guidelines for sedation and analgesia, understanding the continuum depth of

[1] Excerpted from Statement of Granting Privileges for Administration of Moderate Sedation to Practitioners, 2016, of the American Society of Anesthesiologists. A copy of the full text can be obtained from ASA, 1061 American Lane Schaumburg, IL 60173–4973 or online at www.asahq.org

sedation, preoperative fasting guidelines, pharmacology of all medications, monitoring of physiologic variables, and requiring ACLS training. ACLS training is not required for those overseen by a credentialed sedation provider [9].

Deep sedation guidelines are quite different and unique. The ASA mandates that administration of deep sedation should include an anesthesiologist in all cases. Deep sedation should not be applied if the overall goal is to achieve general anesthesia. Those who have been granted privileges for deep sedation must be aware of the differences between deep sedation and general anesthesia. In order to provide deep sedation, practitioners "must demonstrate their ability to [1] recognize that a patient has entered a state of general anesthesia and [2] maintain a patient's vital functions until the patient has been rescued from general anesthesia and returned to an appropriate level of sedation"[2] [10]. The certification requires "formal training program in [1] the safe administration of sedative and analgesic drugs used to establish a level of deep sedation, and [2] rescue of patients who exhibit adverse physiologic consequences of a deeper-than-intended level of sedation." This can be recognized via an ACGME residency or fellowship or by a deep sedation course by the ACCME. An examination must also be passed which covers fasting guidelines, pharmacology, assessment of adequate ventilation, rescue ventilation, ability to intubate with laryngeal mask airway or with endotracheal tube, required hemodynamic monitoring, and ACLS accreditation. Finally, the provider must be approved by the Director of Anesthesia Services in the specific institution as well [10].

Sedation Assessment

In order to assess a patient's depth of sedation, various objective scales such as the Richmond Agitation Sedation Scale (RASS), Riker Sedation Agitation Scale (SAS), Ramsey Sedation Scale (RSS), Minnesota Sedation Assessment Tool (MSAT), Motor Activity Assessment Scale (MAAS), Michigan Opioid Safety Score (MOSS), Pasero Opioid-induced Sedation Scale (POSS), and COMFORT Scale among others have been used and validated [15, 41, 42]. These scales can help monitor patients receive opioids or other sedative for excessive sedation and they may be used to identify and maintain a mild or moderate depth of sedation [41, 42]. For intubated patients, it is recognized that deep sedation may lead to prolonged duration of mechanical ventilation, ICU and hospital LOS, and increased morbidity and mortality, and hence mild and moderate sedation is recommended [43].

In conclusion, with the increasing recognition of opioid-related side effects, especially OIRD in the acute care setting, the onus is on providers to limit the use of opioids by not only adopting opioid sparing pain management strategies but also

[2] Excerpted from Advisory on Granting Privileges for Deep Sedation to Non-Anesthesiologist Physicians, 2017, of the American Society of Anesthesiologists. A copy of the full text can be obtained from ASA, 1061 American Lane Schaumburg, IL 60173–4973 or online at www.asahq.org

implementing monitoring techniques that provide early detection of complications, preferably before they occur. While bedside monitoring by trained personnel is ideal, it is expensive, labor intensive, and personnel dependent. Continuous non-invasive monitoring not only affords an attractive alternative but also suffers significant limitations. A combination of continuous monitoring techniques and clinical assessment tools integrated together with the help of machine learning could be the holy grail of monitoring for OIRD in the acute care setting but would need to be validated. These new systems are built with the intent to diagnose and treat rather than assess for rescue measures. Restricted administration of opioids by certified personnel will further decrease the incidence and promote patient safety. Guidelines and practice advisories by national organizations are continually being updated, taking into account new research and adherence of these guidelines can not only assist practitioners but also prevent patient harm.

References

1. WHO Guidelines for the pharmacological and radiotherapeutic management of cancer pain in adults and adolescents. WHO Guidelines Approved by the Guidelines Review Committee. Geneva. 2018.
2. Practice Guidelines for Acute Pain Management in the Perioperative Setting. An updated report by the American Society of Anesthesiologists Task Force on acute pain management. Anesthe J Am Soc Anesthe. 2012;116(2):248–73.
3. Puntillo KA, Max A, Timsit J-F, Vignoud L, Chanques G, Robleda G, et al. Determinants of procedural pain intensity in the intensive care unit. The Europain® study. Am J Respir Crit Care Med. 2014;189(1):39–47.
4. Gupta RK, Edwards DA. Monitoring for opioid-induced respiratory depression. Anesthe Pat Saf Found Newsl. 2018:(32)70–2.
5. Ayad S, Khanna AK, Iqbal SU, Singla N. Characterisation and monitoring of postoperative respiratory depression: current approaches and future considerations. Br J Anaesth. 2019;123(3):378–91.
6. Anesthesiologists ASo. Continuum of depth of sedation: definition of general anesthesia and levels of sedation/analgesia. Approved by ASA House of Delegates on October 13, 1999, and last amended on October 15, 2014. 2014.
7. Sedation ASoATFo, Non-Anesthesiologists Ab. Practice guidelines for sedation and analgesia by non-anesthesiologists. Anesthesiology. 2002;96(4):1004–17.
8. Care DMA. From moderate sedation/Analgesia (Conscious Sedation). Approved by the ASA House of Delegates on October. 2004;27.
9. Credentialing AHCo. Statement of granting privileges for Administration of moderate sedation to practitioners. In: Anesthesiologists ASo, editor. ; 2016.
10. Administration CoQMaD. In: Anesthesiologists ASo, editor. Advisory on granting privileges for deep sedation to non-anesthesiologist physicians; 2017.
11. Hjermstad MJ, Fayers PM, Haugen DF, Caraceni A, Hanks GW, Loge JH, et al. Studies comparing numerical rating scales, verbal rating scales, and visual analogue scales for assessment of pain intensity in adults: a systematic literature review. J Pain Symptom Manag. 2011;41(6):1073–93.
12. Brochard L, Martin GS, Blanch L, Pelosi P, Belda FJ, Jubran A, et al. Clinical review: respiratory monitoring in the ICU-a consensus of 16. Crit Care. 2012;16(2):219.

13. Barr J, Fraser GL, Puntillo K, Ely EW, Gelinas C, Dasta JF, et al. Clinical practice guidelines for the management of pain, agitation, and delirium in adult patients in the intensive care unit. Crit Care Med. 2013;41(1):263–306.
14. Severgnini P, Pelosi P, Contino E, Serafinelli E, Novario R, Chiaranda M. Accuracy of critical care pain observation tool and behavioral pain scale to assess pain in critically ill conscious and unconscious patients: prospective, observational study. J Intensive Care. 2016;4(1):68.
15. Puntillo K, Pasero C, Li D, Mularski RA, Grap MJ, Erstad BL, et al. Evaluation of pain in ICU patients. Chest. 2009;135(4):1069–74.
16. Overdyk FJ, Dowling O, Marino J, Qiu J, Chien H-L, Erslon M, et al. Association of opioids and sedatives with increased risk of in-hospital cardiopulmonary arrest from an administrative database. PLoS One. 2016;11(2):e0150214.
17. Rijkenberg S, Stilma W, Bosman RJ, van der Meer NJ, van der Voort PHJ. Pain measurement in mechanically ventilated patients after cardiac surgery: comparison of the behavioral pain scale (BPS) and the critical-care pain observation tool (CPOT). J Cardiothorac Vasc Anesth. 2017;31(4):1227–34.
18. Apfelbaum JL, Horlocker TT, Agarkar M, Connis RT, Hebl JR, Nickinovich DG, et al. Practice guidelines for the prevention, detection, and Management of Respiratory Depression Associated with Neuraxialn Opioid Administration: an updated report by the American Society of Anesthesiologists Task Force on Neuraxial opioids and the American Society of Regional Anesthesia and Pain Medicine. Obstet Anesth Dig. 2017;37(1):11.
19. Imhoff M, Kuhls S. Alarm algorithms in critical care monitoring. Anesth Analg. 2006;102(5):1525–37.
20. Sjoding MW, Dickson RP, Iwashyna TJ, Gay SE, Valley TS. Racial Bias in pulse Oximetry measurement. N Engl J Med. 2020;383(25):2477–8.
21. Weinger M. Dangers of postoperative opioids: APSF work- shop and white paper address prevention of postoperative respiratory complications. 2007. p. http://www.apsf.org/newsletters/html/2007/winter/01_opioidsOverdyk.htm.
22. Overdyk FJ, Carter R, Maddox RR, Callura J, Herrin AE, Henriquez C. Continuous oximetry/capnometry monitoring reveals frequent desaturation and bradypnea during patient-controlled analgesia. Anesth Analg. 2007;105(2):412–8.
23. Salottolo K, Carrick M, Johnson J, Gamber M, Bar-Or D. A retrospective cohort study of the utility of the modified early warning score for interfacility transfer of patients with traumatic injury. BMJ Open. 2017;7(5):e016143.
24. Ronen M, Weissbrod R, Overdyk F, Ajizian S. Smart respiratory monitoring: clinical development and validation of the IPI™(integrated pulmonary index) algorithm. J Clin Monit Comput. 2017;31(2):435–42.
25. Maddox RR, Williams CK, Oglesby H, Butler B, Colclasure B. Clinical experience with patient-controlled analgesia using continuous respiratory monitoring and a smart infusion system. Am J Health Syst Pharm. 2006;63(2):157–64.
26. Patino M, Kalin M, Griffin A, Minhajuddin A, Ding L, Williams T, et al. Comparison of postoperative respiratory monitoring by acoustic and transthoracic impedance technologies in pediatric patients at risk of respiratory depression. Anesth Analg. 2017;124(6):1937–42.
27. Van Loon K, Breteler M, Van Wolfwinkel L, Leyssius AR, Kossen S, Kalkman C, et al. Wireless non-invasive continuous respiratory monitoring with FMCW radar: a clinical validation study. J Clin Monit Comput. 2016;30(6):797–805.
28. Khanna AK, Overdyk FJ, Greening C, Di Stefano P, Buhre WF. Respiratory depression in low acuity hospital settings-seeking answers from the PRODIGY trial. J Crit Care. 2018;47:80–7.
29. Sun Z, Sessler DI, Dalton JE, Devereaux P, Shahinyan A, Naylor AJ, et al. Postoperative hypoxemia is common and persistent: a prospective blinded observational study. Anesth Analg. 2015;121(3):709.
30. Hopf HW. Preventing Opioid-Induced Postoperative Hypoxemia: No Simple Answer? Anesth Analg. 2016;123(6):1356–58. https://doi.org/10.1213/ANE.

31. Khanna AK, Sessler D, Sun Z, Naylor A, You J, Hesler B, et al. Using the STOP-BANG questionnaire to predict hypoxaemia in patients recovering from noncardiac surgery: a prospective cohort analysis. BJA: Br J Anaesth. 2016;116(5):632–40.
32. Izrailtyan I, Qiu J, Overdyk FJ, Erslon M, Gan TJ. Risk factors for cardiopulmonary and respiratory arrest in medical and surgical hospital patients on opioid analgesics and sedatives. PLoS One. 2018;13(3):e0194553.
33. Andersen LW, Berg KM, Chase M, Cocchi MN, Massaro J, Donnino MW. Acute respiratory compromise on inpatient wards in the United States: incidence, outcomes, and factors associated with in-hospital mortality. Resuscitation. 2016;105:123–9.
34. Khanna A, Buhre W, Saager L, Stefano PD, Weingarten T, Dahan A, et al. 36: derivation and validation of a novel opioid-induced respiratory depression risk prediction tool. Crit Care Med. 2019;47(1):18.
35. Wildemeersch D, Peeters N, Saldien V, Vercauteren M, Hans G. Pain assessment by pupil dilation reflex in response to noxious stimulation in anaesthetized adults. Acta Anaesthesiol Scand. 2018;62(8):1050–6.
36. Gupta K, Prasad A, Nagappa M, Wong J, Abrahamyan L, Chung FF. Risk factors for opioid-induced respiratory depression and failure to rescue: a review. Curr Opin Anaesthesiol. 2018;31(1):110–9.
37. Khanna AK, Hoppe P, Saugel B. Automated continuous noninvasive ward monitoring: future directions and challenges. Crit Care. 2019;23(1):194.
38. Sessler DI, Saugel B. Beyond 'failure to rescue': the time has come for continuous ward monitoring. Br J Anaesth. 2019;122(3):304–6.
39. Rao VK, Khanna AK. Postoperative respiratory impairment is a real risk for our patients: the intensivist's perspective. Anesth Res Pract. 2018;2018:3215923.
40. Saugel B, Hoppe P, Khanna A. Automated continuous noninvasive ward monitoring: validation of measurement systems is the real challenge. Anesthesiology. 2020;132(3):407–10.
41. Marik PE. Management of pain, agitation and delirium. Evidence-based critical care. Berlin: Springer International Publishing; 2015. p. 197–212.
42. Gehlbach B, Kress J. Pain control, sedation, and use of muscle relaxants. Principles of critical care. 3rd ed. New York: McGraw-Hill; 2005. p. 139–63.
43. Oropello JM, Kvetan V, Pastores SM. Lange critical Care. New York: McGraw-Hill Education; 2016.

Chapter 8
Opioid-Induced Tolerance and Opioid-Induced Hyperalgesia in Critical Illness

Edward A. Bittner, Rachel Steinhorn, and J. A. Jeevendra Martyn

Introduction

Opioids are highly effective analgesics and therefore have been the mainstay of pain control in the ICU. However, they can have many adverse effects, including potential for long-term abuse (Table 8.1). Long-term opioid use leads to tolerance (i.e., decreased efficacy of the analgesic effects of the opioid, which can result in a need for higher and more frequent doses to achieve the same analgesic effect), opioid-withdrawal symptoms during weaning and may contribute to the development of opioid-induced hyperalgesia, a paradoxical hypersensitivity to pain (Fig. 8.1). Hyperalgesia is particularly problematic as pain persists, yet further opioid prescribing is largely futile. Both OT and OIH can contribute to both poorly controlled pain and dose escalation.

OT can develop with opioid exposure during a variety of acute and chronic disease states; however, the magnitude seems exaggerated in critically ill and injured patients, especially those who have sustained major trauma (e.g., burn injury), in patients requiring prolonged mechanical ventilation, and in pediatric patients [1]. The development of OT in critically ill patients is due in part to the large doses of

E. A. Bittner (✉) · R. Steinhorn
Department of Anesthesia, Critical Care and Pain Medicine, Massachusetts General Hospital, Boston, MA, USA

Harvard Medical School, Boston, MA, USA
e-mail: ebittner@partners.org

J. A. Jeevendra Martyn
Harvard Medical School, Boston, MA, USA

Shriners Hospitals for Children, Boston, MA, USA

Massachusetts General Hospital, Boston, MA, USA

J. L. Pascual, T. G. Gaulton (eds.), *Opioid Use in Critical Care*,
https://doi.org/10.1007/978-3-030-77399-1_8

Table 8.1 Clinical issues that arise from opioid use in critically ill patients

Clinical issues
Acute presentation of patient on regular opioid prescription (i.e., not opioid naive)
Pain control difficult
Likely to have pre-existing tolerance, and therefore higher doses might be needed to achieve adequate analgesia
Might have opioid-induced hyperalgesia, and therefore a reduced opioid dose and alternative strategies might be needed
Opioid-naive patient treated with short acting opioid as part of the analgesic regimen
Acute tolerance
Development of opioid-induced hyperalgesia
If rapid cessation, acute opioid withdrawal might occur
Opioids prescribed for pain after ICU discharge
Increased prescribing of opioids for longer post-ICU period leading to sustained use
Dependence (physical and psychological)
Increased potential for drug diversion if opioids not used by patient for whom prescribed

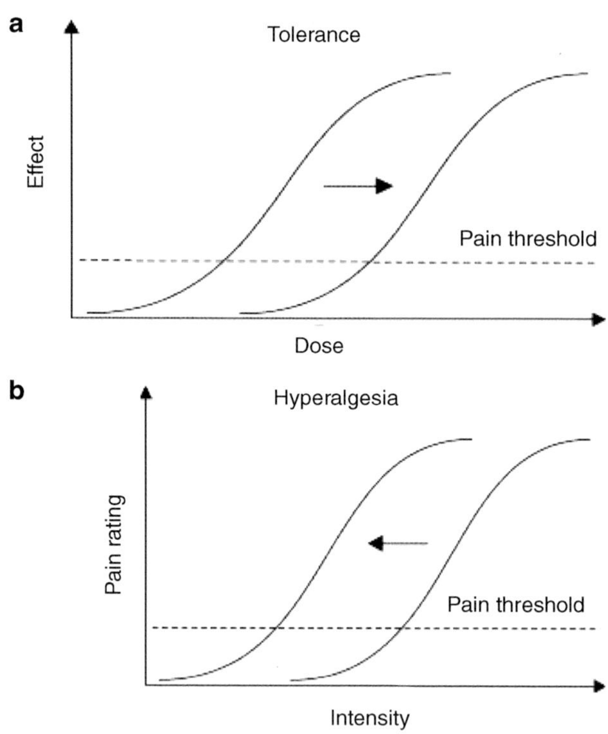

Fig. 8.1 Changes in analgesia and pain resulting from opioid-induced tolerance and hyperalgesia. (**a**) Tolerance to opioid analgesia develops after ongoing exposure to the drug. The same dose of drug administered over time produces less analgesic effect. The rate of onset and extent of tolerance development are variable depending on the individual drug and patient characteristics. Opioid-induced tolerance produces a rightward shift in the dose–response relationship. (**b**) Opioid-induced hyperalgesia describes a paradoxical increase in pain sensitivity resulting from ongoing exposure to opioids. Opioid-induced hyperalgesia produces a leftward shift in the dose–response relationship

opioids needed to control pain as well as the duration of administration. However, the inflammatory response seen in critically ill or injured patients plays an important role in OT. While studies of OIH in humans have largely been limited to volunteers, during the short-term opioid infusions in the perioperative period, in patients receiving methadone substitution therapy, and in patients with chronic pain, it is likely that opioid dose, duration, and the inflammation seen in critically ill or injured patients also play a prominent role in its development.

Critical care clinicians have historically not been overly concerned about OT instead focusing on management of acute life-threatening conditions and their immediate aftermath. It has been assumed that if tolerance develops, it can be overcome by administering more opioids, therefore, even if larger doses have to be given, this would not entail any greater risk to the patient. However, a growing body of evidence suggests that prolonged opioid exposure during critical illness may result in a number of long-term harms including tolerance, addiction, withdrawal, and the possibility for OIH [1]. It is therefore crucial for the critical care practitioner and clinicians caring for survivors of critical illness to be aware of these harmful opioid-associated effects.

This chapter provides an overview of the clinical concepts of OT and OIH as they may play into the management of patients in the ICU setting. The pharmacologic mechanisms of opioids are reviewed, along with the mechanisms leading to the development of OT and OIH. Newer insights into the role of inflammation- and opioid-mediated innate immune responses associated with critical injury and illness are described. Finally challenges in the diagnosis, prevention and treatment of OT and OIT are detailed. By improving understanding of the underlying mechanisms of OT and OIH, it should be possible to develop strategies to better manage pain associated with critical illness and injury, to improve efficacy and safety of opioid use, and to minimize long-term harms.

Opioid Signaling, Sites of Opioid Action, and Pain Pathways

Both natural and synthetic opioids exert their action, at least in part, at the μ opioid receptor, with some having additional activity at other opioid receptors or receptors distinct from the opioid family [2]. The μ receptors are essential for the analgesic actions of opioids, being expressed at key locations within the pain pathway. Their activation suppresses both the reflexive and affective components of pain. The μ receptors are G-protein-coupled receptors (GPCRs) and transmit downstream signals through heterotrimetric Gαβγ-proteins. When an opioid binds to the μ-opioid receptor, the receptor-associated Gαβγ-protein dissociates into Gα and Gβγ subunits. The dissociated G-protein subunits inhibit voltage-gated calcium channels (leading to reduced transmitter release), activate inward-rectifying potassium channels (causing hyperpolarization of the membrane), and inhibit downstream adenylate cyclase enzymes (decreasing cyclic adenosine monophosphate levels). These events reduce excitability and nociception and result in analgesic effects. In addition, activation of μ receptors in the brain's reward circuitry inhibits inhibitory neurotransmission in the ventral tegmental area, reducing the frequency of γ-aminobutyric acid (GABA) inhibitory postsynaptic events, thereby disinhibiting dopaminergic neurons and increasing dopamine release into the striatum and prefrontal cortex. In addition, when an opioid binds to its receptor, it becomes an immediate substrate for phosphorylation by G-protein–coupled receptor kinase (GRK), which leads to recruitment and binding of β-arrestin protein to the receptor. This results in desensitization and sometimes endocytosis of the receptor; each of these events decreases the responses to opioids, inducing tolerance and preventing further analgesic effects. Opioid-receptor signaling terminates when the opioid is displaced from the receptor. After the stimulus (i.e., the agonist) is withdrawn, the desensitized receptor recovers over time (minutes to hours, depending on the agonist), Gα rebinds to Gβγ and once again forms Gαβγ, and the endocytosed receptor is re-expressed on the plasma membrane in a re-sensitized state.

Opioid receptors are distributed throughout the central nervous system, spinal cord, and within peripheral tissue of neural and non-neural origin. Centrally, the periaqueductal gray, locus coeruleus, and rostroventral medulla contain high densities of opioid receptors; opioid receptors are also present in the substantia gelatinosa of the dorsal horn. Transmission of pain sensation (nociception) from the peripheral-tissue injury to the central nervous system occurs through the ascending spinothalamic tract to the thalamus and then to the somatosensory cortex. Descending inhibitory tracts from the brain and other regions, including the rostroventral medulla, modulate nociception. Nociception can be amplified by dorsal-root ganglia and changes in the dorsal horn of the spinal cord. The afferent neurons are sensitized by the sprouting of new axons around the cell bodies of dorsal-root ganglia, as well as by infiltrating macrophages, which release inflammatory substances. Neuron projections from dorsal-root ganglia to the dorsal horn amplify the pain by the release of other pro-nociceptive mediators (e.g., calcitonin gene–related peptide), activation of *N*-methyl-d-aspartate receptors (NMDARs), and the increase in glutamate levels. Second-order neurons transmit these signals upstream to the brain. Injury to tissues results in local and often systemic inflammatory responses, which prime the peripheral sensory neurons and dorsal-root ganglia to exaggerated nociception by up-regulation or modulation of ligand-gated and voltage-gated ion channels. μ-Opioid receptors are newly expressed throughout the nerve membrane. Extravasated circulating leukocytes (e.g., macrophages and lymphocytes) release proinflammatory mediators, further sensitizing the neurons to pain. These leukocytes also release anti-nociceptive endogenous opioid peptides, which bind to the up-regulated opioid receptors on the nerve, attenuating pain.

Effects of Injury on Modulation of Nociception

Most critically ill and injured patients have sustained some form of injury to soft tissues and nerve endings that cause local and often systemic inflammatory responses. These responses launch a cascade of events, including release of proinflammatory substances and activation of *N*-methyl-d-aspartate (NMDA) receptors in the spinal cord [1]. Coinciding with these events are endogenous anti-nociceptive mechanisms that also become operative, such as activation of the inhibitory opioidergic, serotonergic, and noradrenergic pathways [3]. Chemotaxis-mediated extravasation of leukocytes at injured sites secrete endogenous opioid peptides that interact with the injury-induced opioid receptors that are up-regulated along nerve terminals to reduce pain. Moreover, injury-induced reduction of inhibitory control of pain via glycine and γ-aminobutyric acid (GABA) receptors further enhances central sensitization. These local and central changes lead to exaggerated basal and procedural pain, referred to as hyperalgesia (exaggerated pain to painful stimuli, e.g., pin prick) and allodynia (pain to non-painful stimuli, e.g., touch), which are consistent with the body's need to produce essential warning signs and withdrawal responses during pain perception. The injury-induced changes in nociceptive pathways are augmented when there is systemic inflammation, which explains the exaggerated tolerance and opioid dose requirement during critical illness.

Innate Immune Responses to Injury in the Central Nervous System

Injury- or inflammation-related pain can become aggravated or long-lasting, features that cannot be explained by neuronal activation alone. In the central nervous system, the non-neuronal cells (e.g., astroglia and microglia) play a major role in central sensitization. Persistent activation of the spinal cord dorsal horn by the injury-induced barrage of nociceptive input and the associated release of damage-associated molecular patterns (DAMPS) triggers the release of inflammatory mediators (e.g., cytokines) by glial cells that enhance the excitability of adjacent neurons [4]. Although acute stress results in stress-induced analgesia, persistent sympathetic over-activity leads to stress-induced hyperalgesia [5]. Repetitive or ongoing stress can also lead to central and peripheral leukocyte priming and release of inflammatory mediators, which markedly exaggerate pain behaviors. The peripheral immunocytes, which express norepinephrine receptors, respond to the stress-induced catecholamine surge by releasing leukocytes, including monocytes of inflammatory M1 phenotype (as opposed to anti-inflammatory M2 phenotype), which can release inflammatory mediators. Stress-associated glucocorticoid release also functions as DAMPS by promoting glia activation. Superimposition of bacterial inflammation and associated release of pathogen-associated molecular patterns (PAMPS) can cause induction of toll-like receptors (TLRs) in leukocytes with release of inflammatory mediators leading to nociceptor sensitization, evidenced as lower threshold for pain. Clinical evidence also suggests that systemic inflammatory diseases (e.g., rheumatoid arthritis, burn injury) can lead to neuro-inflammation. Neuro-inflammation causes selective breakdown of the blood–brain barrier to inflammatory M1 monocytes, which further exaggerates the neuro-inflammatory responses that modulate mood and nociception [6, 7].

Opioids, even in the absence of systemic inflammation, cause neuro-inflammation by activating TLRs in glia and other immune cells that permeate the blood–brain barrier [8, 9]. Opioids activate TLRs in glial cells in association with exaggerated nociception; antagonism of TLRs or TLR4 knockout in mice does not lead to hyperalgesia, although conflicting results exist [9, 10]. Specific antagonists of each putative inflammatory mediator (e.g. interleukin-1β) have been shown to attenuate OIH. Chronic opioids can further exaggerate the pain responses with development of OIH, creating a vicious cycle of increasing dosage and worsening pain. Clinical observations confirm that OT and OIH in patients with critical illness can be more profound than that experienced in the general population [11, 12]. Other factors that add to central sensitization include age, gender differences, and concomitant inflammatory diseases (e.g., diabetes, cancer, and chemotherapy) [1, 13]. Notably, greater opioid tolerance seems to develop in pediatric patients; this may be related to less inhibition in the dorsal horn and more facilitation by the rostroventral medulla than in adults. Aging exacerbates neuro-inflammation [14]. With increasingly numbers of elderly patients occupying ICU beds, a right-shifted opioid dose–response curve (tolerance) might exist, although this has not been quantified. Thus, there are multiple factors (e.g., inflammation, infection, stress, and use of opioids) as seen in the ICU that can lead to activation of the glia in patients in the ICU and can exaggerate pain behaviors, tolerance, and opioid-induced hyperalgesia, creating a vicious cycle of dose escalation and worsening pain. Thus, tolerance appears to reflect a desensitization of receptor-mediated anti-nociceptive pathways, whereas opioid-induced hyperalgesia involves induction of pro-nociceptive glial–neuronal pathways.

Pharmacologic Mechanisms of OT and OIH

Pharmacokinetics

Altered Opioid Metabolic Clearance or Penetration into Central Nervous System (CNS)

Despite the ubiquitous use of opioids, the pharmacokinetic data on their use in critical illness is very limited. No data support the notion of enhanced opioid clearance due to cytochrome P450 enzyme (CYPE) auto-induction as the mechanism accounting for dose escalation with OT [15]. However, CYPE inducers do increase both CYPE activity and clearance of some drugs (e.g., methadone) resulting in subtherapeutic plasma levels which can be misinterpreted as pharmacodynamic (target organ) tolerance [16]. Similarly, during the hyperdynamic phases of trauma and sepsis, the enhanced elimination kinetics of "flow-dependent" drugs (e.g., fentanyl) could be interpreted as tolerance [17].

Inflammation alters levels of acute-phase-reactant proteins. The acute phase protein relevant to decreased drug action is alpha-1 acid glycoprotein (AAG), which binds to some basic drugs. Methadone has a high affinity for AAG (decreased free fraction), while fentanyl and morphine display minimal AAG binding. Despite minimal fentanyl and morphine binding to AAG, tolerance is still observed in critically ill patients receiving these opioids. Thus, the decreased free fraction that results from AAG binding cannot explain the increased dose requirement seen with all opioids in the ICU. The P-glycoprotein transporter (P-gp) present in brain capillaries controls drug transport out of the central nervous system (CNS). Long-term administration of oxycodone, morphine, and alfentanil, but not methadone, upregulates P-gp expression causing decreased CNS drug penetration and attenuated analgesic effects [16]. Similarly, tumor necrosis factor-α increases expression and activity of P-gp. Together, these observations imply that critical illness-related cytokine release and opioid administration may tighten P-gp-controlled blood–brain barrier permeability with reduced efficiency of some opioids.

Pharmacodynamics

Metabolites Contributing to OT and OIH

When an opioid compound is metabolized, its metabolites can either enhance, antagonize, or have no pharmacologic effects. These features are well exemplified by morphine where the parent drug is active, while its metabolites demonstrate contrasting effects: nor-morphine is inactive, morphine-6-glucuronite (M6G) is more potent than morphine, and morphine-3-glucuronide (M3G) has hyperalgesic effects that antagonize the analgesic effects of morphine and M6G [18]. In conditions such as renal failure which result in accumulation of morphine and its metabolites or with escalating doses of morphine, as seen in the ICU, the markedly increased M3G concentrations can counteract the analgesic potency of morphine and M6G. The M3G hyperalgesic effects occur independent of the MOR, since naloxone does not consistently reverse them. Rather, they seem to be mediated by activation of both microglial (TLRs) and neuronal NMDARs [9]. The magnitude of the contribution of M3G to a deficiency of analgesia is controversial.

Opioid Receptor Signaling Changes During Acute and Chronic Opioid Use

Agonist binding to the μ-opioid receptor results in phosphorylation by GPCR-kinase and recruits β-arrestin protein to the receptor thereby hindering ligand (opioid) access to the μ opioid receptor. This process leads to desensitization or conversion of the μ-opioid receptor from a high-affinity responsive state to a low-affinity decreased signaling state, which partly explains the mechanism underlying acute opioid tolerance. Phosphorylation by other kinases (e.g., protein kinases A and C) and μ opioid receptor endocytosis into the cytoplasm are also implicated in the mechanism of acute tolerance, although contrary evidence that μ-opioid receptor endocytosis mitigates tolerance exists. The particular μ-opioid receptor agonist may also play a role in endocytosis-mitigated tolerance. For example, morphine exposure, which causes tolerance, has little effect on μ receptor endocytosis even with prolonged exposure. By contrast, the synthetic opioid peptide with high μ-opioid receptor specificity DAMGO produces marked receptor endocytosis with little tolerance and therefore the relationship between endocytosis and tolerance is complex [19]. Instead, endocytosis might be required to reverse desensitization, a rapid form of tolerance observed at the cellular level. Desensitized μ-opioid receptors recover with time (minutes to hours, depending on the agonist) after the stimulus is withdrawn. The endocytosed receptors can then be recycled to the cell surface in an active re-sensitized state.

Continued use of opioids produces an exaggerated tolerance to the analgesic effect, which manifests as an escalating dose requirement to maintain analgesia, and subsequently contributes to OIH. Analgesic tolerance develops faster than tolerance to respiratory depression, which explains the increased risk for respiratory arrest with dose escalation in the opioid-tolerant patient. Both duration and dose appear to affect development of OT; opioid infusions seem to induce tolerance faster than intermittent therapy [20]. The rate of onset and extent of OT development is variable depending on the individual drug and patient characteristics. Potent opioids (remifentanil) induce tolerance quicker than less potent ones (meperidine). OT can develop in a shorter time frame, possibly within hours when patients are exposed to high doses (i.e., a phenomenon that classically is referred to as tachyphylaxis). Persistent opioid administration, even in normal subjects, can lead to extreme tolerance and then to paradoxical OIH. The most convincing evidence of OIH is the demonstration of hyperalgesia in drug addicts on maintenance methadone or buprenorphine versus the absence of OIH in matched addicts not receiving opioids. All opioids in clinical and illicit use can lead to OIH. Genetics, environment, and gender also influence OIH, but how these variables influence tolerance and OIH development is unclear.

Prominent signaling changes develop during the continued presence of exogenous or endogenous ligands because the body has intrinsic mechanisms to prevent over stimulation (neuroplasticity). Cellular adaptations during chronic opioid therapy include induction of anti-analgesic (anti-opioid) systems, which portray an adaptive response to persistent opioid agonist-induced inhibitory downstream signaling. The anti-analgesic systems induced include up-regulation and activation of NMDAR, down-regulation of glutamate transporter, and conversion from decreased cAMP to increased cAMP levels. Additional changes associated with OIH include reduction in potassium chloride channel activity, disruption of chloride homeostasis, and increased transduction via TRPV1 [8]. The formation of μ-opioid receptor heterodimers (formed of different opioid receptor subtypes) that bind opioids has also been implicated in the tolerance that develops with chronic opioids [21]. Furthermore, OIH has been demonstrated in triple (μ-, δ-, and κ-) opioid receptor knockout mice; the OIH seems to be mediated by MOR-independent direct interaction with TLRs. Thus, activation of the anti-analgesic system at multiple sites, during chronic opioid therapy, leads to an imbalance between pro-nociceptive and anti-nociceptive pathways and results in mitigation of the analgesic effects, tolerance, as well as OIH.

Evidence and Clinical Significance of OIH in Humans

The problem of OIH has been recognized for over 100 years [22]. While there is extensive preclinical evidence of OIH demonstrating changes in the underlying neurobiology leading to a pro-nociceptive state, there is still debate about the clinical significance of OIH in hospitalized patients. Studies of OIH in humans have largely been limited to volunteers during the short-term opioid infusions, in patients receiving methadone substitution therapy, and in patients with chronic pain and during the perioperative exposure to opioids. The uncertainty regarding the clinical significance of OIH is likely attributable at least in part to the problem that existing often do not make an adequate distinction between increased pain severity and hyperalgesia. Many clinical studies have used only pain scores and opioid consumption as surrogate markers of OIH, which do not consider other potential causes such as inadequate analgesia, changing underlying disease pathology, or tolerance. To make a clinical diagnosis of OIH, a distinction needs to be made between high pain scores and altered sensory processing with allodynia and hyperalgesia. In a systematic review and meta-analysis consisting of 26 studies with 2706 participants, OIH was evident in patients after chronic opioid exposure, but findings were dependent upon pain modality and assessment measures [23]. OIH was more evident in patients with opioid use disorder than in patients with pain which may have implications for patients with critical illness. Small clinical studies, using rigorous assessment measures such as quantitative sensory testing in a range of chronic pain conditions, have shown that opioid use does contribute to hyperalgesia although this effect is enhanced by other factors such as affective state and gender. For example, males who were prescribed opioids show increased hyperalgesia with fentanyl when compared with females, and both showed reduced pressure pain thresholds when compared with healthy controls. Increased thermal sensitivity has also been shown in patients on long-term opioids, even after adjusting for a variety of other factors. This thermal sensitivity may be a consequence of recruitment and sequestration of β-arrestin-2 after μ receptor activation, which has been shown in mice to sensitize transient receptor potential vanilloid (TRPV1) channels to thermal activation.

A systematic review of OIH after surgery consisting of 27 studies with 1494 patients found that higher doses of intraoperative opioid (primarily remifentanil) were associated with an increase in postoperative pain scores and higher 24-hour morphine consumption [24]. A subsequent systematic review of acute OIH and tolerance showed similar findings [25]. Other studies have strengthened this finding, with younger patients seeming to be at increased risk. The explanation for the apparent increased risk of OIH with remifentanil compared with other opioids is unclear but might be related to the fast onset and offset of its action. As indicated previously, the more potent the opioid, the faster the development of tolerance. The high potency of remifentanil is an important contributing factor. It is reasonable to expect that all opioids would function in the same manner, activating pro-nociceptive systems when administered long term, although in recombinant models, remifentanil has been suggested to have additional actions, such as direct activation of

NMDA receptors [26]. It is more likely, however, that it is logistically easier to administer large doses of remifentanil intraoperatively because the context-sensitive half time is so short compared with fentanyl; equivalent doses of fentanyl would likely delay time to extubation. There are also some limited data to suggest that intrathecal opioids can cause OIH although much more study is needed to characterize that route of administration [27]. Importantly, no studies to date have systematically evaluated OIH among critically ill patients or among ICU survivors who commonly suffer from chronic pain.

Identification of Opioid Tolerance and Opioid-Induced Hyperalgesia in Patients

Distinguishing between OT and OIH is challenging but is of clinical importance in patients who require routine or long-term opioid use. In clinical practice, the development of either of these phenomena will result in reduced pain control, with the usual consequence of escalating doses of opioids. Whether the increased opioid requirement is caused by decreasing the potency of the drug because of tolerance or because of lowered pain threshold due to OIH, the clinical effect is the same. If OIH is not appropriately recognized, providers may default to further escalation of opioid doses for pain management, propagating an aggravation of the OIH. Importantly, in the critically ill population many patients may be already using opioid drugs before ICU admission and may have developed tolerance or OIH before they even arrive in the ICU. Patients admitted to the ICU with history of long-term opioids are likely to have aberrant somatosensory responses to painful stimuli. In a large population-based study, opioid use was associated with increased pain sensitivity compared with patients taking non-opioid analgesics [28]. This can reflect OIH, or pre-existing reduction in endogenous pain inhibition, which increases the likelihood of long-term opioid use. In chronic pain patients receiving long-term opioids, dose reduction or cessation can reduce pain sensitivity, with many patients reporting improvements in pain and few experiencing worsening. The implications for acute management of patients on chronic opioid therapy is that, regardless of whether increases in pain sensitivity are due to a pre-existing risk factors, or a consequence of opioid therapy, care must be taken in managing these patients to avoid further opioid-related complications such as OIH.

Clinical criteria for differentiating between OT and OIH have been suggested (Table 8.2) [29]. Key features to assess include the responses to additional opioid and opioid withdrawal, pain quality, location, pain response after healing, timing, and presence of allodynia. With tolerance, an increased opioid dose should be effective in alleviating pain, although high doses may be required to achieve analgesic effects; similarly, a reduction in opioid dose would be expected to produce increased pain (but not hyperalgesia). In contrast, administration of increased opioid dose to a patient with OIH may produce short duration pain relief followed by increased pain

Table 8.2 Distinguishing between opioid tolerance and opioid-induced hyperalgesia

	OT	OIH
Pain response to increased opioid administration	Improved	Worsened
Pain response after removal of pain source (tissue healing)	Improved	Persists
Pain intensity with time/rest	Improved	Increased compared with what initially reported
Pain location	Localized	Diffuse, extending beyond the region of injury or tissue damage
Pain quality	Relieved with higher doses	Lesser quality and harder to pinpoint; noxious stimuli tend to be more painful that would normally be expected
Allodynia	Absent	Present

effects. While OIH-related pain should eventually resolve once treatment with the offending opioid is discontinued, pain resolution from opioid discontinuation in OIH will not be immediate and will require patience. This poses its own challenges for both clinician and patient. To complicate matters further, hyperalgesia resulting from opioid withdrawal is a well-documented phenomenon.

With OT pain tends to be localized and improves with time and reduction in the noxious stimulus (e.g., tissue healing). In contrast, pain associated with OIH is often more diffuse extending beyond the region of injury or tissue damage, is of lesser quality, and noxious stimuli tend to be more painful than would normally be expected. In addition, pain associated with OIH can persist despite removal of the original source of pain or healing of the damaged tissue. As opioid treatment progresses, the pain of OIH may give the impression of becoming more severe than originally reported, despite time, rest, and other measures that would normally allow for a clinically relevant amount of healing. Additionally, allodynia (i.e., a pain response from stimuli which do not normally provoke pain) has been demonstrated in a number of human and animal studies of OIH [30]. Of particular consideration in the assessment of OIH is the way in which clinicians ask their patients to score pain following opioid treatment. The standard numerical scale which is commonly used for pain assessment does not differentiate worsening pain to specific subtypes (e.g., thermal) of noxious stimuli so an assessment of OIH could be missed. It might then be necessary to develop simple mechanical and/or thermal pain testing to determine altered sensitivity to these pain-testing modalities.

Formalized techniques such as quantitative sensory testing (QST) to assess patient responses to defined physical stimuli (thermal and mechanical) may provide a more consistent and objective approach to diagnosing OT versus OIH [31, 32]. While promising in small clinical studies, such approaches have not been systematically studied in ICU patients. Even with QST, the demonstration of hyperalgesia around the surgical site is not necessarily diagnostic of OIH because the tissue response to surgical trauma, with release of inflammatory mediators, can cause peripheral and central sensitization and can be manifested as hyperalgesia. If there is more widespread hyperalgesia well beyond the site of injury, then there is an increased likelihood of OIH. The absence of a simple, objective specific test adds to diagnostic uncertainty, coupled with some overlap in symptoms between OIH, tolerance, acute opioid withdrawal and injury-induced acute neuropathic pain—all of which can occur in the ICU setting. This uncertainty is further compounded by the observation that neuropathic pain often responds poorly to opioids as commonly seen in the critically ill.

Prevention and Treatment

The most effective way to address the problems of OT and OIH is likely to be prevention (Table 8.3). For this reason, it is prudent to minimize opioid administration when possible and utilize alternative analgesia strategies (Table 8.3). It is incumbent on physicians and nurses caring for critically ill patients to carefully evaluate their practice on pain management and adopt an optimal pain management strategy that includes a reduction in noxious stimuli, regular pain assessment, providing adequate analgesia and promoting education regarding sedation and analgesia to the ICU staff. Such mechanistic approaches in combination with multimodal analgesic techniques have been clearly demonstrated to be the most effective pain management strategy to improve outcomes. Peripheral nerve blocks and neuraxial anesthesia can reduce the need for opioids and have an opioid-sparing effect [33]. In addition, drugs such as esmolol and dexmedetomidine can approximate the effect of opioids on heart rate and blood pressure control. However, many critically ill patients will still require opioids acutely, and occasionally, chronically. Most OIH prevention strategies have focused on the glutaminergic system and NMDA receptor activation, both of which are implicated in the development of central sensitization and OIH. Ketamine and methadone have all been shown to attenuate OIH, whereas drugs such as gabapentinoids and α-2 receptor agonists such as clonidine have been shown to attenuate wound hyperalgesia, although there is insufficient evidence to suggest through which mechanism [34]. If intravenous opioid infusion is considered as part of the analgesic regimen, then avoiding high rates of infusion especially remifentanil can reduce risk of OIH.

When a diagnosis of OIH has been made, there are a number of treatment options from which to carefully choose. Provided that the initial painful injury or tissue damage has resolved and the pain persists in spite of—and because of—opioid treatment, the most straightforward approach is to discontinue the offending opioid. This should be done gradually to minimize adverse withdrawal effects. Clinicians should be aware that hyperalgesia may likely worsen early in the discontinuation process. This presents a challenging clinical management situation requiring finding an acceptable balance of analgesia and relief from hyperalgesia upon opioid dose reduction. The clinician may have difficulty convincing the patient with suspected OIH that the medication prescribed to treat pain may have been causing or worsening the pain and that the pain may get worse still before it ultimately resolves.

Table 8.3 Strategies for mitigating OT or OIH

Appropriate use of opioids
Use of valid assessment scales of pain before and during administration of analgesic drugs
Use of intermittent opioid therapy (oral or intravenous) rather than continuous infusions, when possible
Opioid rotation
Minimize use of remifentanil (because of potent induction of opioid-induced hyperalgesia), except when rapid offset of effect is required, as in evaluation of head injury
Minimize use of benzodiazepines (because of delirium and potential opioid-induced hyperalgesia associated with long-term use)
Avoid excessive dose escalation; supplementation of opioid with non-opioid analgesics
Consider addition of methadone to attenuate or delay opioid tolerance
Co-administration of non-opioid analgesics as means to reduce or to potentiate the effects of opioids[a]
N-methyl-d-aspartate receptor antagonists (ketamine).
α2-adrenergic receptor agonists (clonidine or dexmedetomidine),
Gabapentinoids (gabapentin or pregabalin)
Use of nerve blocks to reduce or eliminate the need for opioids
Neuraxial: Thoracic or lumber epidural blocks for thoracic, abdominal, or bilateral leg analgesia
Regional: Brachial plexus block for arm analgesia; femoral or obturator block or both, with or without sciatic nerve block for lower-limb analgesia
Local: Paravertebral block for rib fractures or chest-tube–associated pain transversus abdominis block for lower abdominal surgery
Prevention or reversal of opioid-induced hyperalgesia and opioid-withdrawal symptoms
Tapering of opioid dose when pain score goal is achieved (10–20% dose reduction every 1–4 days)
Use of valid withdrawal assessment scales
Use of adjuncts to opioids (ketamine, dexmedetomidine, or gabapentinoids)
Use of methadone
Reduction of inflammation
Scheduled acetaminophen therapy
Short-term use of ketorolac[b]

Adapted from Martyn et al. [1]
[a]The non-opioid strategies that are listed are usually used in combination with opioids
[b]Other nonsteroidal anti-inflammatory drugs (e.g., ibuprofen) have limited use in the intensive care unit because of cardiovascular, nephrotoxic, and gastrointestinal side effects

If legitimate pain persists and some amount of analgesia with opioids is required, other strategies beyond total opioid discontinuation should be explored with the goal of finding an acceptable balance of analgesia and relief from hyperalgesia upon opioid dose reduction.

Switching from one structural class of opioids to another has been an effective option for mitigating OIH in some studies. Studies to date have demonstrated that OIH is more strongly associated with opioids from the phenanthrene class and conversion to another class may provide resolution of OIH [30]. Codeine, hydromorphone, morphine, and structurally similar opioids undergo glucuronidation as part of their metabolism. Avoidance of an NMDA receptor–activating glucuronide metabolite is possible by switching to an opioid that is structurally unique, such as fentanyl. Guidelines for opioid rotation are empirical and begin with the selection of a safe and reasonably effective starting dose for the new opioid, followed by dose adjustment to optimize the balance between analgesia and side effects [35]. The selection of a starting dose must be based on an estimate of the relative potency between the existing opioid and the new one. Potency differs widely among opioids and among individuals under varying conditions. Therefore to safely and effectively rotate from one opioid to another, the new opioid must be started at a dose that will cause neither toxicity nor abstinence and will be sufficiently efficacious in that pain is no worse than before the change.

Management of OT and OIH should not be viewed as a choice between under-treatment of pain and over-prescribing of opioids. Both extremes should be avoided. Opioid over-prescribing is best controlled by implementation of current clinical practice guidelines with assessment-driven protocols and use of multimodal pain management strategies. Optimal pain management in the ICU should not only focus on acute pain but also aim to prevent the development of chronic pain and the adverse effects of ongoing opioid use. Data extrapolated from studies of perioperative pain demonstrate that appropriate pain control has the potential to prevent the conversion of acute to chronic pain, which should reduce the risk of longer term opioid use after recovery from critical illness [36]. Clinical practice guidelines pertaining to the management of acute, severe pain in critically ill patients have recognized that opioids are a mainstay of a multimodal approach that involves pharmacological and non-pharmacological interventions [37]. These place emphasis and recommendations on non-opioid agents as adjuncts to opioids for severe pain, but the recommendations for these adjuncts are tempered by a lack of higher level evidence supporting their use and concerns related to adverse effects in patients who often have multiple organ dysfunction. It is recommended that pain management in critically ill patients should utilize a protocolized approach that can be tailored to account for an individual's disease process, comorbidities, and pre-existing pain problems. This requires a systematic individualized multimodal pharmacological and non-pharmacological treatment approach that utilizes a multidisciplinary team. The protocolized approach should include regular detailed pain assessments using appropriate tools to evaluate initial pain and response to treatment. Pharmacological strategies should involve the lowest possible dose of opioids that is still effective, with the aim of the earliest possible reduction in the dose and slow transition to non-opioid medications.

The use of opioids should be re-evaluated during ICU discharge and other transitions of care because non-opioid agents may become more viable alternatives as pain severity decreases and organ dysfunction that precluded the use of non-opioids improves [38]. Efforts to control opioid over-prescribing after an ICU stay should be focused on prescribing practices associated with patients' transition of care from hospital to home or other care facility because this where acute-to-chronic use is most likely to occur. These efforts should include avoiding extended release opioid products when treating acute pain states, so opioid doses can be reduced as pain resolves. Appropriate patient counseling is critical because over-prescribing and storage of opioids is common. The electronic health record can be used to help inform prescribing not only through incorporation of prescription monitoring programs but also through computer-generated alerts when prolonged courses of opioids are prescribed [39]. Consideration should be given ICU clinics where pain control and opioid use can be routinely assessed.

Conclusion

Opioids remain the most commonly used analgesics to treat pain in critically ill patients, but carry a significant risk for many adverse effects, contributing to problematic long-term use. Long-term opioid use leads to tolerance which can result in a need for higher and more frequent and may contribute to the development of opioid-induced hyperalgesia. Both OT and OIH can contribute to both poorly controlled pain and dose escalation. OT can develop with opioid exposure during a variety of acute and chronic disease states; the magnitude, however, seems exaggerated in critically ill patients. The development of OT and OIH in critically ill patients is due in part to the large doses of opioids needed to control pain as well as the duration of administration. However, the inflammatory response seen in critically ill or injured patients plays an important role in tolerance and OIH. While the mechanisms underlying inflammatory- and opioid-induced maladaptive pain responses have not been fully elucidated, it is crucial for the critical care practitioner to be aware of the issues of OT, addiction and withdrawal, as well as the possibility for OIH. By improving understanding of the underlying mechanisms and diagnosis, it may be possible to develop strategies to better manage pain associated with critical illness and injury, to improve efficacy and safety of opioid use, and to minimize long-term harms.

References

1. Martyn JAJ, Mao J, Bittner EA. Opioid Tolerance in Critical Illness. N Engl J Med. 2019;380(4):365–78.
2. Pathan H, Williams J. Basic opioid pharmacology: an update. Br J Pain. 2012;6(1):11–6.
3. Ossipov MH, Dussor GO, Porreca F. Central modulation of pain. J Clin Invest. 2010;120(11):3779–87. https://doi.org/10.1172/JCI43766.
4. Ji RR, Chamessian A, Zhang YQ. Pain regulation by non-neuronal cells and inflammation. Science. 2016;354:572–7.
5. Jennings EM, Okine BN, Roche M, Finn DP. Stress-induced hyperalgesia. Prog Neurobiol. 2014 Oct;121:1–18.
6. Wohleb ES, McKim DB, Sheridan JF, Godbout JP. Monocyte trafficking to the brain with stress and inflammation: a novel axis of immune-to-brain communication that influences mood and behavior. Front Neurosci. 2015;8:447.

7. Anderson BJ, Mikkelsen ME. Stressing the brain: the immune system, hypothalamic-pituitary-adrenal axis, and psychiatric symptoms in acute respiratory distress syndrome survivors. Ann Am Thorac Soc. 2017;14(8):39–41.
8. Roeckel LA, Le Coz GM, GavériauxRuff C, Simonin F. Opioid-induced hyperalgesia: cellular and molecular mechanisms. Neuroscience. 2016;338:160–82.
9. Hutchinson MR, Shavit Y, Grace PM, Rice KC, Maier SF, Watkins LR. Exploring the neuroimmunopharmacology of opioids: an integrative review of mechanisms of central immune signaling and their implications for opioid analgesia. Pharmacol Rev. 2011;63:772–810.
10. Waxman AR, Arout C, Caldwell M, Dahan A, Kest B. Acute and chronic fentanyl administration causes hyperalgesia independently of opioid receptor activity in mice. Neurosci Lett. 2009;462:68–72.
11. Bittner EA, Shank E, Woodson L, Martyn JA. Acute and perioperative care of the burn-injured patient. Anesthesiology. 2015;122:448–64.
12. Anand KJ, Willson DF, Berger J, et al. Tolerance and withdrawal from prolonged opioid use in critically ill children. Pediatrics. 2010;125(5):e1208–25.
13. Ji RR, Nackley A, Huh Y, Terrando N, Maixner W. Neuroinflammation and central sensitization in chronic and widespread pain. Anesthesiology. 2018;129(2):343–66.
14. Sparkman NL, Johnson RW. Neuroinflammation associated with aging sensitizes the brain to the effects of infection or stress. Neuroimmunomodulation. 2008;15(4–6):323–30.
15. Schaller SJ, Alam SM, Mao J, et al. Pharmacokinetics cannot explain the increased effective dose requirement for morphine and midazolam in rats during their extended administration alone or in combination. J Pharm Pharmacol. 2017;69:82–8.
16. Kharasch ED. Current concepts in methadone metabolism and transport. Clin Pharmacol Drug Dev. 2017;6:125–34.
17. Han T, Harmatz JS, Greenblatt DJ, Martyn JA. Fentanyl clearance and volume of distribution are increased in patients with major burns. J Clin Pharmacol. 2007;47:674–80.
18. Smith MT. Neuroexcitatory effects of morphine and hydromorphone: evidence implicating the 3-glucuronide metabolites. Clin Exp Pharmacol Physiol. 2000;27:524–8.
19. Pasternak GW, Pan YX. Mu opioids and their receptors: evolution of a concept. Pharmacol Rev. 2013;65(4):1257–317.
20. Dumas EO, Pollack GM. Opioid tolerance development: a pharmacokinetic/ pharmacodynamic perspective. AAPS J. 2008;10:537–51.
21. Costantino CM, Gomes I, Stockton SD, Lim MP, Devi LA. Opioid receptor heteromers in analgesia. Expert Rev Mol Med. 2012;14:e9.
22. Rossbach MJ. Ueber die Gowöhnung an Gifte. Pfluegers Arch Gesamte Physiol Menschen Tiere. 1880;21:213–25.
23. Higgins C, Smith BH, Matthews K. Evidence of opioid-induced hyperalgesia in clinical populations after chronic opioid exposure: a systematic review and meta-analysis. Br J Anaesth. 2019;122(6):e114–26.
24. Fletcher D, Martinez V. Opioid-induced hyperalgesia in patients after surgery: a systematic review and a meta-analysis. Br J Anaesth. 2014;112(6):991–1004.
25. Kim SH, Stoicea N, Soghomonyan S, Bergese SD. Remifentanil-acute opioid tolerance and opioid-induced hyperalgesia: a systematic review. Am J Ther. 2015;22:e62–74.
26. Hahnenkamp K, Nollet J, Van Aken HK, Buerkle H, Halene T, Schauerte S, Hahnenkamp A, Hollmann MW, Strümper D, Durieux ME, Hoenemann CW. Remifentanil directly activates human N-methyl-d-aspartate receptors expressed in Xenopus laevis oocytes. Anesthesiology. 2004;100:1531–7.
27. Cooper DW, Lindsay SL, Ryall DM, Kokri MS, Eldabe SS, Lear GA. Does intrathecal fentanyl produce acute cross-tolerance to i.v. morphine? Br J Anaesth. 1997;78:311–3.
28. Samuelsen PJ, Nielsen CS, Wilsgaard T, Stubhaug A, Svendsen K, Eggen AE. Pain sensitivity and analgesic use among 10,486 adults: the Tromsø study. BMC Pharmacol Toxicol. 2017;18(1):45.
29. Yi P, Pryzbylkowski P. Opioid induced Hyperalgesia. Pain Med. 2015;16(Suppl 1):S32–6.

30. Lee M, Silverman SM, Hansen H, Patel VB. Manchikanti L. a comprehensive review of opioid-induced hyperalgesia. Pain Physician. 2011;14(2):145–61.
31. Mao J. Clinical diagnosis of opioid-induced Hyperalgesia. Reg Anesth Pain Med. 2015;40(6):663–4.
32. Roldan CJ, Abdi S. Quantitative sensory testing in pain management. Pain Manag. 2015;5(6):483–91.
33. Rubio-Haro R, Morales-Sarabia J, Ferrer-Gomez C, de Andres J. Regional analgesia techniques for pain management in patients admitted to the intensive care unit. Minerva Anestesiol. 2019;85(10):1118–28.
34. Hayhurst CJ, Durieux ME. Differential opioid tolerance and opioid-induced Hyperalgesia: a clinical reality. Anesthesiology. 2016;124(2):483–8.
35. Treillet E, Laurent S, Hadjiat Y. Practical management of opioid rotation and equianalgesia. J Pain Res. 2018;11:2587–601.
36. Glare P, Aubrey KR, Myles PS. Transition from acute to chronic pain after surgery. Lancet. 2019;393(10180):1537–46.
37. Devlin JW, Skrobik Y, Gélinas C, et al. Clinical practice guidelines for the prevention and management of pain, agitation/sedation, delirium, immobility, and sleep disruption in adult patients in the ICU. Crit Care Med. 2018;46(9):e825–73.
38. Stamenkovic DM, Laycock H, Karanikolas M, Ladjevic NG, Neskovic V, Chronic Pain BC. Chronic opioid use after intensive care discharge - is it time to change practice? Front Pharmacol. 2019;10:23.
39. Erstad BL. Implications of the opioid epidemic for critical care practice. J Am Coll Clin Pharm. 2019;2:161–6.

Chapter 9
Interaction of Opioids with Sedative Practices in the ICU

Jane Keating, Sandra L. Kane-Gill, and Lewis J. Kaplan

Why Is this Topic Important?

The current opioid epidemic has focused attention on opioid use both in and out of the hospital [1]. While recent progress has been made in decreasing overall opioid-related fatalities, deaths related to the newer synthetic opioids such as carfentanil continue to rise at a rapid rate [2]; Fig. 9.1. The rapid onset of acute respiratory failure and related depressed level of consciousness drives the increasing prevalence of intranasal naloxone rescue therapy by bystanders, and an increase in use by Emergency Medical Services and Emergency Medicine staff [3]. In-hospital opioid administration may be coupled with sedative agent therapy. The combination of an opioid and a sedative – especially a benzodiazepine – greatly magnifies the risk of undesirable and unintended respiratory depression. Moreover, combination therapy may also lead to hypotension that may also depress mentation in a patient who is used to a much higher blood pressure for cerebral blood flow and oxygen delivery [4]. The increased prevalence of obstructive sleep apnea in the clinically severely obese may increase the risk of respiratory depression with opioid therapy in

J. Keating
University of Connecticut, Department of Surgery, Hartford, CT, USA

S. L. Kane-Gill
University of Pittsburgh School of Pharmacy, Department of Pharmacy and Therapeutics, Department of Biomedical Informatics, Pittsburgh, PA, USA

L. J. Kaplan (✉)
Corporal Michael J Crescenz VA Medical Center, Surgical Services, Surgical Critical Care, Philadelphia, PA, USA

Perelman School of Medicine, University of Pennsylvania, Department of Surgery, Division of Trauma, Surgical Critical Care and Emergency Surgery, Philadelphia, PA, USA
e-mail: Lewis.Kaplan@uphs.upenn.edu; Lewis.Kaplan@va.gov

J. L. Pascual, T. G. Gaulton (eds.), *Opioid Use in Critical Care*,
https://doi.org/10.1007/978-3-030-77399-1_9

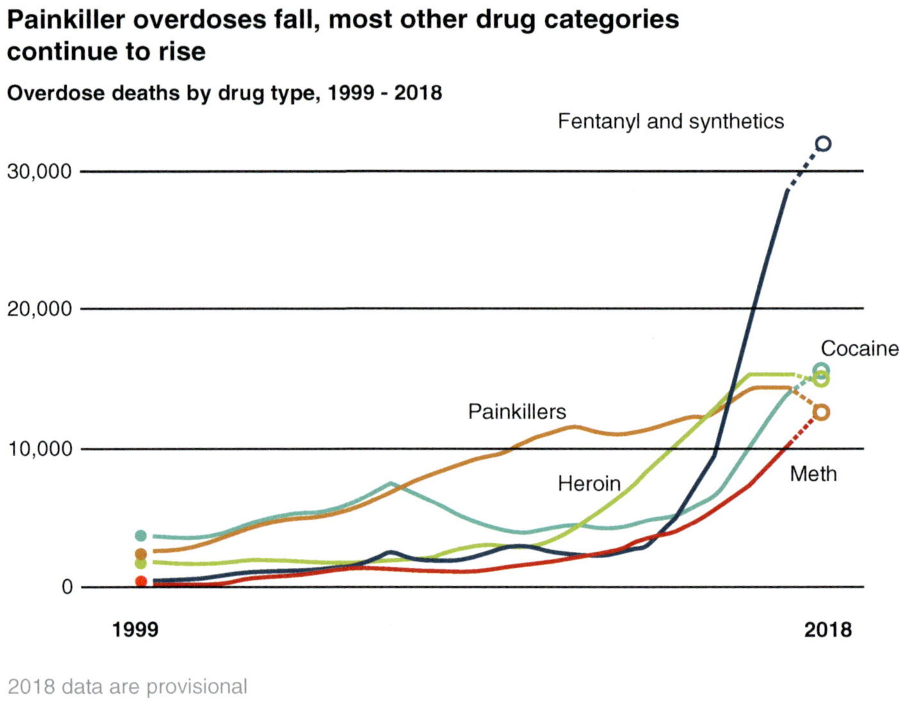

Fig. 9.1 Overdoses in the United States by drug type

isolation or in combination with other agents. Therefore, there is a need for guidance to direct safe opioid use, as well as to avoid iatrogenic injury, prolonged hospital, and ICU length of stay and preventable death.

Opioid Use in Critical Illness

Rather than individual determination of appropriate dosing based entirely upon subjective pain reporting, analgesia dosing is currently driven by pain score scale assessments. Pain score ranges are linked to specific opioid doses and are readily trackable using the modern electronic health record (EHR) [5]. Indeed, hospital evaluation by The Joint Commission identifies the specificity of analgesic ordering to pain scale score range as a process that supports patient safety [6] (see Chap. 7). The need for opioid prescribing may be different between ICUs – an observation that reflects unique patient population needs rather than divergent practice goals. For instance, surgical ICU patients have generally undergone a surgical procedure where new, incisional pain is a prominent feature. In contradistinction, a medical ICU patient population will generally have fewer patients who have undergone surgery and may demonstrate a lesser overt need for analgesia. The converse may be observed with respect to sedation practices, as the MICU may have more of a sedation need for mechanical ventilation, while the SICU may use less sedatives as the greater opioid use may decrease sedative agent requirements. Pediatric ICUs house both medical and surgical patients – much like many community hospital ICUs – and will therefore demonstrate features common to both surgical and medical practices [7]. Regardless, all ICUs will benefit from a structured approach to analgesia and sedation.

Commonly, opioid prescribing practices in the ICU also leverage either routine administration of non-opioid agents, or establish a non-opioid agent prescribing pathway for low level pain scale scores. Both may be successful in reducing overall opioid exposure during critical illness. However, the critically ill may have home chronic opioid use that establishes a need to match their home opioid dosing to prevent withdrawal, as well as additional agent to treat acute pain. Determining an appropriate opioid agent dose may be more challenging in those with chronic pain and chronic opioid use, opioid agonist treatment for addiction with methadone, and those with concomitant psychiatric illness. In these settings, the pharmacodynamic knowledge of a clinical pharmacist is invaluable in targeting and modifying dosing while avoiding adverse drug events [8]. Increasingly, clinical pharmacists are routinely incorporated into critical care teams as key bedside care members, and not solely housed in the facility's pharmacy space for distribution purposes [9].

Opioid Risks in the Critically Ill

Critical illness often impacts physiologic reserve, alters baseline physiology and may impact normal anatomic dynamics including those related to compartment pressure-volume relationships. Accordingly, the well-described reduction in respiratory drive that may accompany opioid administration may be more manifestly exaggerated in the altered host. This observation has led some to recommend routine end-tidal carbon dioxide ($ETCO_2$) monitoring of all patients receiving IV opioid analgesia to more readily detect adverse effects on CO_2 clearance, and trigger rescue therapy; there is little to no data on those receiving oral agents in the hospital [10]. The data underpinning such an approach is limited, and there are a host of confounders that may impact $ETCO_2$ fidelity in the spontaneously ventilating patient including but not limited to: mouth breathing, device malposition, concomitant oxygen therapy with gas stream dilution or washout, device plugging/obstruction or failure, as well as in many facilities, a lack of a central monitoring system establishing alarms only within the patient's room [11]. False alarms appear to be common, but could be viewed as acceptable in the interest of detecting all potentially dangerous events.

High risk populations for adverse events (Fig. 9.2) include those on a continuous infusion of opioid compared to those who receive only demand dosing using a patient controlled analgesia (PCA) device [12]. Higher risk is also observed in those receiving epidural long-acting opioid therapy. The risk profile appears to be reduced in those who

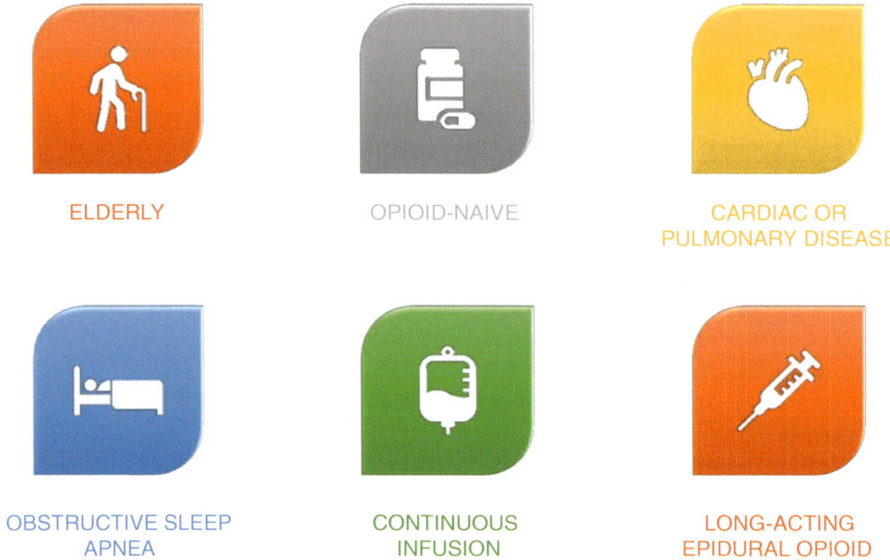

Fig. 9.2 High-risk populations

receive chronic pre-admission opioid therapy as opposed to that of the opioid naïve patient. All opioid receiving patients are at risk for opioid-induced hyperalgesia syndrome which occurs in an unpredictable fashion [13]. Predictably, all opioid receiving patients demonstrate reduced gastrointestinal (GI) motility; routine use of motility supporting and catharsis promoting agents is appropriate [14, 15]. Specific agents such as fentanyl demonstrated idiosyncratic and non-dose dependent adverse effects such as chest wall rigidity syndrome [16].

A risk whose genesis is in the intensive care unit (ICU) but whose expression occurs outside of the ICU, especially for those with prolonged ICU length of stay is unplanned habituation and the creation of a dependent patient population [17, 18]. Therefore, every patient should have a daily evaluation of their analgesic plan, consideration of non-opioid and non-pharmacologic pain management, as well as an opioid de-escalation plan to mitigate this risk. Reducing the overall opioid use as well as reduction or elimination of use once the need for acute therapy has passed strongly argues for a multimodal approach to analgesia, as well as a clinical pathway for routinely encountered patient types [5] (i.e., fast track cardiac surgery, Early Recovery After Surgery pathway colorectal surgery patients).

Emerging Approaches in Acute Pain Management

A truisim is that it is easier to keep a patient out of pain than to rescue them from pain once it is established. Therefore, oral acetaminophen dosing for 24–48 hours prior to an intended procedure is increasingly common [19]. This establishes an acetaminophen level that may be supported by IV acetaminophen intraoperatively, and followed by IV or PO agents through recovery and convalescence as allowed by GI function. Relatedly, the regular use of nonsteroidal anti-inflammatory drugs (NSAIDs) also appears to reduce total opioid requirements. NSAID use requires monitoring of nephrotoxic and bleeding events. While IV ketorolac is the sole agent used for IV administration, there are a plethora of agents for oral use, including some such as meloxicam that have minimal impact on thromboxane-related aspects of the clotting cascade. Indeed, meloxicam has been deemed acceptable for concomitant use with an indwelling epidural catheter in the recently revised guideline from the American Society for Regional Anesthesia (ASRA) [20].

Adjunctive analgesics including gabapentin (strong evidence) and topical lidocaine patches (mixed evidence) also reduce total opioid use [21]. Newer agents such as liposomal bupivacaine enjoy success in nearly eliminating up to 72 hours of analgesic need after procedures that benefit from regional anesthetic techniques such as hand surgery. Other regional anesthetic therapies include temporary local anesthetic infusion pumps – some of which have a variable flow rate as well as a bolus feature for breakthrough pain (On-Q* pain relief system) [22]; as well as the previously mentioned epidural catheter with a continuous or patient-controlled fashion. Paradural catheters and infusions may present more of a technical challenge but appear helpful for acute rib fracture management [23].

In those with chronic pain, ketamine or lidocaine infusions may be excellent in offsetting large dose opioid administration, and may be best undertaken on a pathway; support from an Acute Pain Service may be desirable when utilizing infrequently administered agents. Acupuncture may be utilized as a pain control adjunct as "Battlefield Acupuncture (BFA)" that places "pins" only at specific points on the ear; BFA is not traditional acupuncture but does require a one-day training course supported by a certification process [24]. Select institutions may also offer traditional acupuncture but this modality is uncommonly applied to inpatients. Intraoperative pain prevention has recently utilized cryotherapy applied to intercostal nerves and delivered by an FDA-approved device to mitigate sternotomy pain but is also used during rib fracture stabilization procedures with great success [25].

Complementary approaches including preferred music, a medical musician, aromatherapy, pet therapy, massage therapy, and video gaming all have been employed in efforts to reduce pain, and perhaps with more success, anxiety. Importantly, non-opioid therapeutics are translatable to the post-discharge space where sustained reduction in opioid dosing is realizable, and support multimodality analgesia [26, 27].

Sedation in the ICU

Sedatives are generally employed in the ICU for one of six indications (Fig. 9.3): comfort on mechanical ventilation, as part of multimodal therapy for ICU procedures, continuation therapy to prevent a therapeutic agent withdrawal syndrome,

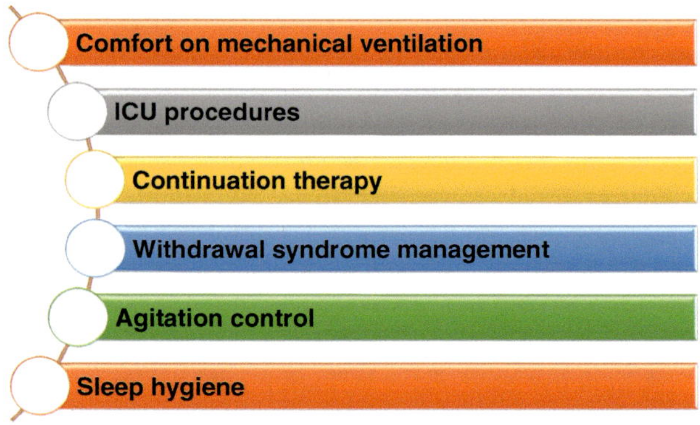

Fig. 9.3 Common sedative uses in the ICU

treatment of alcohol withdrawal syndrome, agitation management, or sleep hygiene support. Other uses occur, but these five capture the majority of uses in US ICUs. Sedative selection commonly depends on the specific goal of sedative therapy, the specific pathway required for metabolism (hepatic versus renal), the duration of need, and interactions with other therapeutic agents – including opioids – and organs, especially in the setting of evolving or established organ failure [28]. Regardless of indication, minimization of sedative agent exposure is preferred to support patient- and family-centered care, reduce adverse drug events, and avoid delirium induction [29]. Of course, conscious sedation is often required for ICU procedures, and generally represents a significant increase in sedation and analgesia compared to the pre-procedure baseline use. Sedation may be induced using a continuous infusion of a short-acting agent such as propofol, or intermittent dosing depending on patient need. Special note is made of the deliberate use of diazepam and phenobarbital for alcohol withdrawal syndrome as this specific indication leverages the drugs long half-life and active metabolites, in the case of diazepam, to reduce the need for ongoing dosing. It is readily apparent that the integrated clinical pharmacist may provide essential support for appropriate agent selection during deliberate sedation of the critically ill.

Sedative Risks in the Critically Ill

All sedative agents may induce respiratory depression, just like opioid agents. Decreased level of consciousness, depressed Glasgow Coma Score, respiratory depression, and acute respiratory failure are all well-chronicled effects. While applied to a therapeutic goal and scoring system such as the Richmond Agitation Sedation Scale (RASS), some agents appear to be associated with delirium induction (benzodiazepines most notably). Moreover, the risk of delirium induction may be higher in the elderly [30]. The reader is cautioned that causation is not always clear, and at present, there are only strong associations. At times, a benzodiazepine remains the therapeutic agent of choice and should be utilized while remaining vigilant for untoward side effects. There appears to be a decreased, but non-zero, risk of habituation compared to opioids after discharge from inpatient care. The major risk with sedatives – besides delirium induction – is that of respiratory depression during spontaneous positive pressure ventilation or independent negative pressure ventilation. Both settings are at increased risk when sedation is accompanied by opioid analgesic therapy [31]. Undesired respiratory depression, especially during spontaneous breathing trials, may be conflated with appropriate decreased minute ventilation in a patient with significant metabolic alkalosis. The elevated pH should physiologically drive the patient to seek a decreased minute ventilation to achieve a more normal pH and medullary proton concentration; reduced sedation will not alter this imperative. These observations are physiologically important for clinical care, but will also impact performance improvement evaluations related to sedative use during ventilator weaning.

Relatedly, the reader should also be aware of the idiosyncratic occurrence of unanticipated bradycardia during propofol infusion termed "propofol infusion syndrome" (PRIS). The bradycardia may be refractory and lead to asystole. Risk factors have been identified and include higher dose infusion (> 4 mg/kg/hr), longer exposure time (> 48 hr), concomitant use of vasopressors or steroids, the presence of a mitochondrial metabolic disorder, traumatic brain injury, rhabdomyolysis, carbohydrate depletion, lipemia, fatty liver syndrome, and metabolic acidosis [32]. Besides infusion cessation, rescue therapy may require renal replacement therapy and on occasion, veno-arterial extracorporeal membrane oxygenation [33]. Not related to the syndrome, but associated with continuous infusion more so than a single dose, is the occurrence of green urine related to propofol administration.

Interaction of Opioids and Sedatives

It is abundantly clear that risk is increased when opioids and sedatives are combined for patient care. This observation should not promote avoiding combining these therapeutic agents, but should instead support vigilance in monitoring for untoward effects, especially in those without an artificial airway and mandatory mechanical ventilation (standing or rescue during an SBT). Opioids and sedatives are generally combined in one of four circumstances (Fig. 9.4): peri-procedural, mechanical ventilation (principally postoperative), post-injury complicated by a withdrawal syndrome or traumatic brain injury, and palliative care around the end-of-life to manage pain and abrogate anxiety.

Not all sedative agents confer the same risk. For example, high risk of acute respiratory failure and hypotension is noted with propofol, but less with dexmedetomidine. Low risk is noted for the typical or atypical antipsychotic agents such as haloperidol or quetiapine, respectively. For every agent, the risk profile is increased when combined with a concomitant opioid; highest risk is for IV continuous infusion but the risk with oral dosing remains non-zero. Increasing use of novel approaches including ketamine by infusion may shift the epidemiology of identified

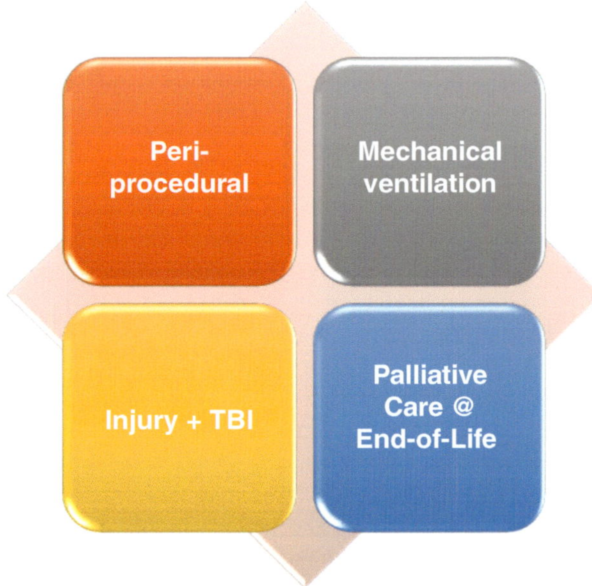

Fig. 9.4 Common uses of opioids and sedatives in the ICU

risk profiles as may the more routine use of multimodal analgesia (i.e., decreased opioid exposure). The impact may be identified during quality improvement assessments of the frequency of hypercarbic and/or hypoxic acute respiratory failure, as well as "failed" spontaneous breathing trials in those receiving both sedatives and opioids as part of their medical management. Of note, duration of therapy and renal and hepatic dysfunction can further intensify the concern for respiratory depression with this combination depending on the agents used.

Sleep Hygiene

Pain notoriously distorts sleep hygiene. Therefore, at a time when respiratory rate is expected to decrease, O_2 saturation often drifts, and a decreased level of consciousness (sleep) is desired, patients may be vulnerable to unrecognized complications of combined therapy [34]. Accordingly, non-pharmacologic therapies are preferred to minimize sedative exposure, especially at a time when analgesic doses may need to be increased to support sleep. Non-pharmacologic approaches include but are not limited to: enforced awake periods during the day, natural light during the day and darkened rooms at night, noise reduction protocols at night, cessation of scheduled tasks at night, minimizing in-room care for the hemodynamically appropriate, as well as white sound generation or preferred music, especially by headphone or ear-bud delivery. Other approaches may also support sleep hygiene, especially reproducing a common pre-sleep sequence of activities or habits in which the patient routinely engages [35].

Pharmacologic support may initially leverage melatonin as this agent does not impact respiratory drive; higher doses – up to 15 mg – may be required in those with elevated catecholamine tone [36]. Other agents, such as antidepressants, and finally atypical antipsychotic agents may be effective when melatonin fails [37]. Regardless of which agent is selected, note is made of the Beer's criteria that should be used in the elderly to avoid untoward medication impact based on age or comorbid condition(s) including diphenhydramine as a sleep aid [38]. One key aspect of deliberate sleep hygiene management is to ensure that new medications that have situational specific use are discontinued on ICU or hospital discharge as one method to avoid polypharmacy, especially in the elderly.

Peri-Procedural Combination Therapy

Unlike procedures that are performed in the Operating Room with the aid of an Anesthesiologist or a Nurse Anesthetist (CRNA) and use general anesthesia, ICU procedures may instead employ deep sedation or moderate sedation [39]. Unique training and credentialing is required to use GA. Special note is made of Anesthesia Intensivists who may use GA in the ICU if the appropriate equipment is brought to the ICU room, parallel to how patients are managed in the GI or cardiology procedure suite. The major use of deep sedation in the ICU is for bedside relaparotomy or re-exploration when there is a temporary abdominal wall closure (TAC) in place, major dressing changes, and airway control – the latter is often combined with a short-acting neuromuscular blocker as well. Deep sedation most commonly employs a continuous infusion of propofol combined with a continuous infusion of opioid such as fentanyl. Moderate sedation is often used for intracranial pressure monitoring device insertion, bronchoscopy, GI endoscopy, transesophageal echocardiography, and cardioversion. An analgesic combined with very little – and occasionally no – sedative is used for central venous pressure (CVP) line insertion, arterial line placement, Peripherally Inserted Central Catheter (PICC) or Midline insertion, and nasal enteral access catheter placement. Monitoring requirements to ensure safety while using deliberate sedation are well-described and are tied to the anticipated duration of action of the administered agents [40].

Mechanical Ventilation

In general, the major need with mechanical ventilation is sedation with a lesser need for analgesia, unless there is concomitant injury, or the patient has undergone a procedure that induces pain (i.e., incisional pain). Procedures specific to mechanical ventilation that may cause pain most notably include suctioning and catheter-associated injury to the sensitive carina. Suctioning also evacuates gas and may create a subjective sensation of suffocation, driving fear around care events. For those on prolonged ventilation, immobility may create pain around body repositioning and when the patient is able to engage in physical therapy; even passive range of motion may create muscular discomfort in the previously minimally mobile patient. Therefore, combination sedative and opioid therapy is common in those on mechanical ventilation, even if the combination is by intermittent dosing.

Recent data from the ICU Liberation taskforce of the Society of Critical Care Medicine notes reduced delirium and coma, days on mechanical ventilation, and mortality when a bundled approach to care is utilized for those receiving mechanical ventilation [41]. The improvements do carry an unanticipated cost – increased reporting of pain. Not surprisingly, more awake patients who may engage in their care will be able to report pain that a more heavily sedated patient could not share. In order to avoid excess sedation, a multimodal approach to pain management is similarly appropriate in this circumstance as well. Nonetheless, recent data suggests that sedation for mechanical ventilation tolerance may exert untoward effects on ventilator cycling and triggering for which the ICU clinician must be vigilant [42]. In particular, sedatives and opioids (at higher sedation levels) were associated with more ineffective inspiratory efforts during exhalation, while sedative only patients demonstrated reduced double cycling. Opioid only administration appeared to be inversely associated with asynchronies. All synchronies were higher in patients who received neither sedation nor analgesia. The data from this study suggest that opioids alone may be a superior method of supporting mechanical ventilation comfort – at least with regard to minimizing asynchronies to which clinicians generally respond.

Post-Injury Patient Care (See Chap. 12)

This topic is complex and embraces a host of variables that drive specific therapy. Analgesia is imperative to manage post-injury pain to a tolerable level, while sedation is useful in managing agitation to facilitate safe care and avoid staff injury during care episodes. The post-TBI patient may manifest episodic hyperadrenergic activity (i.e., hyperadrenergic crisis) that is well managed using a lipophilic beta-blocker such as propranolol. Since propranolol has no impact on respiratory drive, and is administered to a patient with increased catecholamine tone, hypotension is rarely a concern; both issues are of concern with typical sedatives [43]. More commonly, agitation relates to the presence of an oral endotracheal tube, TBI, or alcohol or illicit substance effect or withdrawal syndrome. While the Clinical Institute Withdrawal Assessment (CIWA) protocol seems effective for patients care for outside of the ICU, failure to control alcohol withdrawal symptoms leading to ICU admission should prompt the use of a more intense approach. The MINnesota Detoxification Scale (MINDS) protocol does just that and provides options for three different benzodiazepine-based approaches that may be supplemented with an adjunctive agent such as a barbiturate or ketamine. Care is required in the absence of airway control as barbiturates in particular excel at depressing the respiratory drive and merit caution [44]. The use of sedation to avoid *delirium tremens* may prolong mechanical ventilation due to concerns about airway protection [45].

Diazepam may have a selective advantage in this circumstance as the majority of dosing occurs early in the clinical course to achieve acute control, followed by predictable decreases in sedative effect thereafter [46].

Other notable entities include intracranial hypertension (ICH) and intra-abdominal hypertension (IAH). With ICH, agitation increases intracranial pressure as well as cerebral oxygen consumption making sedation a key element in avoiding preventable secondary brain injury. The accurate determination of intra-abdominal pressure may require sedation, as may the therapeutic reduction in IAP by reducing abdominal wall tone, especially in those at risk of visceral edema or secondary ascites generation (i.e., secondary abdominal compartment syndrome). Therapeutic decreases in Intra-Abdominal Pressure (IAP) enhance venous return to preserve cardiac performance, but also increase blood flow across the kidneys by reducing renal vein hypertension; at times, deep sedation coupled with neuromuscular blockade is required and is consistent with recommendations from WSACS – the Abdominal Compartment Society [47].

Palliative Care at the End-of-Life

Symptom management is essential for those at the end-of-life where comfort and death with dignity are priorities. Analgesics are key in managing pain, and sedatives are excellent at mitigating anxiety or agitation. Both kinds of agents may be combined to achieve an individual patient's goals in this circumstance without concern about dependency induction in the dying patient [48]. Note is made that opioids and sedatives are commonly combined with a variety of other agents – some of which are used in a nonstandard acute medicine fashion for symptom mitigation but are not the subject of this review. One apt example is the use of haloperidol for nausea mitigation. The goal of combining opioids and sedatives in this focused group of patients include avoiding gasping, respiratory distress, or heightened anxiety when the end-of-life is imminent. In this way, combination therapy support patient- and family-centered care, improving the quality of the dying process for both. An overarching principle is that the smallest effective dose of any administered agent should be used in the support of quality of remaining life in a way that is consistent with the patient's explicitly stated or documented goals [49].

Special Circumstances

Maintenance Buprenorphine Products and Perioperative Considerations

There are several FDA-approved buprenorphine/naloxone products including buccal film (Bunavail®), sublingual film and tablet (Suboxone®), and sublingual tablets (Zubsolv®). Buprenorphine products without naloxone are also available including buccal film (Belbuca®), transdermal patch (Butrans®), sublingual tablet

(Subutex®), injectables (Buprenex®, Sublocade®), and a subcutaneous implant (Probuphine®). The first step in acute pain management is understanding the reason for receiving buprenorphine products including treatment of opioid dependence or chronic pain. If buprenorphine is used to treat opioid dependence, then it is imperative to understand the current phase of therapy: (1) induction; (2) stabilization; or (3) maintenance, as this will influence treatment decisions. The patient's current dose and last intake will also help guide therapeutic decision-making. Checking the state's drug monitoring program database could assist with understanding compliance and dosages. Communication with the patient concerning their medical history is key in deciding a management plan.

Managing acute onset, postoperative pain in patients receiving maintenance buprenorphine can be a challenge because of the decreased efficacy of opioids resulting from buprenorphine's high affinity for the mu receptor, long half-life, and partial agonism. While competitive affinity for the mu receptor is a concern, there is some data to suggest that receptors are still available for the binding of opioid agonists in the presence of buprenorphine products [50]. Importantly, maintenance buprenorphine cannot be considered an adequate treatment of acute onset postoperative pain. In general, it is recommended that non-opioid analgesics are provided for mild pain and continuous regional anesthesia, short-acting opioids, or PCA in combination with adjunctive therapies are considered for moderate to severe pain [51]. This approach to severe pain treatment will require diligent monitoring for the occurrence of adverse effects related to combination therapy.

Anticipated Surgery

Opioid-assisted treatment with buprenorphine/naloxone products is a newer approach to patient care and as such acute pain management for patients undergoing therapy lacks an evidence-based approach. Therefore, there is no consensus concerning the discontinuation or continuation of buprenorphine products before anticipated surgeries [51]. The 2004, the US Center for Substance Abuse Treatment recommended discontinuation of buprenorphine therapy [52]. However, as experience increases, expert opinion obtained in a Delphi manner published in 2019 recommends for continuation of therapy, even in combination with acute postoperative opioid agents [53]. Discontinuing buprenorphine therapy is complex and requires detailed planning.

Discontinuing buprenorphine for anticipated surgery ceases drug intake days to weeks before elective surgery. Patients who had their maintenance buprenorphine discontinued preoperatively are expected to require more analgesia for acute postoperative pain management compared to a patient who continues their preoperative therapy and receives postoperative opioids in addition to maintenance buprenorphine. Therefore, patients with buprenorphine products discontinued preoperatively should be considered opioid-tolerant patients requiring more substantial postoperative opioid doses [51]. If a patient discontinues buprenorphine products preoperatively, then it should not be the goal to resume therapy immediately postoperatively while taking other opioids as this could initiate an opioid withdrawal reaction. It is advised that a buprenorphine prescriber be consulted for re-initiation of maintenance therapy after the need for acute pain management using opioid agents has passed.

Unanticipated Surgery

It is more generally accepted to continue buprenorphine for emergent and urgent surgeries because of the lack of time to prepare a patient care plan. Additionally, acute discontinuation may require substantially larger opioid doses that increase the risk for postoperative opioid-induced respiratory depression during the initial 24-hour period after the last buprenorphine dose was ingested. These complexities are why buprenorphine is typically continued for unanticipated surgeries.

Maintenance Opioid Agonist Treatment for Patients Unable to Take Anything by Mouth

Methadone maintenance treatment provided to opioid or heroin dependent patients is increasing in frequency. The increase is largely driven by the current opioid epidemic that the country faces, although other uses include chronic pain management. Methadone is available in a number of formulations at present. Methadone is available as an injectable, tablet, dispersible diskets, solution, and as a concentrated solution. From a surgical perspective, questions arise concerning administration to patients who are directed to take nothing by mouth [54]. It is not ideal to miss any doses of the methadone maintenance treatment as withdrawal symptoms may arise in as little as 72 hours after the last methadone dose. In a diligent effort to avoid missing any doses, methadone can be administered by nasogastric tube, sublingual liquid or intravenously. Changes in the route of administration require consideration of the pharmacokinetic properties of the drug for an equipotent dose; consultation with a pharmacist is advised to avoid dosing error. Like buprenorphine above, continuing methadone maintenance therapy through anticipated and unanticipated surgery is increasingly common. Importantly, be cautious when prescribing a maintenance dose of methadone unless the dose is verified and discussions with the patient/caregiver confirm when the last dose was administered. Interrogation of a state database may be key in confirming details of maintenance therapy.

Methadone and Buprenorphine for Acute Pain Management

Methadone has been proposed as an alternative to morphine for the treatment of acute, postoperative pain and may be administered via PCA. The advantages of methadone over morphine are the lack of an active metabolite and lack of renal elimination [55]. Methadone administered after cesarean section via PCA resulted in similar pain control but less pruritus [56]. These data should be considered exploratory and not to be taken as standard practice nor standard of care.

Despite prevalent thoughts, the partial agonist properties of buprenorphine fail to demonstrate a ceiling effect and an anticipated lesser risk profile compared to standard opioids used for post-operative analgesia. A meta-analysis concluded that buprenorphine, when compared to morphine at equipotent doses for treatment of acute pain in an opioid naïve patient, appears to have similar analgesic effects and adverse effects; some decrease in pruritus was noted [57]. On the other hand, buprenorphine does offer a sublingual route of administration as a potential advantage for a patient with problematic intravenous access. An evolving approach to the use of methadone and buprenorphine for acute management is preoperative or intraoperative administration to reduce postoperative opioid requirements.

COVID-Related Issues

Opioid and sedative administration practices have shifted over the course of the pandemic. During the early period of personal protective equipment (PPE) shortage, when students, many clinicians, and family members were excluded from the hospital in large part, heavy sedation and analgesia was common [58]. That departure from the usual practice of minimized sedation and goal-achieving analgesia helped reduce the number of room entries per shift, limit clinician exposure to a COVID-19 positive patient, and preserve PPE. The recognition of different COVID-19 pneumonia phenotypes drove reduced invasive mechanical ventilation and directly reduced the need for sedation and analgesia compared to the early period of the pandemic known as the "first wave." Eliminating family members from the bedside also likely led to increased sedation, as family member presence helps maintain orientation and participation in daily care [59]. As the first wave waned, PPE supplies increased, and facilities reopened to usual care, opioid and sedation practices have also transitioned to usual dosing approaches. Regular digital connectivity with family members and other loved ones helps support non-pharmacologic approaches to sedation and analgesia. Throughout the pandemic, therapeutic agent shortages were common and aided by having a PharmD as a member of the critical care team to help guide appropriate agent selection, avoid undesirable medication interactions, achieve therapeutic goals, and enhance remote family education [60].

Best Practices for Opioid and Sedative Prescription in the ICU

A number of best practices may be articulated when using either opioids or sedatives in the ICU alone or as part of combination therapy. Eight such recommendations are provided below:

1. Establish an order set for each that clearly describes stepwise titration of agents for analgesia and sedation
2. Articulate and follow a pathway that routinely uses multimodal analgesia and does not rely exclusively or principally on opioid analgesics
3. Re-evaluate the agent and dose and route each day on bedside rounds, in particular in conjunction with an RT (who should be a routine team member)
4. Incorporate a clinical pharmacist into the ICU team to aid with agent selection, therapeutic substitution, and medication reconciliation as well as to avoid post-ICU polypharmacy
5. Train Advanced Practice Providers in sedation and analgesia management as well as the key tenets of Primary Palliative Medicine
6. Incorporate a Palliative Care Medicine physician into the ICU team
7. Routinely use non-pharmacologic approaches to pain management as well as sleep hygiene
8. Evaluate your ICU's performance on a quarterly basis in conjunction with team-member leadership

Conclusions

Both opioid analgesics and sedatives have important roles in critical care medicine management. Delineating a care plan and pathway for the safe and effective use of each agent, separately as well as in combination, is a wise approach for any ICU. Deliberate leveraging of APPs and clinical pharmacists as part of the care team helps support adherence to pathways, provides alternatives to commonly used agents, and may be particularly important for unique populations. Planning to routinely incorporate non-pharmacologic alternatives to opioids and sedatives helps decrease patient risk and improve ICU safety. Every ICU should develop, deploy, and regularly evaluate their performance along this key axis of patient care.

References

1. Nelson LS, Juurlink DN, Perrone J. Addressing the Opioid Epidemic. JAMA. 2015;314:1453–4.
2. Christopher Ingraham. Drug overdoses fell significantly in 2018 for first time in decades, provisional CDC data show. *Washington Post* Available at: https://beta.washingtonpost.com/business/2019/07/17/drug-overdoses-fell-significantly-first-time-decades-provisional-cdc-data-show/. Accessed: 27 Aug 2019.
3. Chamberlain JM, Klein BL. A comprehensive review of naloxone for the emergency physician. Am J Emerg Med. 1994;12:650–60.
4. Becker DE. Adverse Drug Interactions Anesthesia Progress. 2011;58:31–41.
5. Devlin JW, et al. Clinical practice guidelines for the prevention and Management of Pain, agitation/sedation, delirium, immobility, and sleep disruption in adult patients in the ICU. Crit Care Med. 2018;46:e825.

6. Joint Commission Enhances Pain Assessment and Management Requirements for Accredited Hospitals. The Official Publication of Joint Commission Requirements 37, 2–4 (2017).
7. Hauck LC, Bojko T. Opiate weaning in pediatric intensive care patients. Pediatr Crit Care Med. 2001;2:288.
8. Boren, L. L., Locke, A. M., Friedman, A. S., Blackmore, C. C. & Woolf, R. Team-based medicine: incorporating a clinical pharmacist into pain and opioid practice management. PM R. 2019. https://doi.org/10.1002/pmrj.12127.
9. Horn E, Jacobi J. The critical care clinical pharmacist: evolution of an essential team member. Crit Care Med. 2006;34:S46.
10. McCarter T, Shaik Z, Scarfo K, Thompson LJ. Capnography monitoring enhances safety of postoperative patient-controlled analgesia. Am Health Drug Benefits. 2008;1:28–35.
11. Lam T, et al. Continuous pulse oximetry and capnography monitoring for postoperative respiratory depression and adverse events: a systematic review and meta-analysis. Anesth Analg. 2017;125:2019–29.
12. Hagle M, Lehr V, Brubakken K, Shippee A. Respiratory depression in adult patients with intravenous patient-controlled analgesia. Orthop Nurs. 2004;23:18–27.
13. Chu LF, Angst MS, Clark D. Opioid-induced hyperalgesia in humans: molecular mechanisms and clinical considerations. Clin J Pain. 2008;24:479–96.
14. Luthra, P., Burr, N. E., Brenner, D. M. & Ford, A. C. Efficacy of pharmacological therapies for the treatment of opioid-induced constipation: systematic review and network meta-analysis. Gut. 2018. https://doi.org/10.1136/gutjnl-2018-316001.
15. Kurz A, Sessler DI. Opioid-induced bowel dysfunction: pathophysiology and potential new therapies. Drugs. 2003;63:649–71.
16. Roan JP, Bajaj N, Davis FA, Kandinata N. Opioids and Chest Wall rigidity during mechanical ventilation. Ann Intern Med. 2018;168:678.
17. Robertson R, Darsey E, Fortenberry J, Pettignano R, Hartley G. Evaluation of an opiate-weaning protocol using methadone in pediatric intensive care unit patients. Pediatr Crit Care Med. 2000;1:119–23.
18. Kyranou M, Puntillo K. The transition from acute to chronic pain: might intensive care unit patients be at risk? Ann Intensive Care. 2012;2:36.
19. De Oliveira GS, Castro-Alves LJ, McCarthy RJ. Single-dose systemic acetaminophen to prevent postoperative pain: a meta-analysis of randomized controlled trials. Clin J Pain. 2015;31:86–93.
20. Horlocker TT, et al. Regional anesthesia in the patient receiving antithrombotic or thrombolytic therapy: American Society of Regional Anesthesia and Pain Medicine evidence-based guidelines (fourth edition). Reg Anesth Pain Med. 2018;43:263.
21. Lee BH, et al. Pre-emptive and multi-modal perioperative pain management may improve quality of life in patients undergoing spinal surgery. Pain Physician. 2013;16:E217–26.
22. Avanos Pain Management. ON-Q* Pain relief system. Available at: https://avanospainmanagement.com/solutions/acute-pain/on-q-pain-relief-system/. Accessed: 27 Aug 2019.
23. Cheema FA, Chao E, Buchsbaum J, Giarra K, Parsikia A, Stone ME, Kaban JM. State of rib fracture care: a NTDB review of analgesic management and surgical stabilization. Am Surg. 2019;85(5):474–8.
24. Battlefield Acupuncture | Medical Acupuncture. Available at: https://www.liebertpub.com/doi/10.1089/acu.2007.0603. Accessed: 27 Aug 2019.
25. Pishkarmofrad Z, Navidian A, Ahmadabadi CA, Aliahmadi E. Effects of localized cryotherapy on the severity of thoracic pain in patients undergoing coronary artery bypass grafting. Surg Nurs J. 2016;5:22–7.
26. Chlan LL, et al. Effects of patient-directed music intervention on anxiety and sedative exposure in critically ill patients receiving mechanical ventilatory support: a randomized clinical trial. JAMA. 2013;309:2335–44.
27. Bradt, J. & Dileo, C. Music interventions for mechanically ventilated patients. Cochrane Database Syst Rev. CD006902. 2014. https://doi.org/10.1002/14651858.CD006902.pub3

28. Hughes CG, McGrane S, Pandharipande PP. Sedation in the intensive care setting. Clin Pharmacol. 2012;4:53–63.
29. Roberts DJ, Haroon B, Hall RI. Sedation for critically ill or injured adults in the intensive care unit: a shifting paradigm. Drugs. 2012;72:1881–916.
30. Mehta S, et al. Prevalence, risk factors, and outcomes of delirium in mechanically ventilated adults. Crit Care Med. 2015;43:557–66.
31. Ayad S, Khanna AK, Iqbal S, Singla N. Characterisation and monitoring of postoperative respiratory depression: current approaches and future considerations | Elsevier enhanced reader. Br J Anaesth. 2019;123:378–91.
32. Hemphill S, McMenamin L, Bellamy MC, Hopkins PM. Propofol infusion syndrome: a structured literature review and analysis of published case reports. Br J Anaesth. 2019 Apr 1;122(4):448–59.
33. Mirrakhimov AE, Voore P, Halytskyy O, Khan M, Ali AM. Propofol infusion syndrome in adults: a clinical update. Crit Care Res Prac. 2015;2015:1–10.
34. Hardin KA. Sleep in the ICU: potential mechanisms and clinical implications. Chest. 2009;136:284–94.
35. Hu, R. et al. Non-pharmacological interventions for sleep promotion in the intensive care unit. Cochrane Database Syst Rev. 2015; 2015.
36. Melatonin reduces the need for sedation in ICU patients: a randomized controlled trial. Minerva Anestesiologica. 2015; 81:1298–1310.
37. Marshall J, et al. Antipsychotic utilization in the intensive care unit and in transitions of care. J Crit Care. 2016;33:119–24.
38. American Geriatrics Society 2019 Updated AGS Beers Criteria® for potentially inappropriate medication use in older adults. J Am Geriatr Soc. 2019;67:674–694.
39. Green SM, Krauss B. Procedural sedation terminology: moving beyond "conscious sedation". Ann Emerg Med. 2002;39:433–5.
40. Practice Guidelines for Moderate Procedural Sedation and Analgesia 2018A Report by the American Society of Anesthesiologists Task Force on Moderate Procedural Sedation and Analgesia, the American Association of Oral and Maxillofacial Surgeons, American College of Radiology, American Dental Association, American Society of Dentist Anesthesiologists, and Society of Interventional Radiology. Anesthesia. 2018; 128:437–479.
41. SCCM | Home. Society of Critical Care Medicine (SCCM). Available at: https://sccm.org/ICULiberation/Home. Accessed: 27 Aug 2019.
42. de Haro C, et al. Effects of sedatives and opioids on trigger and cycling asynchronies throughout mechanical ventilation: an observational study in a large dataset from critically ill patients. Crit Care. 2019;23:245.
43. Alali AS, et al. Beta-blockers and traumatic brain injury: a systematic review and meta-analysis. Ann Surg. 2017;266:952–61.
44. Rosenson J, et al. Phenobarbital for acute alcohol withdrawal: a prospective randomized double-blind placebo-controlled study. J Emerg Med. 2013;44:592–8.
45. Brotherton AL, Hamilton EP, Kloss HG, Hammond DA. Propofol for treatment of refractory alcohol withdrawal syndrome: a review of the literature. Pharmacotherapy. 2016;36:433–42.
46. Weintraub SJ. Diazepam in the treatment of moderate to severe alcohol withdrawal. CNS Drugs. 2017;31:87–95.
47. Algorithms – WSACS – the Abdominal Compartment Society. Available at: http://www.wsacs.org/foam-resources/education/algorithms.html. Accessed: 27 Aug 2019.
48. Balducci L. Death and dying: what the patient wants. Ann Oncol. 2012;23:56–61.
49. Cherny NI, Portenoy RK. Sedation in the management of refractory symptoms: guidelines for evaluation and treatment. J Palliat Care. 1994;10:31–8.
50. Lembke A, Ottestad E, Schmiesing C. Patients maintained on buprenorphine for opioid use disorder should continue buprenorphine through the perioperative period. Pain Med. 2019;20:425–8.

51. Anderson TA, Quaye A, Ward EN, et al. To stop or not, That Is the Question: Acute Pain Management for the Patient on Chronic Buprenorphine. Anesthesiology. 2017;126:1180–6.
52. Center for Substance Abuse Treatment Clinical Guidelines for the Use of Buprenorphine in the Treatment of Opioid Addiction. Treatment Improvement Protocol (TIP) Series 40. DHHS Publication No. (SMA) 04–3939. Rockville: Substance Abuse and Mental Health; 2004.
53. Goel A, Azargive S, Weissman JS, et al. Perioperative pain and addiction interdisciplinary network (PAIN) clinical practice advisory for perioperative management of buprenorphine: results of a modified Delphi process. British J Anaesthesia. 2019;123:333–42.
54. Alford DP, Compton P, Samet JH. Acute pain Management for Patients Receiving Maintenance Methadone or buprenorphine therapy. Ann Intern Med. 2006;144:127–34.
55. Ebneshahidi A, Akbari M, Mohseni M, Heshmati B, Aghadavoudi O. Efficacy and safety of morphine versus methadone for patient-controlled analgesia: a randomized clinical trial. J Res Med Sci. 2012;1:8–12.
56. Ebneshahidi A., Akbari M. & Heshmati B. Patient-controlled versus nurse-controlled post-operative analgesia after caesarean section. Adv Biomed Res. 1; 2012. https://doi.org/10.4103/2277-9175.94428.
57. White LD, Hodge A, Vlok R, et al. Efficacy and adverse effects of buprenorphine in acute pain management: systematic review and meta-analysis of randomised controlled trials. Br J Anaesthia. 2018;120:688–78.
58. Ah Rhee CJ, Karass M, Abe O, Elshakh H, Kim M, Sajid F, Ju T, Voronina A, Al-Ghrairi A, El Marabti E, Mann J. Self-extubation rate and sedation requirement in covid-19. Chest. 2020;158(4):A634. https://doi.org/10.1016/j.Chest.2020.08.596. Epub 2020 Oct 12. PMCID: PMC7548811.
59. Davidson JE, Aslakson RA, Long AC, Puntillo KA, Kross EK, Hart J, Cox CE, Wunsch H, Wickline MA, Nunnally ME, Netzer G. Guidelines for family-centered care in the neonatal, pediatric, and adult ICU. Crit Care Med. 2017;45(1):103–28.
60. Halpern NA, Kaplan LJ, Rausen M, Yang JJ. Configuring ICUs in the COVID-19 Era: A collection of evolving experiences. https://www.sccm.org/COVID19RapidResources/Resources/Configuring-ICUs-in-the-COVID-19-Era-A-Collection. Accessed 1 Mar 2021.

Chapter 10
Acute Pain Management in Patients with Opioid Dependence

Arthur Kitt and Andrew Kim

Introduction

Opioid *dependence* refers to the state in which a patient requires an exogenous opioid in order to maintain normal physiologic functioning. Thus, if an individual goes a period of time without the drug, he/she would have symptoms of opioid withdrawal. Both the opioid dose and duration required to establish dependence are highly variable, but dependence can occur in opioid naïve patients in as few as 4–8 weeks [1]. *Addiction* is defined as a chronic condition in which an individual uses substances or engages in compulsive behaviors despite harmful negative consequences [2]. While dependence is defined by a physiologic state, addiction refers to a set of behaviors. In the context of opioids, almost all patients who are prescribed chronic opioid therapy become dependent but only some of them—from 2% to 27%—develop addiction [3].

While addiction and dependence are general terms used to describe behavioral and physiologic phenomena, the DSM-V outlines diagnostic criteria for an opioid-specific syndrome called *opioid use disorder* (OUD). The criteria for this disorder involve the occurrence of two of the following items within a 12-month period:

1. Taking larger amounts or taking drugs over a longer period than intended
2. Persistent desire or unsuccessful efforts to cut down or control opioid use
3. Spending a great deal of time obtaining or using the opioid or recovering from its effects
4. Craving, or a strong desire or urge to use opioids
5. Problems fulfilling obligations at work, school, or home
6. Continued opioid use despite having recurring social or interpersonal problems

---

A. Kitt (✉) · A. Kim
Department of Anesthesiology and Critical Care, Hospital of the University of Pennsylvania, Philadelphia, PA, USA
e-mail: Arthur.kitt@pennmedicine.upenn.edu; Andrew.kim2@pennmedicine.upenn.edu

J. L. Pascual, T. G. Gaulton (eds.), *Opioid Use in Critical Care*,
https://doi.org/10.1007/978-3-030-77399-1_10

7. Giving up or reducing activities because of opioid use
8. Using opioids in physically hazardous situations
9. Continued opioid use despite ongoing physical or psychological problem likely to have been caused or worsened by opioids
10. Tolerance (i.e., need for increased amounts or diminished effect with continued use of the same amount)
11. Experiencing withdrawal (opioid withdrawal syndrome) or taking opioids (or a closely related substance) to relieve or avoid withdrawal symptoms

An estimated 2.4 million Americans had OUD in 2015 [4]. Evidence has shown that the use of medication-assisted treatment (MAT) is effective in preventing relapse and lowering the cost of care for patients with OUD [5]. MAT combines the use of medication management with traditional counseling and behavioral therapies to prevent opioid relapse. MAT has been shown to effectively reduce the rates of illicit opioid use as well as all-cause mortality—largely due to decreased deaths related to overdose and suicide [6]. Acknowledging the proven benefits of MAT, public health officials have attempted to increase access to treatment for patients with OUD, and the number of patients on these medications has increased over the last several years.

There are three drugs that the Food and Drug Administration (FDA) has approved for the treatment of OUD—methadone, suboxone, and naltrexone. In 2015, the National Survey on Drug Use and Health estimated that 356,843 patients were treated with methadone, 76,116 patients treated with suboxone, and 13,934 patients treated with naltrexone as medication-assisted treatment for OUD [4]. Thus, roughly 18–20% of patients with OUD were treated with MAT in 2015—a percentage comparable to estimates from 2009 to 2013 [7]. Each of these drugs has unique pharmacodynamics that make them both ideal for use in MAT and challenging to manage when patients on these medications develop acute pain. As covered elsewhere in this text, chronic exposure to opioids leads to qualitative and quantitative changes in opioid receptors and thereby changes in patient response to opioids. Providers must consider many factors when managing a patient with opioid dependence, as they are at increased risk for:

- Opioid withdrawal
- Poor analgesia
- Respiratory depression
- Relapse for opioid use disorder

Since opioid dependent patients are already at increased risk for respiratory depression, providers must consider all additional patient related risk factors, including age > 65, obstructive sleep apnea, chronic obstructive pulmonary disease, cardiac disease, diabetes, and hypertension [8]. Additional sedatives among opioid-dependent patients should be avoided—both because they may decrease respiratory drive and because they may make it more difficult to identify oversedation as an early warning sign for respiratory depression. Providers may consider using continuous respiratory monitoring via continuous pulse oximeter or capnography in high-risk patients.

It is also important for providers caring for opioid-dependent patients to recognize signs of withdrawal. Early signs and symptoms of withdrawal include lacrimation, rhinorrhea, diaphoresis, restlessness, insomnia, and diffuse body and joint aches. Later signs may include tachycardia, hypertension, nausea/vomiting, diarrhea, dehydration, and hyperglycemia [5]. A validated clinical assessment tool used to evaluate the severity of opioid withdrawal is the Clinical Opiate Withdrawal Scale (COWS) [9]. This is an 11-point scale that incorporates physical signs and symptoms of withdrawal that can be used to guide treatment. Patients with mild symptoms may be treated with supportive therapy, such as antiemetics and clonidine. Patients with moderate to severe symptoms may warrant treatment with supplemental opioids [10]. In patients who are opioid dependent, management and prevention of withdrawal is a first step in treatment of acute pain.

Methadone

Methadone is a Drug Enforcement Agency schedule II drug that was invented by German scientists during World War II and approved by the FDA as an analgesic agent in 1947. It was then approved by the FDA for the treatment of opioid use disorder in 1972 and was the only medication designated for this purpose over the next 30 years. It remains by far the most common medication prescribed as MAT in the world and has a been widely shown to reduce death rates, HIV infection rates, unemployment, and rates of illicit opioid use among patients with opioid use disorder [11, 12]. Methadone use as MAT has also been associated with higher rates of retention in outpatient treatment programs. There are many reasons why methadone is successful in the treatment of patients with OUD, most of which arise out of its pharmacokinetic and pharmacodynamic traits.

Pharmacodynamics

Methadone is a synthetic opioid with full mu receptor agonism. It is a racemic mixture of two enantiomers—R-methadone acts as the mu receptor agonist and is more potent, as it has a tenfold higher affinity for opioid receptors than S-methadone [13]. It is unique from other opioids in that part of its clinical effect comes from its noncompetitive antagonism at NMDA receptors. This gives it further analgesic value, as NMDA receptors are involved in the pain signaling pathway. While different in their affinity for mu opioid receptors, both enantiomers have similar activity at the NMDA receptors. In addition to acting on mu opioid and NMDA receptors, methadone also is a potent serotonin and norepineprhine reuptake inhibitor, which further adds to its analgesic properties [14]. Its analgesic activity at the NMDA, serotonin, and norepinephrine receptors in addition to its mu agonism is believed to be the reason methadone can be more effective than other opioids for intractable pain states such as cancer pain [15]. Its potent analgesic activity, extended duration of action, and decreased euphoric and neurotoxic effects all help to make methadone an effective medication in the management of OUD.

Pharmacokinetics

Methadone has a mean 75% bioavailability when taken orally via liquid or tablet but can also be administered intravenously [16]. Methadone can be detected in plasma within 30 minutes of oral ingestion, with peak plasma concentrations noted after 2 to 4 hours followed by a slow and steady decline [17]. Methadone has a long and variable half-life, typically in the range of 8 to 59 hours, but averages 22 hours [16, 18]. Its long duration of action is attributed to extensive plasma protein binding, with approximately 90% of methadone being bound to plasma proteins, including albumin, lipoproteins, and alpha 1 glycoprotein following administration of a therapeutic dose [19, 20]. As alpha 1 glycoprotein is an acute phase reactant, methadone may have decreased efficacy in patients under stress due to an increase in protein binding.

Methadone is metabolized extensively in the liver as well as in the small intestines, though the metabolism of methadone is highly variable. Methadone is metabolized primarily by CYP3A4 and secondarily by CYP2D6, with CYP2D6 preferentially metabolizing R-methadone and CYP3A4 and CYP1A2 metabolizing both the R and S enantiomers [21]. CYP3A4 expression can vary up to 30-fold and genetic polymorphisms of CYP2D6 can result in a range of the rate of metabolism, from poor to rapid [21]. In addition, a wide variety of medications and substances can also induce or inhibit CYP3A4 and CYP2D6 and initiation of methadone itself can induce the CYP3A4 enzyme for a period of 5–7 days leading to low plasma levels initially followed by unexpectedly high levels after a week as the medication dose is increased [21]. The combination of differences in individual expression and polymorphisms of CYP3A4 and CYP2D6 and other medications and substances that affect enzymatic activity, account for the significant inter-individual variability in methadone half-life. Metabolites of methadone typically have little to no pharmacodynamic activity, and because it does not accumulate in patients with renal dysfunction and is minimally extracted with hemodialysis, is generally safe to administer in patients with renal dysfunction [22].

Adverse Effects

The side effects from methadone are qualitatively similar to that of other opioids, including constipation, nausea, cough suppression, respiratory depression, and gonadotropin/ACTH dysregulation. Methadone is distinct from other mu agonists in that it tends to produce less euphoria and sedation [23]. However, when dosed for pain, because the duration of action is shorter than its elimination half-life, patients are at increased risk for respiratory depression and death [21]. Methadone can also prolong the QTc interval, which can cause cardiac arrhythmias such as *torsade de pointes*. This is of particular concern in the setting of high dosages of methadone (greater than 60 mg/day), electrolyte aberrances, the use of IV Methadone (IV formulations contain chlorobutanol which further prolongs QTc intervals), or the concurrent use of a CYP3A4 inhibitor [24]. Thus, caution should be used when patients with a QTc greater than 500 ms are taking methadone or when administered with other drugs that prolong the QTc interval.

Dosing

As an analgesic, methadone has a duration of activity of approximately 4–8 hours [21]. Thus, when given for pain, methadone is typically prescribed two to three times per day. However, when methadone is dosed as MAT to prevent withdrawal or to suppress cravings, it is prescribed once daily. Given the large inter-individual variability in its pharmacokinetics, dosing of Methadone for both pain control and for MAT in patients with OUD is not straightforward and largely depends on the severity of pain and degree of opioid tolerance for each patient. Effective daily methadone doses for MAT typically fall between 60 to 100 mg per day, though higher and lower doses are not uncommon [16, 25]. Some studies have indicated that a higher dose of methadone is associated with lower rates of relapse [25, 26]. When patients are initiated on methadone for MAT, the recommended starting dose is 20 mg per day, which can be increased up to 10 mg per day as needed until the patient no longer has symptoms of withdrawal or cravings [16]. Doses typically should not exceed 60 mg per day in the first week or 100 mg per day in the subsequent week.

When transitioning from other opioids to methadone or vice versa, there is no consensus conversion ratio that has been shown to be uniformly effective. In one published review of studies involving methadone conversions for analgesia, researchers found that the most common ratios used when converting other opioids to methadone was a 4:1, 5:1, and 10:1 morphine equivalent dose ratio [27]. For example, if a 4:1 ratio were employed, a patient on 60 mg per day of oral morphine equivalence would be converted to 15 mg methadone per day. These studies showed a wide variation in terms of analgesic efficacy with these direct conversions [27]. Similarly, when converting methadone doses to oral morphine and other opioids, there is no consensus ratio used that results in equianalgesic potency. This is likely due to the wide variation in individual responses to methadone with regards to metabolism and opioid cross tolerance [27]. Thus, when converting from methadone to other opioids and vice versa, multiple dose adjustments may be required based on clinical effect.

Acute Pain Management

For patients using Methadone for MAT in the setting of OUD, acute pain management during hospitalization—particularly the peri-operative period—can be challenging. Patients with OUD have been shown to have increased sensitivity to pain and lowered pain tolerance compared to opioid naïve patients, and there is a paucity of research and lack of standardized protocols to guide pain control in this clinical context [28]. Whenever possible, a preadmission or preoperative evaluation can be helpful in order to set patient expectations, obtain a thorough pain and OUD history, identify critical medications being used to manage chronic pain, screen for high-risk psychiatric comorbidities, check an EKG to measure QTc interval, and discuss a perioperative pain plan with the patient [29].

For patients on daily methadone for MAT, an attempt should be made to continue the outpatient methadone dose during the hospitalization and during the perioperative period in order to cover physiologic opioid requirements and prevent withdrawal symptoms. Patients should continue their daily methadone dose up to and including the day of surgery. If enteral access is not available postoperatively, intravenous methadone can be substituted with a dose adjustment to account for the 75–80% bioavailability of oral methadone. The methadone can also be divided into three doses administered every 8 hours to assist with analgesia.

If methadone cannot be continued, conversion to another long-acting opioid is advisable. Bearing in mind the highly unpredictable equipotent ratios of methadone to other opioids, it is recommended that one consider a conservative estimate of morphine to methadone ratio from 4:1 to 10:1 [29]. This should be administered with caution and close monitoring of the patient. However, continuation of the outpatient methadone regimen or equipotent long–acting opioid will likely be inadequate in providing relief of the additional pain burden from an acute insult.

Short-acting opioid medications may additionally be required to achieve adequate analgesia, and patient controlled analgesia is one method of administration that has been shown to be effective in this population [29]. Whenever possible, non-pharmacologic interventions and opioid sparing medications should be considered to manage acute pain in these patients. Regional and neuraxial analgesia should be administered when applicable while analgesic adjuncts such as NSAIDs, gabapentin, and NMDA antagonists should be considered if there are no contraindications.

All patients on methadone in the acute pain setting require close monitoring for pain control as well as for side effects with a focus on respiratory depression and sedation. As previously mentioned, consideration for continuous capnography or pulse oximetry monitoring is recommended for patients at high risk for respiratory depression [8]. Discharge planning should include close communication with the outpatient methadone provider to verify discharge medications and inpatient dosing of methadone during the hospitalization. A clear plan for opioid prescriptions at discharge should be provided for the patient. Visiting caregivers and support people can also be utilized to assist with medication adherence.

Buprenorphine

Buprenorphine is a Drug Enforcement Agency Schedule III controlled substance. It is a semisynthetic, highly potent lipophilic opioid derived from the naturally occurring compound thebaine. It has partial agonism and a high binding affinity for the mu opioid receptor and antagonism with high binding affinity for the kappa and delta opioid receptors [30]. Like methadone, it can be used as an analgesic agent or an agent for MAT in patients with OUD. Buprenorphine is available in sublingual (Suboxone, Subutex, Zubsolv), buccal (Bunavail), implantable (Probuphine), and IM injectable (Sublocade) formulations for the treatment of OUD as well as parenteral (Buprenex), buccal (Belbuca), and transdermal (Butrans) formulations for the treatment of acute and chronic pain management [31]. The two forms that will be focused on in this chapter are the two most common forms administered, which are sublingual and transdermal. Sublingual formulations of buprenorphine can be combined with naloxone in a 4:1 ratio to reduce abuse potential that could result from aberrant IV use.

Pharmacodynamics

The effects of its partial agonism and high binding affinity for the mu opioid receptor make buprenorphine both a relatively safe analgesic agent and an ideal medication for use as MAT. Studies have shown that, while buprenorphine is indeed a partial agonist at the mu opioid receptor, there is no ceiling effect on its analgesic effect, which makes it a highly effective analgesic agent [32, 33]. Multiple studies in patients with chronic cancer and noncancer pain conditions have shown that transdermal buprenorphine is effective in relieving pain in a dose-dependent fashion [34, 35]. The efficacy of buprenorphine as an analgesic has been shown to be comparable to full mu opioid agonists in the treatment of chronic low back pain [36]. Because of its partial agonism at mu opioid receptors, there does appear to be a ceiling effect with respiratory depression, but its antagonism at kappa and delta opioid receptors indicate that it may also block the euphoric effects commonly seen with other opioids [33].

Another distinctive feature of buprenorphine is that it has a higher binding affinity for mu opioid receptors than other commonly administered opioids, including a 1.7x higher affinity than hydromorphone, 5.4x higher than morphine, and 6.2x higher than fentanyl [37]. This has multiple consequences when buprenorphine is co-administered with other opioids. The first is that it attenuates the effects of other opioids due to competitive inhibition. One study showed that hydromorphone that was administered after sublingual buprenorphine showed an attenuated clinical effect for up to 98 hours after buprenorphine discontinuation [38]. Another consequence of the higher binding affinity of buprenorphine is that, if it is initiated when patients have been receiving high doses of full mu opioid receptor agonists, buprenorphine will uncouple and replace the full agonist and potentially precipitate opioid withdrawal [28]. In order to prevent this, initiation of treatment with buprenorphine is typically recommended when a patient starts to have withdrawal symptoms after cessation of other opioids. If administered in this context, buprenorphine can then serve to mitigate withdrawal symptoms rather than precipitate them.

Pharmacokinetics

Buprenorphine can be administered in an intravenous, buccal, sublingual, and transdermal form, as bioavailability when taken in an oral formulation is poor [39]. The sublingual and buccal formulations of buprenorphine have a 51% and 28% bioavailability, respectively, although some of the newer buccal formulations cite higher percentages of bioavailability [40]. Transdermal bioavailability of buprenorphine is approximately 15% [30]. Upon entering systemic circulation, buprenorphine is 96% protein bound and then eventually metabolized in the liver to norbuprenorphine by the CYP3A4 enzymatic pathway, which has minimal pharmacodynamic activity [39].

Once buprenorphine binds to mu opioid receptors, its prolonged clinical effect is largely due to its prolonged binding time with the receptor [41]. Elimination of buprenorphine and its by-products occurs primarily through the feces, with 10–30% excreted in the urine [42]. In patients with renal impairment, buprenorphine clearance is roughly equivalent to that of patients with normal renal function and thus dosing and frequency does not need to be significantly adjusted in this population [43]. Patients with significantly impaired liver function have impaired metabolism and clearance of buprenorphine as well as increased bioavailability [44]. Thus, dosing of buprenorphine should be adjusted in patients with severe hepatic impairment.

Each formulation of buprenorphine has a distinct pharmacokinetic profile. The time to maximum plasma concentration for sublingual or buccal buprenorphine ranges from 40 minutes to 3.5 hours [39]. The half-life of sublingual buprenorphine has high variability in its elimination, ranging from 24 to 69 hours [45]. Intravenous buprenorphine has been shown to have an elimination half-life of roughly 5.2 hours [46]. After initiation of transdermal buprenorphine, time until minimum effective plasma concentration ranges from 11 to 21 hours with a half-life of 25 to 36 hours, both factors of which are dependent on dosing [47]. Higher doses of transdermal buprenorphine are associated with faster achievement of effective plasma concentration and longer elimination half-life [47]. In sublingual formulations of buprenorphine with naloxone, the bioavailability of naloxone is roughly 10% [48]. Thus, naloxone has minimal clinical effect when taken in the intended sublingual route. The inclusion of naloxone in the sublingual formulation is to negate any euphoria that buprenorphine can provide if the film were to be tampered with and converted into an injectate. The elimination half-life of sublingual naloxone is approximately 1–2 hours [48].

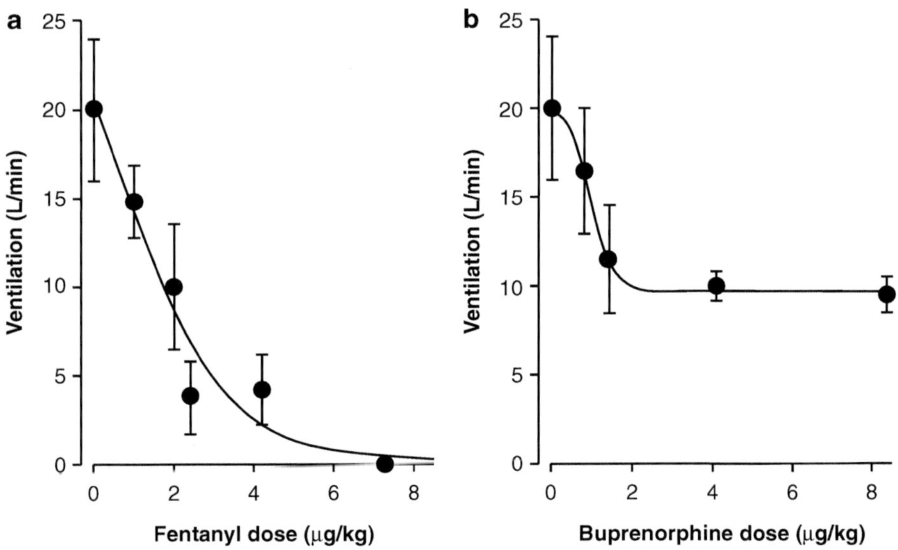

Fig. 10.1 Study showing the dose-response curves for minute ventilation after increasing doses of fentanyl vs buprenorphine [50]

Side Effects

Side effects of buprenorphine are similar to that of other opioids, including sedation, nausea, constipation, and pruritis. While respiratory depression can occur with buprenorphine, such cases have typically been seen when associated with concomitant use of other respiratory depressants such as benzodiazepines [28]. However, as depicted in Fig. 10.1, due to its partial agonism at the mu opioid receptor, buprenorphine has shown to have a ceiling effect for its change on minute ventilation when compared to a full agonist such as fentanyl [49].

As with other opioids, respiratory depression caused by buprenorphine can be reversed with administration of naloxone. However, higher doses of naloxone may be required to partially or fully reverse respiratory depression caused by buprenorphine due to its high binding affinity for the mu opioid receptor [51]. In regards to other side effects, transdermal buprenorphine appears to have lower rates of several side effects than other opioids, including constipation (1%), nausea (4%), and pruritis (0.7%) [52].

Dosing

While there are few validated studies in terms of equianalgesic potency, data available indicate that the ratio of transdermal buprenorphine to oral morphine is 1:110–115 [53]. A retrospective study among cancer and noncancer patients found similar analgesic potency between fentanyl 25 mcg/h patch, 60 mg oral morphine, and 35 mcg/h buprenorphine transdermal patch [53]. When applied via the transdermal route, the most commonly studied doses of buprenorphine for pain are 35 mcg/h and 70 mcg/h. These doses are typically not available in the United States, where transdermal buprenorphine is available as 7.5, 10, 15, and 20mcg/h patches. In regards to sublingual dosing of buprenorphine-naloxone, the typical starting dose used is 4 mg–1 mg every 12 hours and then increased until withdrawal symptoms are abated. Most studies have shown that a minimum dose of 8 mg daily of sublingual buprenorphine is required to abate withdrawal symptoms [54]. In PET studies showing mu opioid receptor availability, 16 mg sublingual doses of buprenorphine were associated with 87–92% occupancy of brain receptors and 32 mg sublingual doses were associated with 94–98% occupancy of mu opioid receptors in the brain [55].

Acute Pain Management

Due to some of its aforementioned unique pharmacologic characteristics, buprenorphine therapy can pose a challenge in the setting of acute pain. Whereas standard recommendations used to be to discontinue suboxone or buprenorphine for patients on chronic therapy 3–7 days prior to elective surgery, the current fund of literature has not shown any clear benefit to doing so [56]. More recent guidelines indicate that acute pain management can be achieved either by continuing buprenorphine or substituting it with other opioids based on context, while others advocate for consistent continuation of buprenorphine therapy through the perioperative period [28, 57–60]. Currently, there is no consensus on how buprenorphine therapy should be managed during the perioperative period.

Discontinuation of buprenorphine 3–7 days prior to surgery and substituting with another opioid such as methadone in theory would allow adequate time for buprenorphine elimination. In this scenario, the effects of other opioids given during the perioperative period would not be attenuated because mu opioid receptors would be available for full agonists to bind to. However, discontinuation of MAT and substitution with other opioids does put the patient at risk for relapse. When substituting other opioids for buprenorphine, it may also be difficult to predict baseline opioid requirements in order to prevent withdrawal symptoms prior to or after surgery for patients on chronic buprenorphine.

If buprenorphine were discontinued, opioids prescribed in the interim should be weaned and discontinued before restarting buprenorphine. This process should be carefully coordinated with the outpatient prescriber—especially if prescribed for MAT—in order to ensure resumption of treatment during a vulnerable time period in the treatment of OUD. One should not underestimate the risks associated with a gap in treatment of buprenorphine MAT, as studies have shown that mortality rate for patients in the first 4 weeks after treatment cessation is particularly high [61].

If the decision is made to continue buprenorphine throughout the perioperative period, or if buprenorphine cannot be discontinued prior to an episode of acute pain, providers must be aware that additional opioids prescribed are likely to have an attenuated effect. If buprenorphine is continued, patients will not have gaps in treatment and are unlikely to have withdrawal symptoms. Additionally, sublingual buprenorphine has been shown to be as effective as morphine as an analgesic when prescribed every 6 hours in the postoperative period [62].

However, higher doses of short-acting opioids than typically prescribed for opioid naïve patients will likely be required with close monitoring for side effects.

If a provider encounters the buprenorphine management conundrum prior to surgery, the issue should be discussed with the patient and his/her support team. The provider should discuss the risks and benefits of continuing and discontinuing buprenorphine during the perioperative period while also addressing any fears or concerns before a treatment strategy is decided upon. One consideration would be the risk of relapse or overdose when transitioning a patient with a history of OUD from buprenorphine to a full agonist. Other concerns the patient may have may include the risk of withdrawal if transitioned off buprenorphine or the risk of poorly controlled postoperative pain if buprenorphine is maintained.

While there is no clear evidence for the superiority of one strategy versus another, several protocols have been proposed for deciding on a management strategy. Most of the perioperative buprenorphine protocols that have been proposed suggest continuing buprenorphine when mild to moderate perioperative pain is expected. If buprenorphine is continued, it may be a more effective analgesic if it is divided into three daily doses. One protocol suggests that buprenorphine should be discontinued if severe perioperative pain is expected and daily buprenorphine dose is greater than 16 mg [31]. In situations when buprenorphine is discontinued, some protocols propose initiating a long-acting opioid such as methadone in order to cover baseline opioid requirements in addition to short-acting opioids as needed [60]. Regardless of whether buprenorphine is continued or discontinued, if moderate to severe pain is expected, multimodal analgesia should be considered. This would include use of regional or neuraxial analgesia when possible and use of analgesic adjunctive medications such as acetaminophen, NSAIDs, ketamine, and gabapentinoids [28]. Close monitoring for signs of withdrawal, cravings, over sedation, and respiratory depression should be implemented.

Naltrexone

Naltrexone is a semisynthetic mu opioid receptor antagonist that was derived from oxymorphone and is used as a treatment as MAT for OUD and alcohol dependence [57]. It is widely available in the United States in two formulations—a daily oral formulation called Revia® and a monthly (every 28 days) intramuscular injectable formulation called Vivitrol®. Naltrexone is useful for MAT in these formulations because, unlike opioid antagonists like naloxone, naltrexone can be orally bioavailable and have an extended half-life. It has been FDA approved for the treatment of alcohol dependence since 1994 and was FDA approved for use in the treatment of

OUD in 1984. The use of naltrexone has been shown to be effective in reducing the euphoria and cravings associated with alcohol use because of its ability to block the endogenous opioid activity involved in the alcohol reinforcement pathway [63]. Similarly, naltrexone blocks euphoric effects associated with any concomitant opioid use. However, through the years, researchers have found there to be poor adherence practices among patients prescribed oral naltrexone for both of these conditions [64]. A Cochrane review showed that oral naltrexone, likely because of its low adherence (28%), showed no difference with placebo in preventing relapse among those with OUD [65]. The monthly intramuscular injectable version of naltrexone was designed to improve treatment adherence. One study showed a 61% adherence rate among patients receiving injectable naltrexone after 1 year and found there to be decreased rates of illicit opioid use [66].

Pharmacodynamics

Naltrexone is distinct from other agents used for MAT in that it is a mu opioid receptor competitive antagonist. It also has partial agonism at kappa opioid receptors [67]. Like buprenorphine, naltrexone also has a high binding affinity for mu opioid receptors. When administered under normal physiologic conditions, naltrexone has minimal clinical effect [63]. Under conditions of physiologic stress and pain, naltrexone can block the effects of endogenous opioids. When exogenous opioids are administered, naltrexone blocks nearly all of their effects when it is administered and has reached a minimum plasma concentration of 1 ng/ml [67]. When the standard 50 mg daily oral dose of oral naltrexone is administered, PET studies have shown that 95% of mu opioid receptors in the brain are occupied, with minimal inter-subject variability [68]. Naltrexone not only inhibits the euphoric and analgesic effects of opioids, administration of naltrexone can precipitate withdrawal symptoms for a patient who recently used opioids. In order to avoid these withdrawal symptoms, initiation of naltrexone therapy is recommended only after a patient has been abstinent from opioids for at least 7–10 days.

While the primary action of naltrexone is to block exogenous and endogenous mu agonist activity, another important physiologic effect of naltrexone treatment is that it can cause increased proliferation and activity of mu opioid receptors. In a study involving male rats, those that received naltrexone infusions for 7 days had increased levels of mu receptor immunoreactivity and binding sites when compared with those that received placebo infusions [69]. The higher rate of mu opioid receptor binding in this state is thought to be due to a change from mu receptors to an active configuration after exposure to naltrexone. Extrapolated to humans, this information indicates that patients on chronic naltrexone therapy are likely to have higher sensitivity to the effects of opioids once naltrexone is eliminated. This must be taken into account when caring for a patient in whom naltrexone was recently discontinued.

Pharmacokinetics

While oral naltrexone has absorption, it undergoes extensive first-pass metabolism—from 5% to 60% [70]. Oral naltrexone reaches a peak effect after 1 hour and has an elimination half-life of 10 hours when used daily for at least 7 days [67]. Intramuscular injectable naltrexone is encapsulated in a biodegradable polymer that slowly degrades after injected. Injectable naltrexone reaches a peak serum concentration after 2 days and has a 5 to 7 day elimination half-life [64]. The plasma concentration of the injectable naltrexone then exhibits a slow decline after 14 days, but appears to reliably maintain a minimally effective concentration for 28 days after it is administered—see Fig. 10.2. Both oral and injectable naltrexone, after metabolized by aldo-keto reductase enzymes in the liver cytosol, produce the active metabolite 6β naltrexol [71]. The metabolite 6-naltrexol exhibits weaker antagonism compared to its parent compound but displays a longer half-life of 12 hours for a single oral dose [72]. It is then eliminated by the kidneys in urine [23]. Because of its active metabolite with weak mu opioid antagonist activity, the activity of naltrexone can be prolonged in patients with renal impairment. The half-life of both oral and injectable naltrexone do not vary significantly between chronic or one time use [64, 70].

Side Effects

Early side effects that are associated with naltrexone induction are those associated with opioid withdrawal, including nausea, diaphoresis, diarrhea, restlessness, etc. Because of increased proliferation of opioid receptors and receptor availability for patients on naltrexone, those who have recently discontinued naltrexone are at increased risk for opioid induced respiratory depression and overdose [5]. Additionally, patients on naltrexone are at risk for drug-induced hepatitis and should have their liver function monitored periodically while on this medication. A common side effect of injectable naltrexone is pruritis or a rash at the injection site [64]. There has been an association between naltrexone treatment and dysphoria, but the mechanism for this is unclear and may be multifactorial [73].

Dosing

Standard doses are applied for both oral daily and monthly intramuscular injectable naltrexone. The standard oral daily dose of naltrexone is 50 mg, but some providers start naltrexone induction with a half-dose of 25 mg to minimize withdrawal symptoms [5]. In some situations, patients are transitioned from a daily to a three times per week regimen but still take 350 mg per week in three divided doses. The standard dosage of intramuscular injectable naltrexone is 380 mg every 4 weeks.

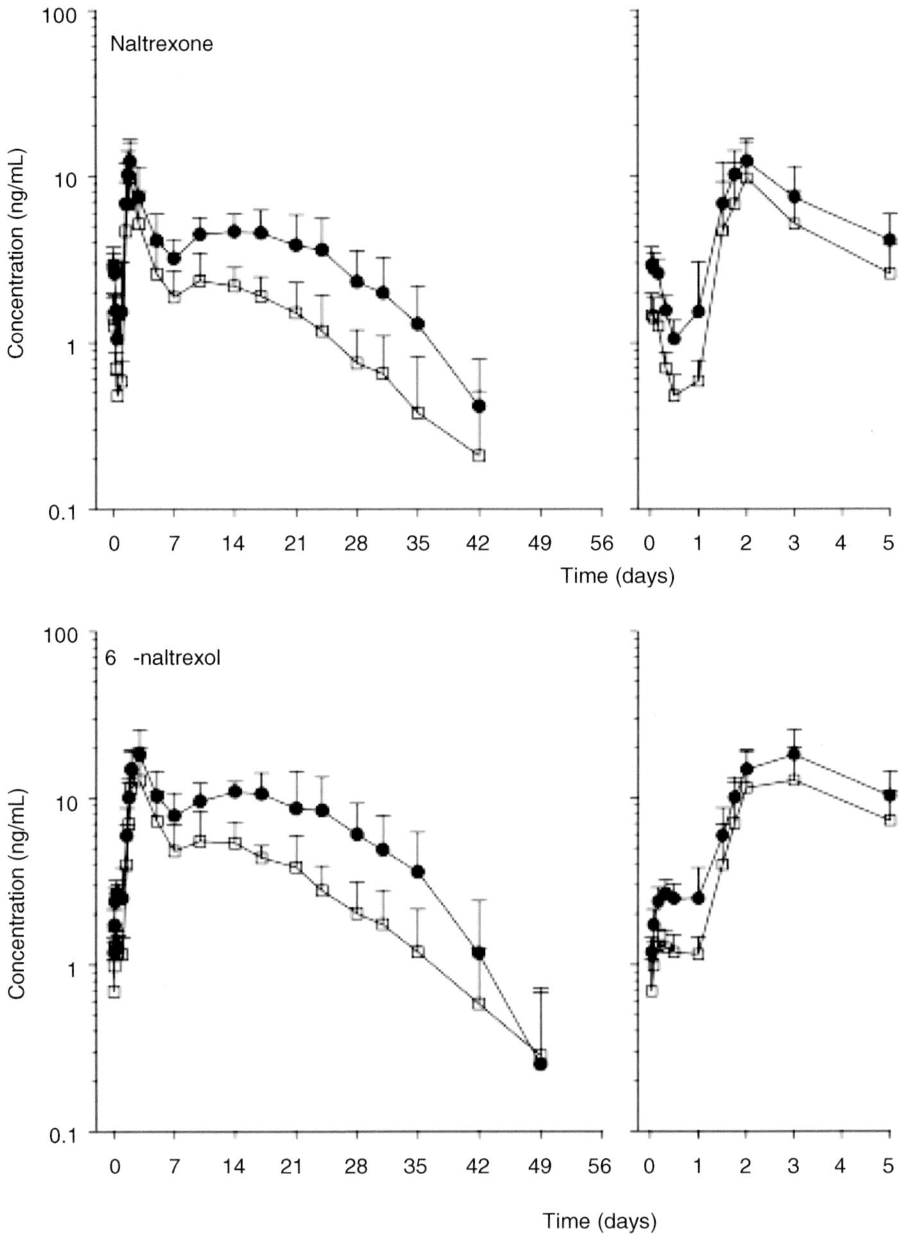

Fig. 10.2 Plasma concentrations of naltrexone and 6β-naltrexone after IM injections of 380 mg (top) and 190 mg (bottom) naltrexone [64]

Acute Pain Management

Unlike with buprenorphine management, if the provider has the opportunity to discontinue oral or injectable naltrexone prior to a painful surgery or insult, they should do so. Oral naltrexone should be discontinued at least 72 hours before a painful surgery or insult, and intramuscular injectable naltrexone should be discontinued for at least 4 weeks [28].

For patients whom naltrexone is able to be discontinued appropriately prior to the painful surgery or insult, providers must be aware that any opioids given may have an exaggerated response due to increased opioid receptors and availability [74]. These patients should not be treated like opioid tolerant patients who require higher doses of opioids to achieve analgesia and have higher thresholds for respiratory depression. Opioid sparing multimodal techniques should be employed in these patients, such as regional or neuraxial analgesia when appropriate and use of non-opioid adjunctive medications.

Once the patients are weaned off of any opioids postoperatively, the patient should then restart naltrexone in either form approximately 7 days after discontinuation to avoid causing withdrawal symptoms. Close coordination of care should be discussed with the patient and his/her outpatient naltrexone provider, including an opioid stop date and a plan to resume MAT.

If the provider has to manage a patient with acute pain who has not stopped their naltrexone, the provider must be very aware of its pharmacodynamics and duration of action. During the period of with expected naltrexone activity—28 days since the last injectable naltrexone or roughly 2–3 days for oral naltrexone—the effect of any additional opioids given will be significantly attenuated. Pain control will be difficult to achieve with opioids and every effort should be made to utilize neuraxial or regional analgesia and analgesic adjunctive medications. Providers must be aware of the timing of naltrexone washout, as the patient may go from exceedingly opioid tolerant to opioid sensitive once the drug is eliminated. Close patient monitoring during this time period is critical to avoid opioid induced respiratory depression. Discussion with the patient and his outpatient naltrexone provider is necessary upon discharge in order to coordinate a plan for resumption of MAT.

Conclusion

Patients who use methadone, buprenorphine, or naltrexone present a unique challenge in the inpatient and acute care setting. Each drug has unique pharmacokinetics and pharmacodynamics that can make it challenging to manage acute pain, prevent withdrawal, and avoid opioid-related adverse events. The strategies for the management of acute pain for patients who regularly take each of these medications—as well as some of their properties—are summarized below.

Methadone:

1. Maintain home/physiologic dose to prevent withdrawal
   (a) Continue daily methadone dose or split into three divided doses
   OR
   (b) Switch to another long-acting opioid, use a MED conversion of 4:1 to 10:1
2. Administer additional analgesia to treat acute pain
   (a) Neuraxial, regional, or site-specific local anesthetic techniques when applicable
   (b) Supplemental short-acting opioids may be required; patient-controlled analgesia may be useful
   (c) Analgesic adjuncts may be administered, such as acetaminophen, NSAIDs, neuroleptics (gabapentin, pregabalin), SNRIs, muscle relaxants, NMDA antagonists
3. If discontinued, may resume at any time while taking into consideration doses of other concurrent opioids.

Buprenorphine:

1. Maintain home/physiologic dose to prevent withdrawal
   (a) Continue home dose of buprenorphine
   OR
   (b) Replace buprenorphine with full opioid agonist, preferentially long acting (e.g., methadone)
2. Administer additional analgesia to treat acute pain
   (a) Neuraxial, regional, or site-specific local anesthetic techniques when applicable.
   (b) Supplemental short-acting opioids may be required but their effects will be attenuated if buprenorphine is present; patient-controlled analgesia may be useful.
   (c) Analgesic adjuncts may be administered, such as acetaminophen, NSAIDs, neuroleptics (gabapentin, pregabalin), SNRIs, muscle relaxants, NMDA antagonists
3. If discontinued, may resume when patient has been weaned down or off of other opioids so as not to precipitate withdrawal.

Naltrexone:

1. Depending on the formulation taken, opioids will be rendered largely ineffective for
   (a) 2–3 days after last PO dose.
   (b) 28 days after last IM dose.

Table 10.1 Characteristics of drugs commonly prescribed for medication-assisted treatment

Drug	Common Formulations	Peak Onset	Half Life	Responsiveness to other opioids
Methadone	Oral, IV	2–4 hours	8–59 hours (average 22)	Opioid tolerant; effects of opioids are additive
Buprenorphine	Sublingual (SL), Buccal, Transdermal (TD)	SL: 40 min – 3.5 hours TD: 11–21 hours	SL: 24–69 hours TD: 25–36 hours	Opioid tolerant; effects of other opioids are additive but attenuated if buprenorphine is still present
Naltrexone	Oral (PO), Intramuscular (IM)	PO: 1 hour IM: 2 days (IM)	PO: 10 hours IM: 5–7 days	Opioid sensitive; effects of other opioids are severely attenuated if naltrexone is still present, but dramatically enhanced once naltrexone is eliminated

AFTER which patients will be highly opioid sensitive

2. Administer additional analgesia to treat acute pain
   (a) Neuraxial, regional, or site-specific local anesthetic techniques when applicable.
   (b) Analgesic adjuncts will likely be necessary, such as acetaminophen, NSAIDs, neuroleptics (gabapentin, pregabalin), SNRIs, muscle relaxants, NMDA antagonists.
3. To restart, must wait at least 7 days after discontinuation of other opioids to restart in order to avoid precipitating withdrawal (Table 10.1).

References

1. Sharma B, Bruner A, Barnett G, Fishman M. Opioid use disorders. Child Adolesc Psychiatr Clin N Am. 2016;25(3):473–87.
2. Definition of Addiction [Internet] American society of addiction medicine. 2019. p. 117–24. Available from: https://www.asam.org/docs/default-source/quality-science/asam's-2019-definition-of-addiction-(1).pdf?sfvrsn=b8b64fc2_2.
3. Ballantyne JC, LaForge KS. Opioid dependence and addiction during opioid treatment of chronic pain. Pain. 2007;129(3):235–55.
4. Cathie E. Alderks PD. Trends in the use of methadone, buprenorphine, and extended-release naltrexone at substance abuse treatment facilities: 2003-2015 [internet]. The CBHSQ Report. Available from: https://www.samhsa.gov/data/sites/default/files/report_3192/ShortReport-3192.html
5. Substance Abuse and Mental Health Services Administration. Medications for opioid use disorder. Treatment Improvement Protocol (TIP) Series 63, Full Document. 2019;(HHS Publication No. (SMA) 19-5063FULLDOC).
6. Degenhardt L, Randall D, Hall W, Law M, Butler T, Burns L. Mortality among clients of a state-wide opioid pharmacotherapy program over 20 years: risk factors and lives saved. Drug Alcohol Depend. 2009;105(1–2):9–15.

7. Saloner B, Karthikeyan S. Changes in substance abuse treatment use among individuals with opioid use disorders in the United States, 2004-2013. JAMA. 2015;314(14):1515–7.
8. Gupta K, Prasad A, Nagappa M, Wong J, Abrahamyan L, Chung FF. Risk factors for opioid-induced respiratory depression and failure to rescue: a review. Curr Opin Anaesthesiol. 2018;31(1):110–9.
9. Wesson DR, Ling W. The clinical opiate withdrawal scale (COWS). J Psychoactive Drugs. 2003;35(2):253–9.
10. Organization. WH. Clinical guidelines for withdrawal management and treatment of drug dependence in closed settings. [Internet]. 2009. Available from: https://www.ncbi.nlm.nih.gov/books/NBK310652/.
11. Peles E, Schreiber S, Adelson M. 15-year survival and retention of patients in a general hospital-affiliated methadone maintenance treatment (MMT) center in Israel. Drug Alcohol Depend [Internet] 2010;107(2–3):141–148. Available from: https://doi.org/10.1016/j.drugalcdep.2009.09.013
12. Farrell M, Ward J, Mattick R, Hall W, Stimson GV, Des Jarlais D, et al. Fortnightly review: methadone maintenance treatment in opiate dependence: a review. BMJ. 1994;309(6960):997.
13. Trescot A. Treatment of chronic pain by medical approaches. Clinical use of opioids. New York, NY: Springer; 2015. p. 99–110.
14. Codd EE, Shank RP, Schupsky JJ. Serotonin and norepinephrine uptake inhibiting activity of centrally acting analgesics: structural determinants and role in antinociception. J Pharmacol Exp Ther. 1995;274:1263–70.
15. Fürst P, Lundström S, Klepstad P, Runesdotter S, Strang P. Improved pain control in terminally ill cancer patients by introducing low-dose oral methadone in addition to ongoing opioid treatment. J Palliat Med. 2018;21(2):177–81.
16. Eap CB, Buclin T, Baumann P. Interindividual variability of the clinical pharmacokinetics of methadone: implications for the treatment of opioid dependence. Clin Pharmacokinet. 2002;41(14):1153–93.
17. Payte JT, Zweben JE. Opioid maintenance therapies. In: Principles of addiction medicine. Chevy Chase: American Societ of Addiction Medicine; 1998. p. 557–70.
18. Walsh LS, Strain EC. Pharmacology of methadone. In: Strain EC, Stitzer ML, editors. The treatment of opioid dependence. Baltimore: Johns Hopkins University Press; 2006. p. 59–76.
19. Brunton L, Parker K. No title. In: Goodman and Gilman's Manual of Pharmacology and Therapeutics. New York: McGraw-Hill; 2008. p. 351–71.
20. Eap C, Cuendet C, Baumann P. Binding of d-, l-, and dl-methadone, and dl-methadone to proteins in plasma of healthy volunteers: role of the variants of alphar1-acid glycoprotein. Clin Pharmacol Ther. 1990;47:338–46.
21. Trescot A. Clinical use of opioids. In: Treatment of chronic pain by medical approaches. New York: Springer; 2015. p. 99–110.
22. Davis MP, Walsh D. Methadone for relief of cancer pain: a review of pharmacokinetics, pharmacodynamics, drug interactions and protocols of administration. Support Care Cancer. 2001;9(2):73–83.
23. Miyoshi HR, Leckband SG. Systemic opioid analgesics. In: Bonica's management of pain. 3rd editio. Philadelphia: Lippincott Williams and Wilkins; 2001. p. 1202–1220.
24. Kornick CA, Kilborn MJ, Santiago-Palma J, Schulman G, Thaler HT, Keefe DL, et al. QTc interval prolongation associated with intravenous methadone. Pain. 2003;105(3):499–506.
25. Strain EC, Bigelow GE, Liebson IA, Stitzer ML. Moderate- vs high-dose methadone in the treatment of opioid dependence: a randomized trial. J Am Med Assoc. 1999;281(11):1000–5.
26. Ling W, Wesson DR, Charuvastra C, Klett CJ. A controlled trial comparing buprenorphine and methadone maintenance in opioid dependence. Arch Gen Psychiatry. 1996;53(5):401–7.
27. Weschules DJ, Bain KT. A systematic review of opioid conversion ratios used with methadone for the treatment of pain. Pain Med. 2008;9(5):595–612.
28. Ward EN, Quaye ANA, Wilens TE. Opioid use disorders: perioperative management of a special population. Anesth Analg. 2018;127(2):539–47.

29. Peng PWH, Tumber PS, Gourlay D. Review article: perioperative pain management of patients on methadone therapy. Can J Anesth. 2005;52(5):513–23.
30. Gudin J, Fudin J. A narrative pharmacological review of buprenorphine: a unique opioid for the treatment of chronic pain. Pain Ther [Internet]. 2020. Available from: https://doi.org/10.1007/s40122-019-00143-6.
31. Quaye AN-A, Zhang Y. Perioperative management of buprenorphine: solving the conundrum. Pain Med. 2019;20(7):1395–408.
32. Pergolizzi J, Aloisi AM, Dahan A, Filitz J, Langford R, Likar R, et al. Current knowledge of buprenorphine and its unique pharmacological profile. Pain Pract. 2010;10(5):428–50.
33. Dahan A, Yassen A, Romberg R, Sarton E, Teppema L, Olofsen E, et al. Buprenorphine induces ceiling in respiratory depression but not in analgesia. Br J Anaesth [Internet]. 2006;96(5):627–632. Available from: https://doi.org/10.1093/bja/ael051
34. Poulain P, Denier W, Douma J, Hoerauf K, Šamija M, Sopata M, et al. Efficacy and safety of transdermal buprenorphine: a randomized, placebo-controlled trial in 289 patients with severe cancer pain. J Pain Symptom Manag. 2008;36(2):117–25.
35. Likar R, Kayser H, Sittl R. Long-term management of chronic pain with transdermal buprenorphine: a multicenter, open-label, follow-up study in patients from three short-term clinical trials. Clin Ther. 2006;28(6):943–52.
36. Steiner DJ, Sitar S, Wen W, Sawyerr G, Munera C, Ripa SR, et al. Efficacy and safety of the seven-day buprenorphine transdermal system in opioid-Naïve patients with moderate to severe chronic low back pain: an enriched, randomized, double-blind, placebo-controlled study. J Pain Symptom Manage [Internet]. 2011;42(6):903–17. Available from:. https://doi.org/10.1016/j.jpainsymman.2011.04.006.
37. Volpe DA, Tobin GAMM, Mellon RD, Katki AG, Parker RJ, Colatsky T, et al. Uniform assessment and ranking of opioid Mu receptor binding constants for selected opioid drugs. Regul Toxicol Pharmacol [Internet] 2011;59(3):385–390. Available from: https://doi.org/10.1016/j.yrtph.2010.12.007
38. Correia CJ, Walsh SL, Bigelow GE, Strain EC. Effects associated with double-blind omission of buprenorphine/naloxone over a 98-h period. Psychopharmacology. 2006;189(3):297–306.
39. Elkader A, Sproule B. Buprenorphine. Clinical pharmaokinetics in the treatment of opioid dependence. Clin Pharmacokinet. 2005;44(7):661–80.
40. Kuhlman JJ, Lalani S, Magluilo J, Levine B, Darwin WD, Johnson RE, et al. Human pharmacokinetics of intravenous, sublingual, and buccal buprenorphine. J Anal Toxicol. 1996;20(6):369–78.
41. Sutcliffe KJ, Henderson G, Kelly E, Sessions RB. Drug binding poses relate structure with efficacy in the μ opioid receptor. J Mol Biol [Internet]. 2017;429(12):1840–51. Available from: https://doi.org/10.1016/j.jmb.2017.05.009
42. Walter D, Inturrisi C. Absorption, disctribution, metabolism, and exretion of buprenorphine in animals and humans. In: Cowan A, Lewis J, editors. Buprenorphine: combating drug abuse with a unique opioid. Wiley-Liss; 1995. p. 113–35.
43. Hand CW, Sear JW, Uppington J, Ball MJ, Mcquay HJ, Moore RA. Buprenorphine disposition in patients with renal impairment: single and continuous dosing, with special reference to metabolites. Br J Anaesth [Internet] 1990;64(3):276–282. Available from: https://doi.org/10.1093/bja/64.3.276
44. Furlan V, Demirdjian S, Bourdon O, Magdalou J, Taburet AM. Glucuronidation of drugs by hepatic microsomes derived from healthy and cirrhotic human livers. J Pharmacol Exp Ther. 1999;289(2):1169–75.
45. Kuhlman JJ, Levine B, Johnson RE, Fudala PJ, Cone EJ. Relationship of plasma buprenorphine and norbuprenorphine to withdrawal symptoms during dose induction, maintenance and withdrawal from sublingual buprenorphine. Addiction. 1998;93(4):549–59.
46. Bullingham R, McQuay H, Porter E, Allen M, Moore R. Sublingual buprenorphine used postoperatively: ten hour plasma drug concentration analysis. Br J Clin Pharmacol. 1982;13(5):665–73.

47. Comparison C, Likar R, Lorenz V, Korak-leiter M, Kager I, Sittl R, et al. Transdermal buprenorphine patches applied in a 4-day regimen versus a 3-day regimen : a single-site , Phase lll. Clin Ther. 2007;29(8):1591–606.
48. Harris DS, Jones RT, Welm S, Upton RA, Lin E, Mendelson J. Buprenorphine and naloxone co-administration in opiate-dependent patients stabilized on sublingual buprenorphine. Drug Alcohol Depend. 2000;61(1):85–94.
49. Dahan A, Yassen A, Bijl H, Romberg R, Sarton E, Teppema L, et al. Comparison of the respiratory effects of intravenous buprenorphine and fentanyl in humans and rats. Br J Anaesth [Internet] 2005;94(6):825–834. Available from: https://doi.org/10.1093/bja/aei145
50. Dahan A. Opioid-induced respiratory effects: new data on buprenorphine. Palliat Med. 2006;20(SUPPL. 1):3–8.
51. Dahan A. Opioid-induced respiratory effects: new data on buprenorphine. Palliat Med. 2006;20:S3–8.
52. Griessinger N, Sittl R, Likar R. Transdermal buprenorphine in clinical practice - a post-marketing surveillance study in 13179 patients. Curr Med Res Opin. 2005;21(8):1147–56.
53. Sittl R, Likar R, Nautrup BP. Equipotent doses of transdermal fentanyl and transdermal buprenorphine in patients with cancer and noncancer pain: results of a retrospective cohort study. Clin Ther. 2005;27(2):225–37.
54. Hjelmström P, Banke Nordbeck E, Tiberg F. Optimal dose of buprenorphine in opioid use disorder treatment: a review of pharmacodynamic and efficacy data. Drug Dev Ind Pharm [Internet]. 2020;46(1):1–7. Available from: https://doi.org/10.1080/03639045.2019.1706552.
55. Greenwald MK, Johanson CE, Moody DE, Woods JH, Kilbourn MR, Koeppe RA, et al. Effects of buprenorphine maintenance dose on μ-opioid receptor availability, plasma concentrations, and antagonist blockade in heroin-dependent volunteers. Neuropsychopharmacology. 2003;28(11):2000–9.
56. Goel A, Azargive S, Lamba W, Bordman J, Englesakis M, Srikandarajah S, et al. The perioperative patient on buprenorphine: a systematic review of perioperative management strategies and patient outcomes. Can J Anesth [Internet]. 2019;66(2):201–217. Available from: https://doi.org/10.1007/s12630-018-1255-3.
57. Harrison TK, Kornfeld H, Aggarwal AK, Lembke A. Perioperative considerations for the patient with opioid use disorder on buprenorphine, methadone, or naltrexone maintenance therapy. Anesthesiol Clin [Internet]. 2018;36(3):345–359. Available from: https://doi.org/10.1016/j.anclin.2018.04.002.
58. Lembke A, Ottestad E, Schmiesing C. Patients maintained on buprenorphine for opioid use disorder should continue buprenorphine through the perioperative period. Pain Med (United States). 2019;20(3):425–8.
59. Jonan AB, Kaye AD, Urman RD. Buprenorphine formulations: clinical best practice strategies recommendations for perioperative management of patients undergoing surgical or interventional pain procedures. Pain Physician. 2018;21(1):E1–12.
60. Alford DP, Compton P, Samet JH. Acute pain management for patients receiving maintenance methadone or buprenorphine therapy. Ann Intern Med. 2006;144(2):127–34.
61. Sordo L, Barrio G, Bravo MJ, Indave BI, Degenhardt L, Wiessing L, et al. Mortality risk during and after opioid substitution treatment: systematic review and meta-analysis of cohort studies. BMJ. 2017;357:j1550.
62. Alizadeh S, Mahmoudi GA, Solhi H, Sadeghi-Sedeh B, Behzadi R, Kazemifar AM. Post-operative analgesia in opioid dependent patients: comparison of intravenous morphine and sublingual buprenorphine. Addict Heal [Internet]. 2015;7(1–2):60–5. Available from: http://www.ncbi.nlm.nih.gov/pubmed/26322212%0A http://www.pubmedcentral.nih.gov/articlerender.fcgi?artid=PMC4530195
63. Unterwald EM. Naltrexone in the treatment of alcohol dependence. J Addict Med. 2008;2(3):121–7.

64. Dunbar JL, Turncliff RZ, Dong Q, Silverman BL, Ehrich EW, Lasseter KC. Single- and multiple-dose pharmacokinetics of long-acting injectable naltrexone. Alcohol Clin Exp Res. 2006;30(3):480–90.
65. Minozzi S, Amato L, Vecchi S, Davoli M, Kirchmayer U, Verster A. Oral naltrexone maintenance treatment for opioid dependence. Cochrane Database Syst Rev. 2011;.
66. Krupitsky E, Nunes EV, Ling W, Gastfriend DR, Memisoglu A, Silverman BL. Injectable extended-release naltrexone (XR-NTX) for opioid dependence: long-term safety and effectiveness. Addiction. 2013;108(9):1628–37.
67. Sudakin D. Naltrexone: not just for opioids anymore. J Med Toxicol. 2016;12(1):71–5.
68. Weerts EM, Kim YK, Wand GS, Dannals RF, Lee JS, Frost JJ, et al. Differences in δ- and μ-opioid receptor blockade measured by positron emission tomography in naltrexone-treated recently abstinent alcohol-dependent subjects. Neuropsychopharmacology. 2008;33(3):653–65.
69. Unterwald EM, Anton B, To T, Lam H, Evans CJ. Quantitative immunolocalization of mu opioid receptors: regulation by naltrexone. Neuroscience. 1998;85(3):897–905.
70. Ferrari A, Bertolotti M, Dell'Utri A, Avico U, Sternieri E. Serum time course of naltrexone and 6β-naltrexol levels during long term treatment in drug addicts. Drug Alcohol Depend. 1998;52(3):211–20.
71. Breyer-Pfaff U, Nill K. Carbonyl reduction of naltrexone and dolasetron by oxidoreductases isolated from human liver cytosol. J Pharm Pharmacol. 2004;56(12):1601–6.
72. Meyer MC, Straughn AB, Lo MW, Schary WL, Whitney C. Bioequivalence, dose-proportionality, and pharmacokinetics of naltrexone after oral administration. J Clin Psychiatry. 1984;45(9):15–9.
73. Crowley TJ, Wagner JE, Zerbe G, Macdonald M. Naltrexone-induced dysphoria in former opioid addicts. Am J Psychiatry. 1985;142(9):1081–4.
74. Sigmon SC, Bisaga A, Nunes EV, O'Connor PG, Kosten T, Woody G. Opioid detoxification and naltrexone induction strategies: recommendations for clinical practice. Am J Drug Alcohol Abuse. 2012;38(3):187–99.

Chapter 11
Management of Opioid Overdoses

Matthew Niehaus, Nicholas Goodmanson, and Lillian Emlet

Background

In 2017, the United States Department of Health and Human Services declared the rapid rise in opioid abuse a public health emergency. Historically, the epidemic began in the early 1990s when pharmaceutical companies launched a large-scale public relations campaign suggesting opioids had no addictive potential [1]. Furthermore, regulatory bodies and physician groups worked to expand the FDA-approved indication of opioid use beyond cancer pain. These campaigns were extremely successful: prescriptions of Oxycontin, a popular long-acting formulation of oxycodone, rose from 670,000 in 1997 to 6.2 million in 2012 [2]. The opioid epidemic has evolved in three waves. First, overdoses in the 1990s were largely due to prescription opioids. Then, in 2010, a surge in opioid overdoses resulted from increased heroin use. Finally, the recreational use of highly potent synthetic opioids, such as fentanyl, resulted in a surge of opioid-related deaths in 2017 and continued increases since [3].

The burden of opioid misuse disorders is staggering. In 2018, 47,600 deaths were attributed to opioid overdose, rising even before the Covid-19 pandemic, to over 81,000 deaths in the 12 months ending May 2020. At the writing of this report, over two million people have been identified as having opioid use disorder (OUD) and

M. Niehaus
Department of Emergency Medicine, University Hospitals Cleveland Medical Center/Case Western Reserve University, Cleveland, OH, USA

N. Goodmanson
Department of Medicine, University of Illinois at Chicago/Advocate Christ Medical Center and Advocate Lutheran General Hospital, Champaign, IL, USA

L. Emlet (✉)
Departments of Critical Care Medicine & Emergency Medicine, VA Pittsburgh Healthcare System/University of Pittsburgh Medical Center, Pittsburgh, PA, USA
e-mail: emlell@ccm.upmc.edu

J. L. Pascual, T. G. Gaulton (eds.), *Opioid Use in Critical Care*,
https://doi.org/10.1007/978-3-030-77399-1_11

10.3 million people have misused at least one opioid prescription [4]. New persistent opioid use is a common complication after elective surgery, with greatest risk for transitioning to long-term use after the fifth day of exposure [5, 6]. Despite efforts by physicians to reduce inpatient and outpatient opioid dosage and prescriptions, OUD continues to be a major threat to public health. In a large retrospective cohort study of 162 hospitals in 44 states between 2009 and 2015 examining over 22 million admissions that included over four million cases requiring ICU care, the number of opioid overdose admissions requiring ICU care increased and their respective mortality also increased [7]. Thus, critical care physicians must be prepared to care for patients with opioid overdoses.

Pharmacology

Opioids exert their physiologic effects by binding to mu, kappa, or delta receptors, which are widely distributed in the body. Mu receptors in the thalamus, amygdala, and dorsal root ganglia are primarily responsible for the analgesic effects of opioids [8]. Brainstem mu receptors mediate respiratory depression by blunting the physiologic response to hypercarbia and hypoxemia. Mu activation in the Edinger-Westphal nucleus causes pupillary constriction [8]. Finally, mu receptors distributed along the gastrointestinal (GI) tract modulate GI dysmotility.

Mu receptor desensitization is responsible for opioid dependence. Unlike endogenous opioids, which exhibit time-limited effects, persistent exogenous opioids cause prolonged activation of the mu receptor and cause receptor desensitization over time. Receptor desensitization manifests clinically as the need for larger and more frequent opioid doses to achieve the desired analgesic and euphoric effects. Mu desensitization is not homogeneous however, and while the nociceptive response is diminutive over time, other clinical effects lag [9]. For example, though escalating opioid doses are needed for euphoric effects, receptor desensitization in brainstem respiratory centers is less pronounced, and thus higher doses significantly increase the risk of fatal respiratory depression.

Because receptor pharmacokinetics are unreliable in overdose, however, toxicity can be unpredictable [8]. For example, consumption of large medication quantities can overwhelm enzymatic pathways and cause erratic drug metabolism. Decreased GI motility can cause prolonged absorption of oral medications. Finally, intravenous use of crushed oral formulations can lead to unpredictable drug absorption and systemic effects.

Initial Management

Opioid intoxication should be considered in all patients who present with altered mental status (AMS), respiratory depression, and miotic pupils. Those at greatest risk include pulmonary disease (COPD/ asthma, restrictive lung diseases, obesity-hypoventilation syndrome, sleep apnea) and chronic end-organ dysfunction (neurologic, renal, and cardiac impairment) resulting in decreased clearance and less physiological reserve for unintentional overdose. In the inpatient setting, clinicians should obtain a detailed medication administration history to look for synergistic effects of other sedatives (benzodiazepines, psychiatric or seizure medications) with opioids. Consideration should be made for embedded electronic medical record (EMR) tools to identify during medication reconciliation transitions out of ICU and at discharge to determine the risk for overdose or serious opioid-induced respiratory depression. An example of this is the Risk Index for Overdose or Severe Opioid-Induced Respiratory Depression (RIOSORD), which evaluates predicted probability of opioid-induced respiratory depression within 6 months stratified over 7 risk classes, in order to guide risk-benefit medication decisions over time for outpatients [10]. Patient-controlled analgesia (PCA) devices increase opioid intoxication risk and should have protocols in place for capnography monitoring. In the Emergency Department (ED), historical data will be sparse, and thus the clinician must maintain a high index of suspicion in all patients with AMS and depressed respirations.

Initial management of patients with opioid intoxication should follow the standard circulation, airway, and breathing (CAB) algorithm. Vital signs should be obtained, and abnormalities addressed promptly. In pulseless patients, advanced cardiac life support (ACLS) should ensue. Because opioid reversal agents are unlikely to be beneficial in cardiac arrest, attention should be paid to chest compressions and airway management [11]. Methadone overdoses are often associated with QT prolongation and *torsades de pointes* ventricular arrythmias. Empiric magnesium supplementation, overdrive pacing, or ECMO should be considered for refractory arrythmias if witnessed in-hospital.

In patients presenting with coma and depressed respirations, airway management is essential. Death from opioid intoxication occurs due to acidosis-induced circulatory collapse from hypoxemia and hypercarbia. Respiratory support should be initiated using noninvasive methods first while attempting to reverse opioid effects. Often, due to the rapid onset of naloxone, bag valve mask (BVM)-assisted respirations are sufficient and invasive procedures (i.e., endotracheal intubation) can often be avoided. Polypharmacy with other CNS depressants increases risk of loss of protective reflexes, aspiration, and respiratory arrest leading to cardiac arrest. Non-cardiogenic pulmonary edema can occur (2–10%) after naloxone administration, seen as hypoxemia and crackles, and clinicians must consider early noninvasive ventilation (NIV), mechanical ventilation, and diuresis [12].

Critically ill patients often arrive with hypoxemic-ischemic neurologic injury following out of hospital respiratory and cardiac arrest. Reperfusion injury following opioid overdose-induced respiratory arrest is more severe than that following sudden cardiac arrest due to primary cardiac arrythmias. The hippocampus, basal ganglia, and globus pallidus are most susceptible to injury, though diffuse leukoencephalopathy of subcortical gray matter can also be seen [13]. Clinicians should implement targeted temperature management in appropriate patients in accordance with current American Heart Association guidelines. Subsequent neuroprognostication using a multimodal assessment should follow at least 72 hours after return to normothermia [14].

Naloxone

Naloxone reverses the clinical effects of opioids through competitive binding of mu opioid receptors. It can be administered intravenously (IV), intranasally, subcutaneously, orally, or by inhalation, although oral and inhalational preparations are infrequently used due to limited bioavailability. There is no standard naloxone dose, and therefore *guidelines recommend administration of the lowest effective dose*, minimizing any potential adverse drug effects [11, 15, 16]. An initial dose of 0.04 mg to 0.4 mg IV should be given, with escalating doses administered every 2 minutes until the desired clinical effect is achieved [16]. No more than 15 mg IV should be given. Non-IV formulations are packaged in 2–4 mg aliquots; thus, the full dose should be given, with convenient intranasal atomizer useful for inpatient rapid response team administration even by nonmedical bystanders. *The goal of naloxone administration is to restore adequate respiratory drive; complete reversal is unnecessary and can precipitate rapid withdrawal.*

The average half-life of naloxone is 60 minutes but ranges from 30 to 90 minutes [16]. Because opioid effects are unpredictable in overdose, intoxication often extends beyond the typical naloxone duration of action. Thus, patients must be observed for 4–6 hours following naloxone administration to ensure that there are no rebound opioid effects. If additional naloxone doses are needed, the patient should be admitted to the intensive care unit (ICU) for at least 24 hours of close monitoring with continuous pulse-oximeter, end-tidal CO2, respiratory rate, and sedation level assessment [17–19]. A continuous infusion of naloxone can provide prolonged opioid receptor antagonism where impending respiratory arrest reoccurs. The infusion rate should start at two-thirds of the effective bolus dose (measured in milligrams per hour) and titrated to respirations [20].

Naloxone is safe. In opioid-naïve patients, common reactions include dose-independent tachycardia and hypertension [16]. Less commonly, non-cardiogenic pulmonary edema has been reported. Though the pathophysiology is poorly understood, naloxone-associated pulmonary edema may be caused by agitation, inhalation against a closed glottis, or a catecholamine surge induced by acute withdrawal [21]. Treatment is supportive and patients may require ventilatory support (e.g., noninvasive or mechanical ventilation). It is therefore essential to administer only the minimum dose needed to restore respiratory drive to prevent withdrawal and ensuing complications.

Subsequent Management

After all acute life-threatening complications of opioid overdose are managed, a complete history and physical exam must be performed. Among inpatients, the likely etiology of opioid intoxication is iatrogenic, and so dose and frequency should be adjusted. Where possible, non-opioid adjuncts for multimodal pain management

Table 11.1 Complications related to opioid overdoses

Neurologic	Hypoxic/anoxic injury
Pulmonary	Non-cardiogenic pulmonary edema
	Aspiration pneumonia/pneumonitis
Cardiovascular	Myocardial infarction
Musculoskeletal	Rhabdomyolysis
	Traumatic injuries (falls, fractures)
	Compartment syndrome
Gastrointestinal/Genitourinary	Acute kidney injury
	Acute liver injury
Environmental	Hypothermia

(acetaminophen, nonsteroidal anti-inflammatory, NMDA receptor antagonists, alpha-2-adrenergic agonists, gabapentinoids, regional nerve blocks, acupuncture) should be used (see other chapters). In the absence of secondary injury due to the overdose (i.e., anoxia), patients with iatrogenic opioid intoxication often require only dose adjustment. Often additional medications are ingested during polypharmacy overdoses, and with delayed gastric emptying and metabolism, an extension of observation time may be required.

If presenting initially from the ED however, a more extensive work up is needed. Secondary complications must be considered, including fractures due to falls and rhabdomyolysis due to prolonged immobility or cardiac arrest, among others (Table 11.1). A comprehensive physical exam should be pursued to evaluate for sources of ongoing intoxication (e.g., opioid patches), a secondary survey for obvious traumatic injuries or deformities, and tight muscle compartments that may indicate compartment syndrome and evolving rhabdomyolysis. Hypothermic patients should be warmed. Co-ingestion is common, and so toxicology screens, acetaminophen, salicylate, and alcohol levels should be measured. Screening for hepatitis and HIV should be pursued in high-risk patients such as IV drug users. An electrocardiogram (EKG) is needed to rule out cardiac ischemia and to evaluate waveform (QTc) intervals, which are commonly deranged in co-ingestions. Clinical condition should dictate additional diagnostic testing, including laboratory measurements and imaging. Comprehensive supportive critical care of the opioid overdose patient is summarized in Table 11.2.

Disposition

If additional doses of naloxone are required, patients should be admitted to the ICU. Due to erratic absorption and manifestation of respiratory depression, symptomatic patients should thus be observed for longer monitoring for respiratory insufficiency. All patients should be counseled on the dangers of opioid use prior to discharge and offered rehabilitation treatment through structured motivational

Table 11.2 Summary treatment recommendations

Organ System	Potential	Treatment Pearls
Neurologic/ Psychiatric	Hypoxic brain injury Withdrawal syndromes Psychiatric disorders	Standard Post-Cardiac Arrest Recommendations (AHA) Monitoring for withdrawal symptoms as they develop Medication reconciliation of psychiatric medications & resuming if able Psychiatry consultation as applicable
Pulmonary	Ventilatory depression Non-cardiogenic pulmonary edema Aspiration pneumonitis Respiratory failure	Naloxone 0.04 mg IV, double dose if no response until 0.4 mg IV, initial bolus dose is to clinical response of improved respiratory rate or neurologic awakening If respiratory/ cardiac arrest 2 mg IV or intranasal Continuous infusion 2/3 of initial dose/ hour [16, 20] Noninvasive ventilation for pulmonary edema as usually resolves within 24–48 hours Refractory hypoxemia of pneumonitis may respond to high-flow nasal cannula first Endotracheal intubation & mechanical ventilation with lung-protective ventilation for refractory ventilatory, neurologic, or hypoxic respiratory failure Daily spontaneous sedation weaning trials
Cardiovascular	Acute coronary syndrome Arrythmias	Trend troponin Transthoracic echo Continuous telemetry Electrolyte repletion Ca Mg K Phos Toxicology screen for QTc prolongating medications polypharmacy ingestions
Gastrointestinal	Ileus	Nasogastric tube decompression Stress ulcer prophylaxis if mechanically ventilated
Renal	Acute kidney injury Rhabdomyolysis	Resuscitate crystalloid fluids Prevent further hypotension or nephrotoxins
Metabolic	Hyperglycemic stress response DVT prophylaxis	Maintain euglycemia
Infectious	Evaluation for fever & infection Prevention of secondary infection	Cultures as appropriate Antibiotics and de-escalation as appropriate
Disposition	Social determinants of health	Social Work consult for screening & support

interviewing techniques (e.g., Screening, Brief Intervention, and Referral to Treatment (SBIRT) or Brief Negotiation Interview (BNI)). After nonfatal overdose, treatment with buprenorphine can be safely initiated in the emergency department or inpatient setting. Buprenorphine is a partial agonist at the mu-opioid receptor and antagonist at the kappa receptor that provides some intrinsic pain control yet has a ceiling effect for respiratory depression. It is restricted, Class III controlled substance that requires additional training for prescribing clinicians. Clinicians should counsel IV drug users on clean needle use, needle exchange programs, safe injection sites, and pre-exposure prophylaxis (PrEP) to protect against HIV. Intranasal naloxone kits should be provided at discharge to all patients who survive nonfatal opioid overdose. Risk reduction should be the primary goal of all clinicians caring for patients with opioid use disorders.

In summary, opioid misuse and overdose is a common clinical entity treated in the intensive care unit, usually due to respiratory failure and secondary trauma or complications. Multiple organs can be involved as a result of opioid toxicity, and supportive critical care is the mainstay of treatment. Recovery can be complicated by neuropsychiatric and psychosocial complexity, and involvement of Addiction Medicine, Social Work services, and Pain Medicine specialists may be required to find optimal control of delirium, pain, and medical critical illness.

References

1. Van Zee A. The promotion and marketing of Oxycontin: commercial triumph, public health tragedy. Am J Public Health. 2009;99(2):221–7.
2. Hwang C, Chang H, Alexander G. Impact of abuse-deterrent OxyContin on prescription opioid utilization. Pharmacoepidemiol Drug Saf. 2014;24(2):197–204.
3. Jones M, Viswanath O, Peck J, Kaye A, Gill J, Simopoulos T. A brief history of the opioid epidemic and strategies for pain medicine. Pain Ther. 2018;7(1):13–21.
4. The Opioid Epidemic by the Numbers [Internet]. HHS.gov. 2019 [cited 9 November 2019]. Available from: https://www.hhs.gov/opioids/sites/default/files/2019-11/Opioids%20Infographic_letterSizePDF_10-02-19.pdf
5. Deyo RA, Hallvik SE, Hildebran C, et al. Association between initial opioid prescribing patters and subsequent long-term use among opioid-naïve patients: a statewide retrospective cohort study. J Gen Intern Med. 2017;32:21–7.
6. Brummett CM, Waljee JF, Goesling J, et al. New persistent opioid use after minor and major surgical procedures in US adults. JAMA Surg. 2017;152(6):e170504.
7. Stevens JP, Wall MJ, Novack L, Marshall J, Hsu DJ, Howell MD. The critical care crisis of opioid overdoses in the United States. Ann Am Thorac Soc Dec. 2017;14(12):1803–9.
8. Boyer E. Management of Opioid Analgesic Overdose. N Engl J Med. 2012;367(2):146–55.
9. White J, Irvine R. Mechanisms of fatal opioid overdose. Addiction. 1999;94(7):961–72.
10. Zedler BK, Saunders WB, Joyce AR, Vick CC, Murrell EL. Validation of a screening risk index for serious prescription opioid-induced respiratory depression or overdose in a US commercial health plan claims database. Pain Med. 2018;19:68–78.
11. Vanden Hoek T, Morrison L, Shuster M, Donnino M, Sinz E, Lavonas E, et al. Part 12: Cardiac arrest in special situations: 2010 American Heart Association Guidelines for cardiopulmonary resuscitation and emergency cardiovascular care. Circulation. 2010;122(18_suppl_3):S829–61.
12. Lavonas EJ, Dezfulian C. Impact of the opioid epidemic. Crit Care Clin. 2020;36:753–69.
13. Dinicu AI, Chaudhai A, Kayyal S. Diffuse subcortical white matter injury and bilateral basal ganglia neuronal loss after acute opioid overdose. Neuroradiol J. 2020;33(3):267–70.
14. Panchal AR, et al. 2020 American Heart Association guidelines for cardiopulmonary resuscitation and emergency cardiovascular care: part 3: adult basic and advanced life support. Circulation. 2020;142:S366–468.
15. Lavonas E, Drennan I, Gabrielli A, Heffner A, Hoyte C, Orkin A, et al. Part 10: special circumstances of resuscitation. Circulation. 2015;132(18 suppl 2):S501–18.

16. Rzasa Lynn R, Galinkin J. Naloxone dosage for opioid reversal: current evidence and clinical implications. Therap Adv Drug Safety. 2017;9(1):63–88.
17. Taenzer AHPJ, McGrath SP, et al. Executive summary: opioid-induced ventilatory impairment (OIVI): Ime for change in the monitoring strategy for postoperative PCA patients. Anesthesiology. 2010;112 https://www.apsf.org/videos/monitoring-for-opioid-induced-ventilatory-impairment-oivi-video/.
18. Chou R, Gordon DB, de Leon-Casasola OA, et al. Management of Postoperative Pain: A Clinical Practice Guideline From the American Pain Society, the American Society of Regional Anesthesia and pain medicine, and the American Society of Anesthesiologists' committee on regional anesthesia, executive committee, and administrative council. J Pain. 2016;17(2):131–57.
19. Jungquist CR, Correll DJ, Fleisher LA, et al. Avoiding adverse events secondary to opioid-induced respiratory depression: implications for nurse executives and patient safety. J Nurs Adm. 2016;46(2):87–94.
20. Nelson LS, Olsen D. Chapter 36: Opioids. Goldfrank's Toxicologic Emergencies, 11e.
21. Schwartz JA, Koenigsberg MD. Naloxone-induced pulmonary edema. Ann Emerg Med. 1987;16(11):1294–6.

Chapter 12
Use of Opioid Analgesics in Postsurgical and Trauma Patients

Daniel R. Brown and Mark R. Pedersen

Introduction

One of the primary objectives for patients admitted to the intensive care unit (ICU) following surgery or traumatic injury is optimal pain control. Not only is adequate analgesia a component of compassionate care, it is essential for maintaining satisfactory hemodynamics and respiratory function. It is also necessary for effective physical therapy and rehabilitation following injury and/or operative intervention. Opioids have long been the mainstay of analgesia in postsurgical and trauma patients, and appropriate selection of opioid analgesics is one of the pillars of effective analgesia. However, equally important is to establish reasonable expectations for pain control, understand the key transition points for shifting from parenteral to enteral analgesics, and recognize the risk for dependence and addiction to these medications following a patient's discharge from the ICU and subsequently the hospital. Additionally, multiple studies have shown that opioid analgesic prescribing practices in the postoperative setting vary widely and lack standardization thus placing patients and providers at risk for over and under prescribing narcotics.

D. R. Brown (✉)
Department of Anesthesiology and Perioperative Medicine, Mayo Clinic, Rochester, MN, USA
e-mail: brown.daniel@mayo.edu

M. R. Pedersen
Department of Anesthesia, University of Iowa, Iowa City, IA, USA
e-mail: mark-pedersen@uiowa.edu

J. L. Pascual, T. G. Gaulton (eds.), *Opioid Use in Critical Care*,
https://doi.org/10.1007/978-3-030-77399-1_12

Pain Assessment

Pain is frequently undertreated in the ICU which can result in serious physiologic and psychologic sequelae for patients [1, 2]. Uncontrolled postoperative pain or following a traumatic injury has been associated with increased sympathetic activity and physiologic stress [1, 2]. It has also been shown to cause long-term psychological effects such as post-traumatic stress disorder and post-intensive care syndrome [2]. The primary method of assessment of pain in postsurgical and trauma patients is by using a patient's own self-report of pain intensity. However, frequently patients in the ICU are unable to communicate that they have untreated pain. In these settings it is useful to utilize validated pain assessment scores. The critical care pain observation tool (CPOT) is a frequently used pain scale in the ICU. This tool has four fields that include: facial expressions, body movements, muscle tension, and ventilator compliance (or voice use in non-intubated patients). Each domain has a score range of 0–2 with a possible score variation of 0–8, with a score of 2 indicating a patient has uncontrolled pain and may benefit from analgesic administration. The Behavioral Pain Scale (BPS) is an additional validated pain assessment tool in the ICU. This scale has three domains which include: facial expression, upper limb movements, and compliance with mechanical ventilation. Both of these scores have been validated as reliable assessments of pain in patients who are unable to verbalize or communicate pain severity [2].

Expectation Management

There is evidence that opioid use following surgical procedures is reduced if reasonable expectations for postoperative pain management have been established preoperatively [3, 4]. Many patients present to the ICU following elective and semi-urgent procedures that would have benefited from pre-procedural counseling about realistic pain management goals following surgery. This is not necessarily the role of the intensive care provider, though this is an excellent opportunity to influence the patient experience by collaborating with surgical colleagues. Often this is a component of the pre-procedural or pre-anesthetic evaluation.

It is important for providers to recognize that many patients' expectations are that they will suffer no pain at all. Patient and provider definitions of controlled pain frequently differ. Analgesic administration has in large part been driven by the assessment of pain based on patient subjective report. The inclusion of pain as the "fifth vital sign" was associated with patients requesting, and receiving, increased amount of opioid analgesics [5]. This approach became increasingly utilized in response to an *Institute of Medicine* report that analgesia in cancer patients was routinely not adequate [5]. This method of monitoring and treating pain has often been associated with unrealistic patient expectations of pain control. It is also widely regarded as a significant factor contributing to the opioid epidemic [5]. Assessing pain strictly from a subjective patient report and through observation of vital signs can lead to significant overdosing of opioid pain medications. Unfortunately, certain routinely used hospital quality indicators still favor liberal administration of analgesics in response to a pain score, even though this may not be in the patient's best interest [5].

Many patients will present to the ICU emergently, some with neurological impairment, others, having already sustained traumatic injury or undergone an emergent surgical procedure. In such patients, establishing analgesic expectations may be difficult. A consistent approach by the entire care team is needed to set and maintain appropriate expectations as well as develop and modify analgesic plans. Providing the expectation that pain will be controlled to the best extent possible which will allow patients to participate in their care and therapy is reasonable and should be addressed early on with patients and their families following surgery or traumatic injury.

Dependence and Addiction

This topic is discussed in depth in other parts of this book. However, appropriate prescription and administration of opioids to ICU patients warrants a discussion of the screening techniques and a consideration of the risk of addiction. The National Institute on Drug Abuse, as well as many state medical boards, provides screening tools to assess risk for future opioid dependence and potential for addiction. One such tool, provided by the National Institute on Drug Abuse, has five domains that include: a family history of substance abuse (including alcohol and prescription medications), personal history of substance abuse, a history of sexual abuse, age, and psychological disease [6]. A patient who scores 3 or less on this assessment is considered low risk for developing opioid dependence issues. A patient who scores greater than 8 is considered high risk for developing dependence issues [6]. Critically-ill, postoperative, and trauma patients will all have a need for opioids for adequate analgesia. However, careful consideration of the type of opioid prescribed, the duration of therapy, and supplementing analgesia with non-opioid adjuncts is highly recommended as part of an effort to reduce opioid abuse and tolerance.

Protocols and Variability in Practice

Initiating opioid therapy in a patient who has undergone surgery or suffered a traumatic injury requires consideration of the type of surgery or extent of injury, a patient's prior use of opioids, and a clear assessment of anticipated course of recovery. A large multicenter review of postoperative opioid prescribing practices reported that there is significant variation in amounts of oral morphine equivalents prescribed postoperatively for identical procedures [7]. Similar findings have been shown in multiple studies [8, 9], highlighting the poor standardization in the prescription of opioid analgesics and in the management of postoperative pain.

Given the identification of this wide variation in prescribing practice, and the significant morbidity and mortality associated with inappropriate opioid administration, many advocate for definitive standardization of opioid prescriptions in the postoperative setting. One strategy has been to limit the opioids prescribed, forcing the patient to be re-assessed when seeking ongoing prescriptions.

Effects of Opioid Use Prior to Surgery or Traumatic Injury

Patients can present to surgical or trauma ICUs with a history of long-term opioid use. Providers must be vigilant and elicit any history of long-term opioid use as there are important potential adverse physiologic and psychologic effects that may ultimately result. Patients may have tolerance to opioid analgesics which may necessitate increased doses, in turn subsequently placing these patients at increased risk for respiratory depression and delirium [10, 11]. Use of a multimodal analgesic regimen is paramount in these settings to reduce the need for opioid escalation. Additionally, long-term effects of opioids can be associated with hyperalgesia in postoperative patients or following injury [10, 11]. Gastrointestinal effects, including constipation and nausea, may also result from long-term opioid use and can exacerbate postoperative or post-traumatic ileus [10, 11]. Respiratory system effects include central and obstructive sleep apnea and CO_2 retention. Chronic opioid use can also cause suppression of the hypothalamic-pituitary-adrenal axis. Opiates have been shown to affect the release of all hormones including adrenocorticotropic hormone, which can cause a relative adrenal insufficiency, in turn influencing the normal host immune response of critically ill patients [10, 11].

Physiologic Effects of Uncontrolled Pain

Severe pain can cause significant physiologic derangements and can induce psychological distress and impairment. Uncontrolled pain can induce sympathetic activity that can result in tachycardia, hypertension, and increased myocardial oxygen demand, potentially inducing myocardial ischemia [1, 12]. Pain from surgical incisions in the thorax and abdomen can impair diaphragm function resulting in altered pulmonary mechanics, tachypnea, atelectasis, and impaired gas exchange [1, 12]. Impaired sleep, delirium, and agitation can result from uncontrolled pain and may be associated with long-term sequalae [1, 12]. Finally, pain has also been shown to cause immunosuppression, increased protein catabolism, and impair wound healing [1, 10–12].

Premedication and Opioid-Sparing Analgesics (Table 12.1)

The use of non-opioid analgesics preoperatively such as acetaminophen, gabapentin, and nonsteroidal anti-inflammatory drugs (NSAIDs) has also been shown to improve postoperative pain control and reduce the use of opioid analgesics after surgery.

Mild to moderate pain in the ICU can be effectively treated with acetaminophen. When used in conjunction with opioids, acetaminophen has been shown to reduce the need for opioids in the postoperative setting [12–14]. Some studies have also shown a reduction in ICU length-of-stay, and delirium incidence and duration with the use of scheduled acetaminophen administration [13, 14]. Intravenous (IV) and oral formulations are available. Intravenous acetaminophen has not been shown to be superior to enteral formulations given its high availability via enteral absorption [15]. If a patient is able to absorb enteral medications, the enteral route of administration is preferred given the significantly lower cost per dose. Acetaminophen has a maximum dose of 4 g in a 24-hour period to prevent risk of liver injury. Special considerations to maximum daily dose are needed when administering this drug to patients with impaired liver function or a history of alcohol ingestion.

NSAIDs produce analgesia via inhibition of cyclooxygenase [1, 12]. This can provide significant analgesia and antipyretic effects. As a class these drugs have been shown to significantly reduce the amount of opioids administered in the postoperative setting; however, they can have significant side effects and should be cautiously used in critically ill patients [1]. NSAID side effects include risk for gastrointestinal bleeding and nephrotoxicity, morbidities common in the critically ill [1, 12, 16]. There has also been controversy regarding NSAID use in patients suffering traumatic fractures as these agents have been associated with impaired bone healing and remodeling [17]. The evidence for this is not robust and has been called into question recently. Ketorolac is an IV NSAID that can be used postoperatively and is metabolized in the liver and excreted in the kidney so the dose may need to be adjusted or held in patients with hepatic and renal impairment [1]. Prolonged use of ketorolac for greater than five days is not recommended as this increases the risk of gastrointestinal bleeding significantly as well as at operative sites [1, 12].

Gabapentin, pregabalin, and carbamazepine are effective medications for the treatment of neuropathic pain [1, 12]. Use of these medications in the ICU has been shown to reduce the total opioid dose administered after surgery. Unfortunately, these drugs must be administered enterally. Also, these drugs have several drawbacks including sedation and impaired cognition, and their use should be with caution in patients at risk for postoperative cognitive dysfunction and delirium [1, 12]. Clinicians should be aware that abrupt discontinuation of these medications may be associated with withdrawal symptoms.

Ketamine is an n-methyl-d-aspartate (NMDA) receptor antagonist. There is also evidence that ketamine acts at mu, kappa, and delta opioid receptors [12, 18]. Ketamine has several properties that make it a good adjunct to opioids in

Table 12.1 Opioid adjuncts commonly used in the ICU

	Intermittent dosing	Infusion dose	Mechanism of action	Metabolism	Critical illness considerations
Acetaminophen [62]	650 mg–1000 mg q6h	N/A	Cyclooxygenase inhibitor, no anti-inflammatory action	Hepatic glucuronidation/CYP oxidation	Do not exceed 4 g/day. May need reduced dosing in patients with hepatic dysfunction
Ketorolac [63]	30 mg q6h(IV)	N/A	Cyclooxygenase inhibitor	Hepatic glucuronidation	Avoid in GI bleeding and patients with AKI/ESRD
Gabapentin [64]	Start 100–300 mg TID may uptitrate	N/A	Unclear, high affinity binding to calcium channels in CNS inhibiting excitatory neurotransmission	Renal clearance, unmetabolized	Reduced dose in kidney dysfunction, potential for sedation
Ketamine [65]	0.1–0.5 mg/kg q6h	0.1–0.5 mg/kg/min	NMDA receptor antagonism	Hepatic N-dealkylation	Direct myocardial depression. Caution in patients with heart failure
Dexmedetomidine [66]	N/A	0.2–2 mcg/kg/hr	Alpha receptor agonism; 1600:1 alpha2:alpha1	Hepatic glucuronidation/CYP oxidation	Caution in patients with bradycardia/ myocardial dysfunction

postoperative and trauma ICU patients. It has sympathomimetic properties that give it a favorable hemodynamic profile and has been shown to augment cardiac output in healthy patients [1, 12]. The effects of ketamine on respiratory function are advantageous for patients in the ICU as it acts as a bronchodilator, and there is minimal respiratory depression associated with analgesic doses of ketamine [1, 12]. Ketamine has been used for many years in burn patients. It has been shown to reduce hyperalgesia and allodynia associated with thermal injuries [19]. For many years, the military has used ketamine as part of a multimodal analgesic regimen for wounded or injured soldiers [20]. Its perioperative use in cardiac surgery patients has further demonstrated a reduction in opioid use and potentially a reduction in the rate of chronic post-sternotomy pain [17]. In patients who have undergone major abdominal surgery, ketamine has also been shown to reduce postoperative opioid requirements and it is thought that this effect may also promote the earlier return of bowel function [21, 22]. There is also strong evidence for the opioid-sparing property of ketamine in patients who have a history of chronic pain with significant opioid use prior to surgery [23].

Although ketamine has shown significant promise and there are many advantages to its use, there are also certain drawbacks to its administration in critically ill patients. Despite the favorable hemodynamic profile there is controversy over ketamine's direct effects on the myocardium. Some investigators have suggested it depresses myocardial function in patients with longstanding congestive heart failure [24]. Furthermore, ketamine increases pulmonary vascular resistance and may be problematic in patients with concomitant pulmonary arterial hypertension [25]. Additionally, ketamine-related tachycardia can be detrimental to patients with severe valvular stenosis or coronary artery disease as it will increase myocardial oxygen demand [1, 12, 24]. It is unclear if these effects are significant at analgesic doses. Ketamine is also a potent sialogogue and secretion burden can become significant following its administration [19]. Ketamine has also been shown to be associated with unpleasant psychoactive effects including hallucinations and emergence delirium [1, 12]. Lastly ketamine has long been associated with increased intracranial pressure, though the clinical significance of this has been called into question in recent years [26].

Dexmedetomidine is an alpha-2 receptor agonist that has sedating and analgesic properties with a favorable hemodynamic profile, though minimal respiratory depression but with some risk of bradycardia [12, 27]. Dexmedetomidine causes analgesia at multiple sites of action, including in the locus ceruleus and inhibition of pain signals through the dorsal horn of the spinal cord. Dexmedetomidine also inhibits the release of norepinephrine from presynaptic terminals and prevents the transmission of pain signals across synapses. Due to these analgesic properties, dexmedetomidine has been studied in multiple surgical populations and shown to reduce opioid consumption as well as pain intensity in patients postoperatively [27].

Regional Anesthesia

There are many regional anesthetic techniques that can provide effective pain control for a patient undergoing a surgical procedure or who has suffered traumatic injury. The use of epidural anesthesia can reduce the use of opioids in postsurgical patients including cardiac, thoracic, intra-abdominal, and orthopedic surgeries [27–30]. Patients who sustain traumatic injuries to the chest and/or abdomen can also see a reduction in opioid consumption when epidural analgesia is used [31]. The benefits of this type of analgesia must be weighed against the risks of the frequent need and use of anticoagulants for venous thrombosis prophylaxis. Careful timing of initiation and discontinuation of neuraxial anesthesia must consider anticoagulation dosing and administration. Additionally, the use of neuraxial regional techniques may cause hypotension as they can block sympathetic nervous system output in the spine with resulting splanchnic vasodilation.

Methadone

Methadone is a unique opioid. For much of its existence it has found its primary use as a treatment for heroin addiction [32]. However, the opioid epidemic has generated new interest in its use in the perioperative setting. Methadone is available in enteral and parenteral formulations. Of the opioids used in clinical practice, it has the longest half-life with enteral formulations estimated to last between 15 to 55 hours while IV methadone between 8 and 59 hours [32, 33]. When administered at doses of 20–30 mg, the effective duration of analgesia can be from 24 to 36 hours [33]. The principal mechanism of action is similar to other opioids, acting on central and peripheral mu_1 receptors. However, further investigation has shown that it also antagonizes the NMDA receptor [32, 33]. Additionally, methadone has been shown to decrease reuptake of serotonin and norepinephrine [32, 33], see Chaps. 3 and 4.

Opioids with shorter half-lives have the problem of wide variability in plasma concentrations. Even with the use of patient controlled analgesia (PCA) pumps, patients in the ICU and other postoperative settings can range between inadequate analgesia and significant overdosage side effects of opioids such as respiratory depression.

Given the unique properties of methadone and the persistent reporting of inadequate analgesia in the postoperative period, methadone is of great interest in treating acute pain. Studies in patients undergoing complex spine surgery have shown that methadone administration at induction of anesthesia is effective in reducing postoperative opioid use [34]. Investigation into the role of methadone in cardiac surgery patients has shown similar results [35]. In these patients, methadone has been shown to significantly reduce overall use of opioids postoperatively and improve pain scores as compared to patients who instead received fentanyl as the sole analgesic during surgery. Investigations have demonstrated that methadone can be effective in preventing the development of hyperalgesia and allodynia [36]. Additionally, methadone has been shown to decrease opioid tolerance and has been effective in the treatment of neuropathic pain which may develop in the postoperative period [32]. These benefits are thought to be mediated via the antagonism of the NMDA receptor [32, 33].

Despite potential benefits of methadone in the perioperative setting, it nonetheless also has a side effect profile similar to other opioids including respiratory depression, delayed gastric emptying, urinary retention, pruritus, and urticaria [32]. Like other narcotics such as fentanyl, methadone is also associated with development of serotonin syndrome, perhaps related to serotonin reuptake and metabolism [32, 33]. Additionally, methadone can prolong the QT interval placing patients at risk for ventricular arrhythmias, particularly when used in combination with other drugs that prolong the QT interval such as certain antiemetics and antidepressants [32, 33]. An electrocardiogram should be obtained on all patients prior to initiation of methadone therapy.

Opioids Conventionally Used in the Acute Post-Traumatic and Postoperative Period (Table 12.2)

Pain following surgery or traumatic injury follows a different course than some other types of pain (chronic pain, fibromyalgia). The peak pain intensity is on postoperative day 0 and 1. It is expected that as time progresses from the initial insult, the severity of pain and analgesic requirements will decrease. Currently, the mainstay of analgesia in the postoperative and traumatic injury setting is the use of opioid analgesics as part of a multimodal pain regimen. As a class, narcotics reliably provide effective analgesia and have a favorable hemodynamic profile. In the immediate post-injury or postoperative setting IV opioids with rapid onset are preferred, given the acuity and severity of pain these patients will be experiencing as well as concerns regarding drug absorption barring enteral or transcutaneous routes of administration.

Fentanyl is a synthetic opioid with a rapid onset of action making it favorable following surgery or traumatic injury [1, 11]. Fentanyl has an approximately 50-fold greater potency as compared to morphine [1]. When given as a single bolus dose, the duration of action of fentanyl is relatively short, only lasting 25–30 minutes [1, 11]. However, continuous fentanyl infusions can be used when a patient will need continuous sedation and is likely to require analgesia, such as in postoperative and trauma patients who will remain intubated for a prolonged period. The concept of context sensitive half-life is important in this setting. Due to the high lipid solubility of fentanyl, it will accumulate in tissues throughout the body. As a result, increased duration of infusions will result in increased duration of effects, including sedation and respiratory depression even persisting after the infusion is discontinued. Fentanyl can be used as an analgesic in patients who are hemodynamically unstable

Table 12.2 Dosing and considerations of IV opioids commonly used in the ICU [1, 33, 57, 58, 59, 60, 61]

	Morphine	Hydromorphone	Fentanyl	Methadone	Remifentanil
IV bolus dose	2–4 mg	0.5–2 mg	25–100 mcg	5–20 mg	N/A
Infusion dose	1–10 mg/hr	0.5–5 mg/hr	50–20 mcg/hr	N/A	0.5–5 mcg/kg/hr
Hemodynamic effects	May cause hypotension	Negligible, may cause hypotension	Negligible	QTc prolongation, potentially arrhythmogenic	Bradycardia
Use in renal failure	Do not use	Dosing adjustments required	Safe to use	Safe to use	Safe to use
Use in Hepatic Failure	Dosing adjustment required	Dosing adjustments required (50% dose)	Dosing adjustment required, may cause encephalopathy	Increased half-life	No dosing adjustment, may cause encephalopathy
Time to Onset	<10 min	<10 min	<1 min	20–30 min	<5 min
Duration of Action(Bolus)	2–3 hours	2–3 hours	30 min	10–36 hours	N/A

as it has little effect on circulation. Fentanyl is safe for use in patients with end-stage renal disease or acute kidney failure as it is cleared through hepatic metabolism [1, 11]. However, dosing adjustments will be required in patients with impaired liver function.

Remifentanil is another synthetic opioid that is described as being ultra-fast acting. It has a half-life of 5–10 minutes and is metabolized by plasma esterases with no active metabolites [1, 11]. It is typically used as an infusion and can be infused for extended durations with little increase in duration of action. Remifentanil has the potential drawback of producing hyperalgesia if it is suddenly discontinued without initiation of other analgesic therapy [1, 11]. It can also cause significant bradycardia and, therefore, should be used with caution in patients at risk for heart block or who are on concurrent beta blockade.

Morphine has many qualities that make it less desirable for use in the ICU. Morphine has an active metabolite, morphine-6-glucuronide, that can accumulate in patients with renal impairment and cause central nervous system and respiratory depression [1, 11]. Additionally, morphine may cause histamine release which is not ideal in hemodynamically unstable patients [1, 11].

Hydromorphone is a semisynthetic opioid that is slightly more potent than morphine and has a similar time to onset. The duration of action is 2–3 hours for a single bolus dose [1, 11]. There is little histamine release associated with hydromorphone administration with less effects on hemodynamics as seen with morphine. Hydromorphone has had a history of dosing errors owing to its increased potency over morphine. Also, there is the potential for accumulation of its active metabolite (hydromorphone-3-glucuronide) in kidney failure which can be neurotoxic, though this is significantly less of a concern than with morphine administration [1, 11].

Oxycodone is an enteral opioid that binds mu and kappa receptors [37]. Both immediate and extended release formulations are available. Immediate release is most appropriate in postsurgical or trauma patients given its quick onset of action within 10–15 minutes [37]. A single dose can be effective for 3–6 hours [37]. Oxycodone has similar side effects to other opioids including respiratory depression and constipation. However, similar to hydromorphone, there is little histamine release with oxycodone administration [37].

Meperidine is a synthetic opioid derivative and has little modern use in postoperative or traumatic injury analgesia [1, 38]. Meperidine is metabolized to an active metabolite, normeperidine, that can accumulate and induce seizures in experimental models [38]. The primary use for meperidine is in the control of shivering thought to be mediated via its effects on the kappa opioid receptor and alteration of the thermoregulatory set point [38].

Tramadol is an analgesic that has a mixed mechanism of action. It is a moderate mu opioid receptor agonist that also acts centrally to block the reuptake and enhance the effects of serotonin [39, 40]. This combined mechanism of action results in less respiratory depression than pure mu agonist analgesics [39]. Additionally, serotonin antagonist antiemetics have been reported to reduce the efficacy of tramadol in the postoperative period [41].

Fentanyl, morphine, remifentanil, and hydromorphone can be delivered by PCA which can be implemented when a patient regains the ability to guide their own analgesic therapy. PCA offers several benefits in the acute postoperative or traumatic injury setting. There is a more reliable plasma level of analgesic due to more regular administration, as well as ease of nursing workload and increased patient satisfaction [42].

As patients regain ability to tolerate enteral administration of medications they should also have less associated traumatic injury or surgical pain. There will be an increased distinction between pain at rest and pain with activity such as coughing and pulmonary hygiene as well as with therapy and rehabilitation. In this subacute phase of pain, enteral analgesics are a reasonable transition from basal IV narcotic infusions and PCA. Timing of administration of medication in this phase of care is important given the delayed analgesic effect associated with enteral administration. This delay should be anticipated by bedside providers and appropriate timing of analgesic administration with physical therapy and rehabilitation services will increase patient satisfaction and their ability to participate in these important activities. Various narcotics are available in transdermal and intranasal routes of administration. The pharmacokinetics of these routes of administration are less favorable for critically ill patients. Hydromorphone and morphine are available in enteral formulations. Multiple dosages and formulations of these drugs are available that include immediate and extended release. They are available as tablets, liquids, and suppositories. The side effect profile remains similar to the IV forms.

Drug Metabolism of Opioids: Consideration of Specific Populations

Opioids are metabolized in the liver and excreted via the kidneys. Each can differ in the way in which they undergo metabolism. Studies of population pharmacokinetics have found differences in opioid metabolism when stratified by age, sex, and ethnicity [40]. CYP-mediated oxidation accounts for metabolism of most opioids. Variation in CYP enzyme function derived from differences in age, sex, and genetic variation, as well as concomitant drug administration has the potential to result in significant drug-drug interaction [40], see Chap. 4. In addition to individual differences in drug metabolism activity, hepatic and renal function are frequently impaired in the critically ill. It is exceedingly difficult to predict the extent to which patients in the ICU will metabolize opioids [40]. Given that many patients in the ICU can have an extensive medication administration regimen, careful titration of any opioid to safe clinical effect is paramount.

Some opioids used in the ICU can have clinically active metabolites. Morphine and hydromorphone are frequently used to treat postoperative and post-trauma pain; both have active metabolites. Morphine is converted to morphine-6-glucuronide as well as morphine-3-glucuronide [40]. These active metabolites can accumulate in patients with end-stage renal disease and cause respiratory depression, gastrointestinal side effects, and increased sedation. Tramadol must be metabolized to its active metabolite to have full clinical effect. Tramadol and its active metabolite both have μ receptor activity; however, the Tramadol parent compound also affects serotonin and norepinephrine uptake [40]. Fentanyl and methadone are both metabolized by the CYP enzyme system. While this places them at high risk for causing drug interactions with medications metabolized via these pathways, they do not produce clinically active metabolites [40].

In the future, as understanding of the genetic variation in drug metabolism is improved and the impact of environmental factors and critical illness is clarified, personalized drug regimens could be implemented to provide maximal therapeutic benefit with minimal side effects [43]. However, this is in the distant future, and currently critically ill patients require careful and active bedside titration and understanding that these variations exist and one opioid may not be as effective as another for a given patient and a given pain profile.

Specific Cases and Considerations

Sternotomy is the most common wound following cardiac surgery and poorly controlled sternotomy pain can contribute to poor pulmonary function and nonadherence to rehabilitation therapy in the postoperative setting [44]. Sternotomy pain has multiple aspects that make it a particularly painful incision and predispose to chronic pain. First, the sternum is often re-approximated using sternal wires; however, in the early postoperative period, there can still be significant sheer of the sternum when a patient breaths deeply or coughs [45]. Additionally, sternal wires have been implicated in developing significant amounts of pain following cardiac surgery in the acute and chronic phases. Both the sheer effects and the role of sternal wires' impact on sternotomy pain have been attenuated by the introduction of rigid fixation devices [45]. The pharmacologic management of sternotomy pain has shifted to a multimodal model of pain control. Administration of long-acting methadone preoperatively, combined with immediate release oxycodone or hydromorphone postoperatively, in addition to acetaminophen, lidocaine patches and GABA analogues are commonly employed perioperatively for the management of sternotomy pain [35, 46]. NSAIDs should be used with caution in this patient population who are at increased risk for acute kidney injury. Regional analgesia techniques, specifically epidural analgesia, are controversial in cardiac surgery [46]. The medically induced coagulopathy from heparin administration during cardiopulmonary bypass and frequent need for continued anticoagulation postoperatively make timing of placement and removal of epidural catheters difficult. Additionally, thoracic epidural analgesia has not been convincingly shown to be superior to multimodal pharmacologic management of pain following cardiac surgery [2, 47].

Thoracotomy, like sternotomy, can have significant impact on patient respiratory and physical function following surgery. Trauma to the intercostal muscles and nerves during surgery can cause significant pain in both acute and chronic phases of recovery [48]. Some studies have found that up to 50% of patients will develop chronic pain following a thoracotomy [48]. Analgesia for thoracotomy is similar to that for sternotomy, utilizing a multimodal regimen outlined above. However, regional analgesia can play a much larger role in thoracotomy pain management with options that include epidural analgesia, intercostal, and paravertebral nerve blocks [49].

Laparotomy for intra-abdominal surgery can also be associated with poor pulmonary hygiene and nonadherence to rehabilitation following abdominal surgery [50]. However, it is also associated with an increased incidence of postoperative ileus. Incidence of ileus following abdominal surgery can be up to 40%, and perioperative opioid use can contribute to the development of paralytic ileus [51]. Thus, the management of postoperative laparotomy pain must balance pain control with the risk for ileus. Reducing opioid administration through the use of non-opioid adjuncts including regional analgesia, acetaminophen, GABA analogs, and ketamine can effectively control pain and reduce the risk of ileus following surgery [51].

Challenges of COVID-19

The COVID-19 pandemic has posed a variety of challenges in caring for critically ill patients. The disease remains poorly understood, and as a result, optimal sedation and analgesia is yet to be defined. Many reports, mainly describing clinical experience, seem to indicate that patients with COVID-19 ARDS have significantly increased sedation and analgesic requirements [52, 53]. One retrospective review of COVID-19 patients has shown analgesia requirements to be up to threefold higher when patients require mechanical ventilation than previously studied ARDS populations [53]. At the time this review was written, there were no data on changes in analgesic requirements attributable to COVID-19 in postsurgical and trauma patients. Perhaps insight will be gained utilizing data from research consortiums that have developed during the pandemic to better understand COVID-19.

ICU Discharge

Many patients will likely need to continue opioid analgesia therapy through the duration of their ICU stay following surgery or a traumatic injury. As patients progress through their recovery, their opioid therapy should progress with them and the assessment of a patient's analgesic regimen should be part of the decision to downgrade them from the ICU. Providers should have a standard protocol ensuring patients are discontinued from high-potency, rapid-onset opioids prior to leaving the ICU. Studies have shown that many medications including antipsychotics and stress ulcer prophylaxis medications prescribed while the patient was critically ill are unknowingly continued throughout hospitalization and upon discharge [51, 54, 55]. Recent data have shown similar trends with opioids [56]. Assessment of patient analgesic needs as the critical illness and immediate insult resolves should result in a discontinuation of analgesics when no longer necessary.

Summary

Patients presenting to a postsurgical or trauma ICU have a myriad of concerns in managing their analgesia and careful consideration of an appropriate opioid regimen is essential to effectively managing their critical illness. Uncontrolled pain can result in increased physiologic derangement as well as predispose patients to long-term physical and psychological disturbances. Appropriately assessing patient pain, through validated assessment tools and the ability to participate in rehabilitation are more appropriate than solely relying on subjective patient reports of pain. There is significant variation in the prescribing practices for opioids following surgery which can result in inadequate or excessive opioid administration. Appropriate assessment, in concert with protocols for managing acute pain, may help to reduce prescribing variation. Additionally, it is advisable that appropriate patients initiated on opioid therapy undergo screening for risk of dependence and addiction. Patients may present to the ICU with longstanding opioid use prior to surgery or traumatic injury. Chronic opioid use prior to presentation may impact baseline physiology and may increase requirements for opioids in the acute setting. Many patients will present to surgical ICUs following interventions that will require effective analgesia for appropriate respiratory function as well as participation in rehabilitation therapies. There are many adjuncts that can be employed in the perioperative setting that can be used to reduce opioid consumption and their associated side effects. Use of less conventional, long-acting opioids in the perioperative setting can help to decrease the use of high-potency, rapid-onset opioids. Regional and non-opioid analgesics have also been shown to reduce opioid requirements. As a patient recovers from their insult and prepares to transition out of the ICU, it is important that a careful review of prescribed medications including opioids is performed. Patients should not continue the most potent opioids as they progress to the next level of care and prepare for discharge. Non-opioid adjuncts may be sufficient for controlling pain in these settings and should be favored.

References

1. Czosnowski Q, Whitman C. Sedatives, analgesics and neuromuscular blockade in the ICU. In: Roberts PR, Todd SR, editors. Comprehensive critical care: adult. 2nd ed. Mt. Prospect: Society of Critical Care Medicine; 2017. p. 453–6.
2. Severgnini P, Pelosi P, Contino E, Serafinelli E, Novario R, Chiaranda M. Accuracy of critical care pain observation tool and behavioral pain scale to assess pain in critically ill conscious and unconscious patients: prospective, observational study. J Intensive Care. 2016;68(4). https://doi.org/10.1186/s40560-016-0192.
3. Apferlbaum JL, Chen C, Mehta SS, Gan TJ. Postoperative pain experience: results from a national survey suggesting postoperative pain continues to be undermanaged. Anesth Analg. 2003;97(2):534–40.
4. Bialosky JE, Bishop MD, Cleland JA. Individual expectation: an overlooked but pertinent factor in the treatment of individuals experiencing musculoskeletal pain. Phys Ther. 2010;90:1345–55.

5. Rummans TA, Burton MC, Dawson NL. How good intentions contributed to bad outcomes: the opioid crisis. Mayo Clin Proc. 2018;93:344–50.
6. Webster LR, Webster R. Predicting aberrant behaviors in opioid-treated patients: preliminary validation of the opioid risk too. Pain Med. 2005;6:432–42.
7. Thiels CA, Anderson SS, Ubl DS, Hanson KT, Bergquist WJ, Gray RJ, et al. Wide variation and overprescription of opioids after elective surgery. Ann Surg. 2017;266(4):564–73.
8. Hill MV, McMahon ML, Stucke RS, Barth RJ Jr. Wide variation and excessive dosage of opioid prescriptions for common general surgical procedures. Ann Surg. 2017;265(4):709–14.
9. Eid AI, DePesa C, Nordestgaard AT, Kongkaewpaisan N, Lee JM, Kongwibulwut M, et al. Variation of opioid prescribing patterns among patients undergoing similar surgery on the same acute care surgery service of the same institution: time for standardization? Surgery. 2018;164(5):926–30.
10. Chou R, Turner JA, Devine EB, Hansen RN, Sullivan SD, Blazina I, et al. The effectiveness and risks of long-term opioid therapy for chronic pain: a systematic review for a National Institutes of Health Pathways to Prevention Workshop. Ann Intern Med. 2015;162(4):276–86.
11. Baldini A, Von Korff M, Lin EH. A review of potential adverse effects of long-term opioid therapy: a practitioner's guide. Prim Care Companion CNS Disord. 2012;14(3):PCC.11m01326. https://doi.org/10.4088/PCC.11m01326.
12. Narayanan M, Venkataraju A, Jennings J. Analgesia in intensive care: part 1. BJA Educ. 2016;16(2):72–8.
13. Subramaniam B, Shankar P, Shaefi S, Mueller A, O'Gara B, Banner-Goodspeed V, et al. Effect of intravenous acetaminophen vs placebo combined with propofol or dexmedetomidine on postoperative delirium among older patients following cardiac surgery: the DEXACET randomized clinical trial. JAMA. 2019;321(7):686–96.
14. Pettersson PH, Jakobsson J, Owall A. Intravenous acetaminophen reduced the use of opioids compared with oral administration after coronary artery bypass grafting. J Cardiothorac Vasc Anesth. 2005;19(3):306–9.
15. Hickman SR, Mathieson KM, Bradford LM, Garman CD, Gregg RW, Lukens DW. Randomized trial of oral versus intravenous acetaminophen for postoperative pain control. Am J Health Syst Pharm. 2018;75(6):367–75.
16. Yang Y, Young JB, Schermer CR, Utter GH. Use of ketorolac is associated with decreased pneumonia following rib fractures. Am J Surg. 2014;207:566–72.
17. Pountos I, Georgouli T, Calori GM, Giannoudis PV. Do nonsteroidal anti-inflammatory drugs affect bone healing? A critical analysis. Scientific World Journal. 2012;2012:606404. https://doi.org/10.1100/2012/606404.
18. Mazzeffi M, Johnson K, Paciullo C. Ketamine in adult cardiac surgery and the cardiac surgery intensive care unit: an evidence-based clinical review. Ann Card Anaesth. 2015;18(2):202–9.
19. McGuinness SK, Wasiak J, Cleland H, Symons J, Hogan L, Hucker T, Mahar PD. A systematic review of ketamine as an analgesic agent in adult burn injuries. Pain Med. 2011;12(10):1551–8.
20. Lyon RF, Schwan C, Zeal J, Kharod C, Staak B, Petersen C, Rush SC. Successful use of ketamine as a prehospital analgesic by pararescuemen during Operation Enduring Freedom. J Spec Oper Med. 2018;18(1):70–3.
21. Kaur S, Saroa R, Aggarwal S. Effect of intraoperative infusion of low-dose ketamine on management of postoperative analgesia. J Nat Sci Biol Med. 2015;6(2):378–82.
22. Brinck ECV, Tiippana E, Heesen M, Bell RF, Straube S, Moore RA, Kontinen V. Perioperative intravenous ketamine for acute postoperative pain in adults. Cochrane Database Syst Rev. 2018;12:CD012033. https://doi.org/10.1002/14651858.CD012033.pub4.
23. Gorlin AW, Rosenfeld DM, Ramakrishna H. Intravenous sub-anesthetic ketamine for perioperative analgesia. J Anaesthesiol Clin Pharmacol. 2016;32(2):160–7.
24. Kakazu C, Lippman M, Hsu D. Ketamine: a positive-negative anesthetic agent. BJA. 2016;117(2):267.
25. Strumpher J, Jacobsohn E. Pulmonary hypertension and right ventricular dysfunction: physiology and perioperative management. J Cardiothorac Vasc Anesth. 2011;25:687–704.

26. Chang L, Raty S, Ortiz J, Bailard N, Mathew S. The emerging use of ketamine for anesthesia and sedation in traumatic brain injuries. CNS Neurosci Ther. 2013;19(6):390–5.
27. Yu SB. Dexmedetomidine sedation in ICU. Korean J Anesthesiol. 2012;62(5):405–11.
28. Ziyaeifard M, Azarfarin R, Golzari SE. A review of current analgesic techniques in cardiac surgery. Is epidural worth it? J Cardiovasc Thorac Res. 2014;6(3):133–40.
29. Guay J, Kopp S. Epidural analgesia for adults undergoing cardiac surgery with or without cardiopulmonary bypass. Cochrane Database Syst Rev. 2019;3:CD006715. https://doi.org/10.1002/14651858.CD006715.pub3.
30. Cummings KC III, Zimmerman NM, Maheshwari K, Cooper GS, Cummings LC. Epidural compared with non-epidural analgesia and cardiopulmonary complications after colectomy: a retrospective cohort study of 20,880 patients using a national quality database. J Clin Anesth. 2018;47:12–8.
31. Peek J, Beks RB, Kingma BF, Marsman M, Ruurda JP, Houwert RM, et al. Epidural analgesia for severe chest trauma: an analysis of current practice on the efficacy and safety. Crit Care Res Prac. 2019;Article ID:4837591. https://doi.org/10.1155/2019/4837591.
32. Brown R, Kraus C, Fleming M, Reddy S. Methadone: applied pharmacology and use as adjunctive treatment in chronic pain. Postgrad Med J. 2004;80(949):654–9.
33. U.S. Food and Drug Administration. Methadone hydrochloride injection, USP. https://www.accessdata.fda.gov/drugsatfda_docs/label/2016/021624s006lbl.pdf. 2016. Accessed 23 Nov 2019.
34. Murphy GS, Szokol JW, Avram MJ, Greenberg SB, Shear TD, Deshur MA, et al. Clinical effectiveness and safety of intraoperative methadone in patients undergoing posterior spinal fusion surgery: a randomized, double-blinded, controlled trial. Anesthesiology. 2017;126(5):822–33.
35. Murphy GS, Szokol JW, Avram MJ, Greenberg SB, Marymont JH, Shear T, et al. Intraoperative methadone for the prevention of postoperative pain: a randomized, double-blinded clinical trial in cardiac surgical patients. Anesthesiology. 2015;122(5):1112–22.
36. Murphy G, Szokol J. Intraoperative methadone in surgical patients: a review of clinical investigations. Anesthesiology. 2019;131:678–92.
37. Sadiq NM, Dice TJ, Mead T. Oxycodone. (Updated 2019 Sep 21). In: StatPearls [Internet]. Treasure Island: StatPearls Publishing. https://www.ncbi.nlm.nih.gov/books/NBK482226/. Accessed 13 Feb 2020.
38. Yasaei R, Saadabadi A. Meperidine. (Updated 2019 Oct 9). In: StatPearls [Internet]. Treasure Island: StatPearls Publishing. https://www.ncbi.nlm.nih.gov/books/NBK470362/. Accessed 13 Feb 2020.
39. Dhesi M, Maani CV. Tramadol. (Updated 2019 Oct 21). In: StatPearls [Internet]. Treasure Island: StatPearls Publishing. https://www.ncbi.nlm.nih.gov/books/NBK537060/. Accessed 13 Feb 2020.
40. Smith HS. Opioid metabolism. Mayo Clin Proc. 2009;84(7):613–24.
41. Stevens AJ, Woodman RJ, Owen H. The effect of ondansetron on the efficacy of postoperative tramadol: a systematic review and meta-analysis of a drug interaction. Anaesthesia. 2015;70(2):209–18.
42. Palmer PP, Miller RD. Current and developing methods of patient-controlled analgesia. Anesthesiol Clin. 2010;28(4):587–99. https://doi.org/10.1016/j.anclin.2010.08.010.
43. Li B, He X, Jia W, Li H. Novel applications of metabolomics in personalized medicine: a mini-review. Molecules. 2017;22(7):1173–83.
44. Bordoni B, Marelli F, Morabito B, Sacconi B, Severino P. Post-sternotomy pain syndrome following cardiac surgery: case report. J Pain Res. 2017;10:1163–9.
45. Allen KB, Icke KJ, Thourani VH, Naka Y, Grubb KJ, Grehan J, et al. Sternotomy closure using rigid plate fixation: a paradigm shift from wire cerclage. Ann Cardiothorac Surg. 2018;7(5):611–20. https://doi.org/10.21037/acs.2018.06.01.
46. Zubrzycki M, Liebold A, Skrabal C, Reinelt H, Ziegler M, Perdas E, Zubrzycka M. Assessment and pathophysiology of pain in cardiac surgery. J Pain Res. 2018;11:1599–611.

47. Svircevic V, Passier MM, Nierich AP, van Dijk D, Kalkman CJ, van der Heijden GJ. Epidural analgesia for cardiac surgery. Cochrane Database Syst Rev. 2013;(6). https://doi.org/10.1002/14651858.CD006715.pub2.
48. Karmakar MK, Ho AM. Postthoracotomy pain syndrome. Thorac Surg Clin. 2004;14(3):345–52.
49. Ng A, Swanevelder J. Pain relief after thoracotomy: is epidural analgesia the optimal technique? Br J Anaesth. 2007;98(2):159–62.
50. Ahmed A, Latif N, Khan R. Postoperative analgesia for major abdominal surgery and its effectiveness in a tertiary care hospital. J Anaesthesiol Clin Pharmacol. 2013;29(4):472–7.
51. Lubawski J, Saclarides T. Postoperative ileus: strategies for reduction. Ther Clin Risk Manag. 2008;4(5):913–7.
52. Adams CD, Altshuler J, Barlow BL, Dixit D, Droege CA, Effendi MK, Heavner MS, Johnston JP, Kiskaddon AL, Lemieux DG, Lemieux SM, Littlefield AJ, Owusu KA, Rouse GE, Thompson Bastin ML, Berger K. Analgesia and sedation strategies in mechanically ventilated adults with COVID-19. Pharmacotherapy. 2020;40(12):1180–91. https://doi.org/10.1002/phar.2471. Epub 2020 Nov 20.
53. Kapp CM, Zaeh S, Niedermeyer S, Punjabi NM, Siddharthan T, Damarla M. The use of analgesia and sedation in mechanically ventilated patients with COVID-19 acute respiratory distress syndrome. Anesth Analg. 2020;131(4):e198–200. https://doi.org/10.1213/ANE.0000000000005131. PMID: 32675640; PMCID: PMC7373364.
54. Tomichek JE, Stollings JL, Pandharipande PP, Chandrasekhar R, Ely EW, Girard TD. Antipsychotic prescribing patterns during and after critical illness: a prospective cohort study. Crit Care. 2016;20(1):378–85.
55. Wohlt PD, Hansen LA, Fish JT. Inappropriate continuation of stress ulcer prophylactic therapy after discharge. Ann Pharmacother. 2007;41(10):1611–6.
56. Collier C, Finoli L. Evaluation of opioids at transition of care from intensive care unit in opioid-naïve patients. Crit Care Med. 2019;47(1):652.
57. Murphy PB, Barrett MJ. Morphine. [Updated 2019 Oct 9]. In: StatPearls [Internet]. Treasure Island: StatPearls Publishing; 2020. Available from: https://www.ncbi.nlm.nih.gov/books/NBK526115/.
58. Abi-Aad KR, Derian A. Hydromorphone. [Updated 2019 Sep 10]. In: StatPearls [Internet]. Treasure Island: StatPearls Publishing; 2020. Available from: https://www.ncbi.nlm.nih.gov/books/NBK470393/.
59. Ramos-Matos CF, Lopez-Ojeda W. Fentanyl. [Updated 2019 Oct 3]. In: StatPearls [Internet]. Treasure Island: StatPearls Publishing; 2020. Available from: https://www.ncbi.nlm.nih.gov/books/NBK459275/.
60. Dean M. Opioids in renal failure and dialysis patients. J Pain Symptom Mange. 2004;28(5):497–504. Published 2004 Nov.
61. Soleimanpour H, Safari S, Shahsavari Nia K, Sanaie S, Alavian SM. Opioid drugs in patients with liver disease: a systematic review. Hepat Mon. 2016;16(4):e32636. Published 2016 Mar 6.
62. Gerriets V, Nappe TM. Acetaminophen. (Updated 2019 Dec 15). In: StatPearls [Internet]. Treasure Island: StatPearls Publishing. https://www.ncbi.nlm.nih.gov/books/NBK482369/. Accessed 13 Feb 2020.
63. Mahmoodi AN, Kim PY. Ketorolac. (Updated 2019 Nov 6). In: StatPearls [Internet]. Treasure Island: StatPearls Publishing. https://www.ncbi.nlm.nih.gov/books/NBK545172/. Accessed 13 Feb 2020.
64. Yasaei R, Katta S, Saadabadi A. Gabapentin. (Updated 2020 Jan 20). In: StatPearls [Internet]. Treasure Island: StatPearls Publishing. https://www.ncbi.nlm.nih.gov/books/NBK493228/. Accessed 13 Feb 2020.
65. Reel B, Maani CV. Dexmedetomidine. (Updated 2019 Jun 18). In: StatPearls [Internet]. Treasure Island: StatPearls Publishing. https://www.ncbi.nlm.nih.gov/books/NBK513303/. Accessed 13 Feb 2020.
66. Rosenbaum SB, Palacios JL. Ketamine. (Updated 2019 Feb 21). In: StatPearls [Internet]. Treasure Island: StatPearls Publishing. https://www.ncbi.nlm.nih.gov/books/NBK470357/. Accessed 13 Feb 2020.

Chapter 13
Long-Term Effects of Pain and Opioid Use in the ICU

Mary Ann Hernando and Mark E. Mikkelsen

Introduction

Many critically ill patients admitted to an intensive care unit (ICU) will experience moderate-to-severe pain during their admission [1, 2]. This includes pain at rest [3] and pain experienced during common ICU procedures [4]. As a result, adequate treatment of pain is a recognized priority in critical care medicine.

Survivors of critical illness, a population that is growing due to advances in care, often experience chronic pain. In the context of the coronavirus disease 2019 (Covid-19) pandemic, the disease due to severe acute respiratory syndrome coronavirus 2 (SARS-CoV-2), these issues have never been more salient.

While there is growing recognition of chronic pain after ICU admission, fundamental questions remain unanswered. Specifically, is acute pain during critical illness related to the chronic pain that survivors experience? Does this chronic pain, combined with frequent exposure to opioids in the critical care setting, present a risk for post-ICU opioid dependence? As critical care delivery in the twenty-first century is designed to improve both short- and long-term outcomes, these are vital questions for the bedside provider.

In this chapter, we review international pain guidelines and the long-term implications of current pain management practices in the ICU. We then explore the epidemiology of pain following critical illness, with a focus on chronic pain that

M. A. Hernando
Perelman School of Medicine at the University of Pennsylvania, Philadelphia, PA, USA

Internal Medicine, Columbia University Irving Medical Center, New York, NY, USA

M. E. Mikkelsen (✉)
Perelman School of Medicine at the University of Pennsylvania, Philadelphia, PA, USA

Division of Pulmonary, Allergy, and Critical Care Medicine, Perelman School of Medicine at the University of Pennsylvania, Philadelphia, PA, USA
e-mail: mark.mikkelsen@uphs.upenn.edu

J. L. Pascual, T. G. Gaulton (eds.), *Opioid Use in Critical Care*,
https://doi.org/10.1007/978-3-030-77399-1_13

Table 13.1 Non-pharmacologic interventions and non-opioid pharmacologic adjuvants recommended in clinical practice guidelines to mitigate pain and opioid use in the ICU [5]

Non-pharmacologic interventions	Non-opioid pharmacologic adjuvants
Music therapy	Acetaminophen
Massage	Nefopam
Cold therapy	Low-dose ketamine
Relaxation techniques	Neuropathic pain medications (e.g., gabapentin)

develops or worsens after an ICU admission. We then consider the impact of chronic post-ICU pain on quality of life and evaluate the existing data regarding changes in opioid use after critical illness. Finally, we conclude by discussing strategies to prevent and mitigate chronic post-ICU pain.

International Pain Guidelines and Current Practices

In 2018, the Society of Critical Care Medicine published its updated Clinical Practice Guidelines for the Prevention and Management of Pain, Agitation/Sedation, Delirium, Immobility, and Sleep Disruption (PADIS) in Adult ICU Patients [5]. The pain management recommendations emphasize a multimodal approach to analgesia that includes non-pharmacologic interventions and non-opioid pharmacologic adjuvants as strategies to reduce opioid use and minimize the risks associated with opioid exposure (Table 13.1) [5]. These guidelines also recommend protocol-based pain assessment and management using standardized pain assessments (e.g., behavioral pain scale (BPS) or critical-care pain observation tool (CPOT)) to facilitate sedation minimization and, explicitly, to reduce opioid consumption [5].

Despite this emphasis on non-opioid alternatives and adjuncts for the treatment of pain in critically ill patients, opioids remain the mainstay of pain management in the ICU. Opioids are also frequently used in critically ill patients to enhance sedation, improve mechanical ventilation synchrony, and reduce agitation, with many patients receiving continuous opioid infusions for prolonged periods of time during their ICU stay [6]. In one retrospective study of 286 US acute care facilities, 56% of nonsurgical patients admitted to an ICU received opioids during their admission [7]. This high exposure to opioids in the ICU raises concern for the potential of ICU-acquired opioid dependence and subsequent long-term opioid-related morbidity.

Life After the ICU

In addition to concerns for ICU-acquired opioid dependence, critical illness has also been associated with the development of chronic pain [2, 8–10]. As advances in critical care medicine have led to increased survival, there has also been a growing awareness among critical care providers of the long-term impairments that follow critical illness, sometimes termed "survivorship" ailments.

Post-Intensive Care Syndrome (PICS) refers to the series of impairments in cognition, mental health, and physical health that survivors of critical illness commonly endure [11]. Fifty-six percent of survivors of critical illness experience a new and lasting impairment in one or more of these domains, with 21% continuing to experience two or more impairments one year after their critical illness [12]. These impairments contribute to the reductions in health-related quality of life and inability to return to employment that afflict many survivors.

As the understanding of life after critical illness matures, chronic pain has emerged as an important, life-altering, functionally incapacitating condition. Chronic pain may contribute to PICS, and vice versa. It remains unclear whether chronic pain results from acute pain experienced in the ICU and/or residual inflammation exacerbated by disuse and functional impairment [6, 13]. Notably, the presence of chronic pain following critical illness may serve to further aggravate the risk of opioid use and dependence among ICU survivors. An understanding of these suspected long-term consequences of acute ICU pain and opioid use in the ICU is needed to inform the judicious use of opioids in the critical care setting.

Epidemiology of Chronic Pain After Critical Illness

Chronic pain is common among survivors of critical illness [2, 8–10]. In a 2019 review of nine studies evaluating chronic post-ICU pain, the prevalence of chronic pain among ICU survivors ranged from 33% to 73% [14], with an incidence of moderate to severe pain of 45% in one study [10]. A separate, narrative review similarly found prevalence rates that varied substantially [2].

Yet, it is not entirely clear what proportion of patients has pain that is directly attributable to their past critical illness. Most studies of chronic post-ICU pain did not assess patients' baseline chronic pain status, leaving open the possibility that patients reporting chronic post-ICU pain may have had some measure of chronic pain that predated their ICU stay.

Few studies have sought to address this question. In one study of 47 ICU survivors participating in a post-ICU recovery program, 66% reported new pain that had not been present prior to their ICU admission [8]. Another study of 207 ICU survivors found that, 6 months after a medical or surgical ICU stay, 16.3% of patients who had no preexisting chronic pain developed a chronic pain condition that they attributed to their ICU admission, while another 16.8% had chronic pain prior to admission but reported new sources of chronic pain following their ICU stay [10]. Combined, one-third of patients in the study reported chronic ICU-related pain specifically [10].

The results of these studies suggest that most patients experience new pain after their ICU admission, with as many as one-third reporting persistent (i.e., chronic) pain at 6 months [8–10]. The declining prevalence could reflect symptom improvement over time, survivor bias, or both. While some post-ICU pain may be unrelated to the ICU admission, either as preexisting pain or new pain attributable to other causes, a substantial proportion is believed by patients to be new and specifically attributable to their ICU stay. However, a number of confounding factors may be at play in self-reported pain assessments, such as poor patient recall of pain prior to their ICU admission and the presence of new functional impairments following critical illness that may impact perceptions of pain.

The etiology of chronic pain following critical illness is not fully understood. Several possible mechanisms for this acute-to-chronic pain transition have been proposed [6]. One potential mechanism is that sustained activation of peripheral nociceptive fibers during acute pain may lead to eventual structural remodeling of the central nervous system with subsequent hyperactivity that manifests as chronic pain [13]. Additional theories regarding the mechanisms that underlie the transition from acute to chronic pain include interaction between the immune system and central nervous system during the sickness response, as well as alterations in emotional and cognitive processing that impact pain affect [15].

Apart from the acute-to-chronic pain transition, common sequelae of critical illness may also serve as additional mediators of chronic post-ICU pain. Functionally limiting joint contractures, for example, are relatively common. In one study, contractures were found in 39% of ICU patients at the time of transfer out of the ICU, and were associated with limited range of motion and pain [16, 17]. This provides another possible mechanism for the new chronic pain that many ICU survivors experience, and presents an important opportunity for further research and intervention.

For patients who experience chronic pain following an ICU admission, the shoulder joint is the most frequently affected joint [8, 9]. This may be the result of prolonged immobility of the shoulder joint during critical illness due to the location of central lines, ventilator tubing, and other equipment, as well as pressure placed on the shoulder during common nursing procedures such as rolling [9]. Other common sites of pain include the trunk, back, upper limb, and head [8]. Notably, 39% of patients presenting with new chronic post-ICU pain have pain at more than one site [8].

Relatively few studies have attempted to identify risk factors associated with the development of chronic pain following critical illness. Some noted risk factors include severe sepsis [9], admission for trauma or surgery [18], acute respiratory distress syndrome (ARDS) [19], and increasing patient age [9]. Other factors such as ICU length of stay and days of mechanical ventilation have not been found to be predictive of post-ICU pain [10, 20]. Data is lacking on whether acute pain intensity and/or duration during an ICU stay is associated with chronic post-ICU pain conditions [14].

Given the frequent overlap between postoperative patients and patients admitted to the ICU, findings from studies of risk factors for chronic pain and/or chronic postsurgical pain may help shed light on possible additional risk factors for chronic pain following critical illness [8]. A 2016 review of risk factors for the development of chronic postsurgical pain proposed an extensive framework that included patient-related, psychosocial, preoperative, intraoperative, and postoperative variables associated with a higher likelihood of chronic pain [13]. This included risk factors such as severity or duration of pain, female gender, preoperative opioid use, and patient anxiety and depression [13]. These variables present opportunities for further investigation to determine whether they may in fact be risk factors for the development of chronic post-ICU pain as well.

Impact of Chronic Post-ICU Pain

Chronic post-ICU pain contributes to the decreased quality of life seen in survivors of critical illness, with 60% of patients with chronic post-ICU pain reporting moderate to severe impairments in daily life, family activities, and work [10]. Among survivors of severe accidental injuries, those with chronic post-ICU pain were more likely to have a physical disability and inability to work as a result of their critical illness than those without chronic pain [21]. Notably, while chronic pain in general is known to be associated with anxiety and depression, studies of chronic post-ICU pain in particular have yet to find this association [22].

While the consequences of post-ICU pain are severe and long-lasting, recent data suggests that the impact of these impairments on patients' daily functioning may decrease over time. In one study of patients with new chronic post-ICU pain, the mean Brief Pain Inventory (BPI) interference score at baseline assessment was 6.5, representing a high level of interference in daily activities [8]. The two domains with the highest level of interference secondary to chronic pain were "enjoyment of life" and sleep [8]. Notably, though pain severity did not improve at 1 year, pain interference did improve with a reduced mean BPI interference score of 4.5 [8]. This suggests that patients suffering from chronic post-ICU pain achieve some return of their ability to carry out their daily activities despite steady pain levels. This may be due to the development of coping strategies to better manage their pain, an improved sense of self-efficacy over time [8], and/or reflect adaptation, resilience [23], and post-traumatic growth [24].

Patterns of Opioid Use Among ICU Survivors

As noted previously, the frequent use of opioids in the ICU has raised concern for the potential of ICU-acquired opioid dependence and subsequent long-term opioid-related morbidity among survivors of critical illness. As a result, a small number of studies have attempted to evaluate whether or not there is in fact increased opioid use among ICU survivors.

In a retrospective review of 2595 adult patients admitted to the ICU of one tertiary care center, 76.9% were nonusers, 16.9% were intermittent opioid users, and 6.2% were chronic opioid users 3 months prior to admission [25]. At discharge, the proportion of nonusers had increased to 87.8% while intermittent users and chronic users decreased to 8.6% and 3.6%, respectively [25]. Finally, at 4 years of follow-up the proportion of nonusers had further increased to 95.6%, with intermittent users dropping to 2.6% and chronic users dropping to 1.8% [25]. This represents a statistically significant change in the distribution of patients among the three categories of opioid usage before and after their ICU admission, with an increase in nonusers and decrease in both intermittent and chronic users after their ICU stay [25]. Therefore, this study did not find an increase in chronic opioid use following ICU admission. Notably, pre-admission opioid use and prolonged hospital length of stay were associated with chronic opioid use in the study, while age, gender, type of patient (medical vs surgical), and ICU length of stay were not [25].

A separate population-based cohort study of all adult ICUs in Ontario, Canada, sought to evaluate patterns of opioid use following critical illness for the subset of elderly patients who were chronic opioid users prior to their admission [26]. Among the 19,584 patients studied, the median daily dose of opioids filled prior to admission was 32.1 g of morphine equivalent [26]. At 6 months following hospital discharge, 22% of patients had filled a prescription for a higher daily morphine equivalent, 19.8% were unchanged, 21.5% had filled a prescription for a lower daily morphine equivalent, and 36.7% had no prescription filled [26]. These findings suggest that among chronic opioid users, at least among those who survive to 6 months, ICU admission is not associated with an increase in opioid use at 6 months following discharge [26]. Taken together, the two studies described in this section appear to refute the notion that exposure to opioids in the ICU increases the risk of ICU-acquired opioid dependence among adult nonusers or leads to escalating opioid doses among elderly chronic opioid users.

Prevention and Mitigation of Chronic Post-ICU Pain

Because chronic post-ICU pain is a common consequence of critical illness, one that interferes with daily function and quality of life [8–10], strategies to prevent and mitigate chronic post-ICU pain are urgently needed to improve outcomes for ICU survivors. Given the role of acute pain in the development of chronic post-ICU pain, adequate pain management is an essential component of chronic pain prevention [6, 13]. Despite this, only 35.5% of ICU patients have their pain assessed by a physician, and fewer still are assessed using a validated pain assessment tool [27]. Accurate and frequent pain assessment in the ICU is needed to promptly treat acute pain and decrease the likelihood that chronic pain will develop.

While opioids remain the mainstay of acute pain management in the ICU, their use must be balanced against the risk of adverse effects as well as the potential for subsequent ICU-acquired opioid dependence and morbidity. An individualized pain management plan that uses a multimodal analgesia approach as recommended in the PADIS guidelines [5] is therefore needed to achieve this goal. Such an approach should incorporate non-opioid analgesics as well as non-pharmacologic pain management interventions such as music, massage, and relaxation techniques to reduce the need for opioids and minimize the risk of adverse effects (Table 13.1) [5]. For

Table 13.2 The ABCDEF (A2F) bundle elements [28–31]

A	Assess, prevent, and manage pain
B	Both spontaneous awakening trials and spontaneous breathing trials
C	Choice of analgesia and sedation
D	Delirium: assess, prevent, and manage
E	Early mobility and exercise
F	Family engagement and empowerment

patients at risk of joint contractures, which may function as a mediator of chronic post-ICU pain, preventive steps should be taken to minimize the risk that contractures will develop. This may include interventions such as the use of steroids which have been shown to have a protective effect against joint contractures, though further research in this area is still needed [16].

At present, in the absence of an evidence-base to rely upon to mitigate post-ICU chronic pain, we encourage use of the recommended ABCDEF (A2F) bundle. The bundle (Table 13.2) encourages care practices that align with PADIS clinical practice guidelines and foster care delivery designed to limit the immobility, sedation, and brain dysfunction that contribute to the development of PICS and its related consequences [28–31]. Among the realized benefits of the A2F bundle is a greater degree of functional independence after critical illness, a finding that may translate into less post-ICU chronic pain. Specifically, emphasizing early mobility and physical therapy for patients in the ICU may contribute to the prevention of chronic post-ICU pain [8]. Future research is needed to test this important potential benefit of the A2F bundle, adopted by the Society of Critical Care Medicine as the centerpiece of the ICU Liberation collaborative.

For patients who do develop chronic post-ICU pain, outpatient follow-up paired with referral to a specialized pain clinic can ensure that patients receive adequate analgesia tailored to their needs [14]. Follow-up should also include appropriate screening, counseling, and management of any other PICS associated impairments that may be present, such as cognitive impairment [32], anxiety [33], depression [33], and impairments in activities of daily living [34, 35]. The growing rise of post-ICU clinics presents a promising model for the delivery of comprehensive care for survivors of critical illness [36]. However, regardless of where patients receive their follow-up care, providers must ensure that they are conducting thorough medication and functional reconciliation to identify patients who have been continued on opioids or who may be receiving higher doses of opioids than they had been prior to their ICU stay and to identify patients with new, functional impairments [35].

Conclusion

In summary, critically ill patients often experience pain both at rest and during standard ICU procedures. This acute ICU pain has been associated with the development of chronic pain in survivors of critical illness, leading to significant interference in daily functioning and decreased quality of life. Prevention of chronic post-ICU pain requires appropriate ICU pain assessment and management using a multimodal analgesia model as one element of the evidence-based ABCDEF bundle recommended to improve short- and long-term outcomes for critically ill patients. With opioids continuing to play a large role in ICU pain management, providers must take care to use opioids judiciously in order to avoid adverse events and reduce the theoretical risk of ICU-acquired opioid dependence. While existing studies suggest that opioid use in the ICU does not pose an obvious risk of increased chronic opioid use after the ICU stay, additional studies are needed to further characterize the long-term consequences of opioid use in the critical care setting.

References

1. Puntillo KA, Arai S, Cohen NH, et al. Symptoms experienced by intensive care unit patients at high risk of dying. Crit Care Med. 2010;38(11):2155–60.
2. Kemp HI, Laycock H, Costello A, Brett SJ. Chronic pain in critical care survivors: a narrative review. Br J Anaesth. 2019;123(2):e372–84.
3. Chanques G, Sebbane M, Barbotte E, et al. A prospective study of pain at rest: incidence and characteristics of an unrecognized symptom in surgical and trauma versus medical intensive care unit patients. Anesthesiology. 2007;107:858–60.
4. Puntillo KA, Max A, Timsit JF, et al. Determinants of procedural pain intensity in the intensive care unit. The Europain® study. Am J Respir Crit Care Med. 2014;189:39–47.
5. Devlin JW, Skrobik Y, Gelinas C, et al. Clinical practice guidelines for the prevention and management of pain, agitation/sedation, delirium, immobility, and sleep disruption in adult patients in the ICU. Crit Care Med. 2018;46:825–73.
6. Puntillo KA, Naidu R. Chronic pain disorders after critical illness and ICU-acquired opioid dependence: two clinical conundra. Curr Opin Crit Care. 2016;22(5):506–12.
7. Herzig SJ, Rothberg MB, Cheung M, et al. Opioids and opioid-related adverse events. J Hosp Med. 2014;2:73–81.
8. Devine H, Quasim T, McPeake J, et al. Chronic pain in intensive care unit survivors: incidence, characteristics and side-effects up to one-year post-discharge. J Rehabil Med. 2019;51(6):451–5.
9. Battle CE, Lovett S, Hutchings H. Chronic pain in survivors of critical illness: a retrospective analysis of incidence and risk factors. Crit Care. 2013;17(3):R101.
10. Baumbach P, Gotz T, Gunther A, et al. Prevalence and characteristics of chronic intensive care-related pain: the role of severe sepsis and septic shock. Crit Care Med. 2016;44:1129–37.
11. Needham DM, Davidson J, Cohen H, et al. Improving long-term outcomes after discharge from intensive care unit: report from a stakeholders' conference. Crit Care Med. 2012;40(2):502–9.
12. Marra A, Pandharipande PP, Girard TD, et al. Co-occurrence of post-intensive care syndrome problems among 406 survivors of critical illness. Crit Care Med. 2018;46(9):1393–401.
13. Pozek JJ, Beausang D, Baratta JL, Viscusi ER. The acute to chronic pain transition: can chronic pain be prevented? Med Clin N Am. 2016;100(1):17–30.
14. Stamenkovic DM, Laycock H, Karanikolas M, et al. Chronic pain and chronic opioid use after intensive care discharge - is it time to change practice? Front Pharmacol. 2019;10:23.
15. Kyranou M, Puntillo K. The transition from acute to chronic pain: might intensive care unit patients be at risk? Ann Intensive Care. 2012;2:36.
16. Clavet H, Hébert PC, Fergusson D, et al. Joint contracture following prolonged stay in the intensive care unit. CMAJ. 2008;178(6):691–7.

17. Skalsky AJ, McDonald CM. Prevention and management of limb contractures in neuromuscular diseases. Phys Med Rehabil Clin N Am. 2012;23(3):675–87.
18. Granja C, Teixeira-Pinto A, Costa-Pereira A. Quality of life after intensive care – evaluation with EQ-5D questionnaire. Intensive Care Med. 2002;28:898–907.
19. Dowdy DW, Eid MP, Dennison CR, et al. Quality of life after acute respiratory distress syndrome: a meta-analysis. Intensive Care Med. 2006;32(8):1115–24.
20. Timmers TK, Verhofstad MHJ, Moons KGM, et al. Long-term quality of life after surgical intensive care admission. Arch Surg. 2011;146:412.
21. Jenewein J, Moergeli H, Wittmann L, et al. Development of chronic pain following severe accidental injury: results of a 3-year follow-up study. J Psychosom. 2009;66:119–26.
22. Katz J, Rosenbloom BN, Fashler S. Chronic pain, psychopathology, and DSM-5 somatic symptom disorder. Can J Psychiatry. 2015;60:160–7.
23. Maley JH, Brewster I, Mayoral I, et al. Resilience in survivors of critical illness in the context of the survivors' experience and recovery. Ann Am Thorac Soc. 2016;13(8):1351–60.
24. Rendon J. Upside: the new science of post-traumatic growth. New York: Touchstone; 2016.
25. Yaffe PB, Green RS, Butler MB. Is admission to the intensive care unit associated with chronic opioid use? A 4-year follow-up of intensive care unit survivors. J Intensive Care. 2017;32(7):429–35.
26. Wang HT, Hill AD, Gomes T, et al. Opioid use after ICU admission among elderly chronic opioid users in Ontario: a population-based cohort study. Crit Care Med. 2018;46(12):1934–42.
27. Kemp HI, Bantel C, Gordon F, et al. Pain assessment in INTensive care (PAINT): an observational study of physician-documented pain assessment in 45 intensive care units in the United Kingdom. Anaesthesia. 2017;72:1–12.
28. Girard TD, Kress JP, Fuchs BD, et al. Efficacy and safety of a paired sedation and ventilator weaning protocol for mechanically ventilated patients intensive care (Awakening and Breathing Controlled trial): a randomised controlled trial. Lancet. 2008;371(9607):126–34.
29. Schweickert WD, Pohlman MC, Pohlman AS, et al. Early physical and occupational therapy in mechanically ventilated, critically ill patients: a randomized, controlled trial. Lancet. 2009;373(9678):1874–82.
30. Barnes-Daly MA, Phillips G, Ely EW. Improving hospital survival and reducing brain dysfunction at seven California community hospitals: implementing PAD guidelines via the ABCDEF bundle in 6,064 patients. Crit Care Med. 2017;45(2):171–8.
31. Pun BT, Balas MC, Barnes-Daly MA, et al. Caring for critically ill patients with the ABCDEF bundle: results of the ICU liberation collaborative in over 15,000 adults. Crit Care Med. 2019;47(1):3–14.
32. Pandharipande PP, Girard TD, Jackson JC, et al. Long-term cognitive impairment after critical illness. N Engl J Med. 2013;369:1306–16.
33. Desai S, Law T, Bienvenu J, Needham D. Psychiatric long-term complications of intensive care unit survivors. Crit Care Med. 2011;39(12):2790.
34. Hopkins RO, Suchyta MR, Kamdar BB, et al. Instrumental activities of daily living after critical illness: a systematic review. Ann Am Thorac Soc. 2017;14(8):1332–43.
35. Mikkelsen ME, Still M, Anderson BJ, et al. Society of critical care medicine's international consensus conference on prediction and identification of long-term impairments after critical illness. Crit Care Med. 2020;48(11):1670–9.
36. Haines KJ, McPeake J, Hibbert E, et al. Enablers and barriers to implementing ICU follow-up clinics and peer support groups following critical illness: the Thrive Collaboratives. Crit Care Med. 2019;47(9):1194–200.

Chapter 14
Special ICU Populations: Opioids in Neurocritical Care

Meghan M. Caylor and Ramani Balu

Overview of Sedation and Analgesia Practices in Neurocritical Care

As with other critically ill patients, brain-injured patients require sedation and analgesia for multiple purposes including, but not limited to, the facilitation of mechanical ventilation, treatment of pain associated with procedures and routine ICU care, and for minimizing anxiety. In accordance with the most recent Society of Critical Care Medicine (SCCM) Pain, Agitation/Sedation, Delirium, Immobility and Sleep Disruption (PADIS) guidelines, the practice of using light sedation targets has generally been adopted in the neurocritical care population, including incorporation of analgosedation and general avoidance of benzodiazepine sedatives in favor of non-benzodiazepine options such as propofol and dexmedetomidine [1–3]. However, because the landmark studies that paved the way for these recommendations largely excluded patients with primary neurologic injuries, the impact of these sedation practices and corresponding outcomes in patients with brain injury remains poorly understood [4–7].

In addition to their general uses that are common for all critically ill patients, sedation and analgesia are often required in neurocritical care to minimize the impact of routine ICU care on secondary brain injury. For example, common scenarios encountered in the ICU—such as coughing or gagging on endotracheal tubes, tracheal suctioning, or episodes of acute pain or anxiety—can precipitate acute

M. M. Caylor (✉)
Department of Pharmacy, Hospital of the University of Pennsylvania, Philadelphia, PA, USA
e-mail: meghan.caylor@pennmedicine.upenn.edu

R. Balu
Division of Neurocritical Care, Department of Neurology, Perelman School of Medicine, University of Pennsylvania, Philadelphia, PA, USA
e-mail: ramani.balu@pennmedicine.upenn.edu

J. L. Pascual, T. G. Gaulton (eds.), *Opioid Use in Critical Care*,
https://doi.org/10.1007/978-3-030-77399-1_14

elevations of intracranial pressure (ICP) to critical levels in patients with poor intracranial compliance. Alternatively, the hemodynamic side effects of sedatives and analgesics, such as bradycardia and hypotension, may decrease cerebral perfusion and negate any advantages of their use [8, 9].

On the other hand, the requirements of sedation and analgesia must also be balanced with the need to detect minute changes in neurological examination which indicate new or worsening intracranial processes that potentially require rapid intervention. Brain-injured patients require frequent neurologic assessments, and the desire to minimize sedation (which can interfere with these assessments) presents a unique challenge in this ICU population. Fear of masking a patient's subtle signs of neurologic deterioration with sedating agents may also lead to undertreatment of pain, thus creating an ever conflicting need for balancing patient comfort with quality neurologic assessment.

On the opposite end of this spectrum, deep sedation with pharmacologic coma must at times be employed in the treatment of certain pathologic states [9]. Indeed, notable exceptions to the application of light sedation in the neurocritical care setting include the treatment of intracranial hypertension, status epilepticus, and use of continuous neuromuscular blockade for refractory intracranial hypertension, acute respiratory distress syndrome (ARDS), and management of shivering in targeted temperature management (TTM). With the exception of status epilepticus, optimization of analgesia with the use of opiate infusions is considered a standard component of the regimen employed for deep sedation, in addition to use of hypnotic sedatives such as propofol or midazolam. Deep sedation should generally be reserved for use when a clear indication exists and where short-term benefits to the brain are deemed to outweigh the long-term risks.

Assessment of Pain in Patients with Acute Brain Injury

Assessment of pain in patients in neurocritical care represents a particular challenge, since both impairments of consciousness and aphasia can confound standardized assessment tools [10]. Indeed, damage to cortical networks involved in pain perception after brain injury may significantly alter the need for pain control. However, the fact that such patients generally continue to exhibit physiological responses (such as tachycardia, elevated blood pressure, and increased ICP) to painful stimuli highlights the need for tools that can accurately assess pain in brain-injured patients. The Behavioral Pain Scale (BPS) and Critical Care Pain Observation Tool (CPOT) have the highest validity and reliability in patients without brain injury who are unable to self-report pain [1, 11, 12]. Based on small validation studies, their use in neurocritical care is endorsed by both SCCM and the Neurocritical Care Society (NCS) [1, 13]. Larger scale validation and potential refinement of the scales for optimal use in patients with neurologic injuries is needed; however, both the BPS and CPOT seem to be useful tools to systematically evaluate pain in brain-injured patients [14–17].

In survivors of brain injury who develop chronic disorders of consciousness—including persistent vegetative state (VS, also termed unresponsive wakeful syndrome, UWS) and minimally conscious states (MCS)—the inability to communicate and uncertainty about the capacity to consciously perceive pain makes pain assessment extremely challenging [18, 19]. Neuroimaging studies in patients with MCS suggest that cortical responses may be preserved and probably permit the processing and perception of pain; however, similar studies in VS/UWS patients have demonstrated severe impairment in function and connectivity of these pathways [19–21]. Nevertheless, there exists the possibility that a subset of patients with VS/UWS may also retain cortical processing and potentially the ability perceive pain [19, 22]. Thus, a reliable scale to assess for potential pain/nociception responses in these patients is undoubtedly important to providing compassionate care.

The Nociception Coma Scale (NCS) was developed for use in patients with prolonged coma and severe disorders of consciousness. After initial validation, the NCS was further refined by removing the visual response subcategory, which was found to be unchanged in response to noxious stimuli, giving way to the newer NCS-Revised (NSC-R). Similar to the CPOT and BPS-NI (BPS–Non-Intubated), the NCS-R assesses behaviors in categories related to facial expression, motor movements, and vocal responses (Table 14.1) [12, 23, 24]. Importantly, the maximum potential score in VS/UWS patients is lower than in MCS due to the intrinsic limitations of their lower level of consciousness. The NCS-R has since been validated in several small studies, demonstrating a reliable increase in score when patients are exposed to painful stimuli as compared to non-noxious stimuli [18, 24, 25]. Although it is still not possible to know whether the detection of nociceptive responses correlates to subjective pain sensation in an individual patient, the development of the NCS-R represents an important step in objective assessment and quantification in this setting.

Overview of Cerebrovascular Physiology and Hemodynamics

The brain has high energy demands and receives approximately 20% of the cardiac output. Under normal circumstances, cerebral blood flow (CBF) is tightly matched to cerebral metabolic demands, and increases as the cerebral metabolic rate of oxygen consumption ($CMRO_2$) trigger increases in CBF. However, after acute brain injury, perfusion may not be adequate to meet cerebral metabolic demands. In such instances, secondary brain injury occurs [26, 27].

CBF depends linearly on the cerebral perfusion pressure (CPP) and inversely on the cerebrovascular resistance (CVR). Thus, changes in either CPP or CVR can have profound impacts on CBF. In brain-injured patients, CPP equals the difference between mean arterial pressure (MAP) and ICP. Increases in ICP can therefore deleteriously reduce CPP and lead to ischemia. Increases in systemic partial pressure of CO_2 (pCO_2), which most often occur due to reductions in respiratory drive, can lead to pH-dependent vasodilatation of cerebral arterioles. Normally, hypercapnia leads to increases in CBF by decreasing CVR. However, in brain-injured patients, the increased

Table 14.1 Comparison of the Nociception Coma Scale-Revised with other critical care behavioral pain assessment scales

Scoring Domains	Behavioral Pain Assessment Tools					
	BPS-NI		CPOT		NCS-R	
Facial expression	**1**	Relaxed	**0**	Relaxed	**0**	None
	2	Partially tightened	**1**	Tense	**1**	Oral reflexive movement/ startle response
	3	Fully tightened	**2**	Grimacing	**2**	Grimace
	4	Grimacing			**3**	Cry
Motor movements	**1**	No movement of upper limbs	**0**	No movements/ neutral position	**0**	None/flaccid
	2	Partially bent	**1**	Protection	**1**	Abnormal posturing
	3	Fully bent with finger flexion	**2**	Restlessness/ agitation	**2**	Flexion withdrawal
	4	Permanently retracted			**3**	Localization
Verbal	**1**	Vocalization	**0**	Normal vocalization	**0**	None
	2	Moaning ≤3 min	**1**	Sighing, moaning	**1**	Groaning
	3	Moaning >3 min	**2**	Crying out, sobbing	**2**	Vocalization
	4	Verbal complaint or breath holding			**3**	Verbalization (unintelligible)
Muscle tension (CPOT only)			**0**	Relaxed		
			1	Tense, rigid		
			2	Very tense or rigid		
Pain score range	**3–12**		**0–8**		**0–9**	
Threshold score for presence of significant pain/ nociception	≥6		≥3		Unknown ≥4 in MCS or ≥3 in VS/UWS in the validation study; ≥2 in a subsequent study	

Adapted from [12, 23–25]

BPS-NI Behavioral Pain Scale – non-intubated, *CPOT* Critical Care Pain Observation Tool, *MCS* minimally conscious state, *NCS-R* Nociception Coma Scale-Revised, *VS/UWS* vegetative state/ unresponsive wakeful syndrome

cerebral blood volume that occurs after hypercapnia-induced vasodilation can markedly increase ICP, leading to decreased CPP and reductions in CBF. Hyperventilation can similarly decrease ICP through pH-dependent vasoconstriction. While this increases CPP, it will also lead to marked increases in CVR and ultimately decreased CBF and ischemia. For these reasons, maintaining pCO_2 consistently within normal range is a major goal when caring for brain-injured patients [26, 27].

Table 14.2 Comparison of properties of opioids and sedative agents impacting cerebral physiologic parameters

	Mechanism of Action	$CMRO_2$	ICP	CPP and MAP	Comments
Opioids (fentanyl, morphine)	μ-opioid receptor agonist	↔	↔ / ↑	↔ / ↓	Bolus opiates may transiently ↑ICP in response to ↓ MAP Prevent/reduce elevations in ICP by treating pain and blunting response to noxious stimuli
Propofol	$GABA_A$ agonist	↓↓	↓↓	↓/↓↓	Therapy for status epilepticus; typically the agent of choice for sedation in elevated ICP unless hemodynamic instability (use midazolam)
Benzodiazepines (midazolam bolus/ infusion)	$GABA_A$ agonists	↓↓	↓	↓	Therapy for intracranial hypertension and status epilepticus (alternative to propofol)
Dexmedetomidine	α_2-adrenergic agonist	↔ / ↓	↔	↓/↓↓	Used for sedation in a similar fashion as other ICU populations
Ketamine	NMDA-receptor antagonist	↓	↔ / ↓	↔ / ↑	Emerging therapy for refractory status epilepticus (high dose)
Barbiturates (pentobarbital, thiopental)	$GABA_A$ agonists	↓↓↓	↓↓↓	↓↓↓	Last-line therapy for refractory intracranial hypertension and status epilepticus

References: [8, 9, 28–34]

$CMRO_2$ cerebral metabolic rate of oxygen, CPP cerebral perfusion pressure, *ICP* intracranial pressure, *MAP* mean arterial pressure

Changes in cerebral perfusion pressure can also directly alter cerebrovascular tone through pressure-dependent cerebral autoregulation pathways. Reductions in CPP lead to arteriolar vasodilation, while increases in CPP lead to vasoconstriction. Cerebral autoregulation thus serves to maintain near constant levels of CBF in the face of wide fluctuations in CPP [26, 27].

Sedative medications used in neurocritical care can markedly alter cerebral metabolic demand, ICP, respiratory CO_2 production, and MAP. These changes can induce profound alterations in cerebral hemodynamics, and it is important to know the effects of these different medications on cerebrovascular physiology (Table 14.2).

Bolus Dosing of Opioids and ICP

A 2011 systematic review of randomized controlled trials of sedation in patients with severe traumatic brain injury (TBI) found a negative, though transient, impact of bolus opioids (administered over $\leq$5 minutes) on cerebral hemodynamics [28].

In this review, four small randomized studies compared the use of IV bolus doses of morphine 0.07–2 mg/kg, fentanyl 2–10 mcg/kg, sufentanil 0.37–1 mcg/kg, and alfentanil 100 mcg/kg administered over 1–6 minutes. Three of the four studies found that moderate to high opioid boluses resulted in significant increases in ICP from baseline (range of maximum increase, 3–9 mm Hg) [35–37]. The mechanism for ICP elevations after bolus opioid administration in these studies is largely thought to be the result of a cerebral autoregulatory response to a decrease in MAP, where cerebral vasodilation occurs in order to restore cerebral perfusion.

In contrast, a fourth study by Lauer and colleagues showed that slower bolus infusion of opioids (fentanyl, morphine, or sufentanil over 5 minutes, titrated to a maximal 5% decrease in MAP) resulted in no significant increases in ICP in any group [38]. Another study by Werner and colleagues not included in the systematic review found that ICP was unchanged after administration of a sufentanil 3 mcg/kg bolus when MAP was maintained with a norepinephrine infusion, but was significantly higher in the group of patients who became hypotensive despite vasopressor administration [39]. Overall, these studies suggest that a reduction in MAP leads to ICP elevation after rapid opioid boluses, rather than an intrinsic drug-related mechanism being the underlying contributor.

None of the above studies found significant differences between specific agents and change in ICP or MAP. However, higher doses, which resulted in greater decreases in MAP, were shown to produce greater increases in ICP [28, 35–38].

In summary, although bolus doses of opioids can potentially increase ICP, these elevations seem to be driven by decreases in MAP. Thus, the effect of opioids on ICP can be mitigated by moderating the opioid bolus administration rate in order to minimize systemic hypotension. Given the class effect of opioids to produce respiratory depression, maintaining minute ventilation to prevent elevations of $PaCO_2$ would also be an additional important consideration, as hypercarbia would also be expected to increase ICP through cerebral vasodilation.

General Approach to Selection of Analgesic Regimens

In patients requiring close neurologic monitoring due to high risk or concern for impending neurologic deterioration, short-acting agents may be ideal. In this setting, the use of small, frequent bolus doses of IV fentanyl is common. However, due to its high lipophilicity, fentanyl administered as repeated bolus doses or as a continuous infusion can result in accumulation and a prolonged duration of effect. Remifentanil represents an enticing option for analgesia in the neurocritical care setting, as its ultra-short half-life allows rapid awakening for neurologic exams when the infusion is paused. This was demonstrated in a multi-center study that compared an analgesia-based sedation protocol using remifentanil and propofol to a hypnotic-based sedation protocol using either fentanyl or morphine in addition to propofol. Sedation was titrated to a deep sedation goal in all patients. Ultimately, all groups required similar propofol doses during the first three study days (approximately 30–40 mcg/kg/min). However, the study demonstrated that when sedation was paused for examinations, time to neurological assessment was significantly shorter with remifentanil, occurring on average 18 and 25 minutes sooner compared to the fentanyl and morphine arms, respectively; they found no differences between groups in duration of mechanical ventilation or adverse events [2]. Despite the advantage in ability to perform more timely neurologic assessments with remifentanil, its widespread use in the ICU setting is currently curtailed by its cost in relation to other available agents such as fentanyl.

Morphine remains a commonly used agent worldwide; however, its use continues to decline in neurocritical care due to its multiple undesirable properties as compared to other agents—these include a relatively longer half-life, predisposition to accumulation in renal failure due to its renally cleared active metabolite (morphine-6-glucuronide), and elevated risk of adverse hemodynamic effects due to impact on histamine release. However, as detailed below, morphine has a specific place in therapy in the treatment of paroxysmal sympathetic hyperactivity (commonly known as "storming"), where it is considered the IV opiate of choice.

Bolus doses of an IV opioid agent can be repeated as needed based on assessments of pain (numeric rating scale, BPS, CPOT), while maintaining light sedation and limiting hemodynamic responses to noxious stimuli such as endotracheal suctioning, which may cause or exacerbate elevations in ICP. When bolus administration is insufficient, a continuous infusion of fentanyl or remifentanil may be initiated and titrated to similar goals, or in the case of a requirement for deep sedation, to a minimal pain score (e.g., BPS 3–5/12), with additional titration of a sedative agent beyond this [8, 9].

Use of Opioids in Specific Neurocritical Care Disease States

Sedation and Shivering Management in Targeted Temperature Management

Collectively termed targeted temperature management, TTM, the use of induced hypothermia (targeting a body temperature of 32 °C to <36 °C) and controlled normothermia (36–37 °C) for neuroprotection after cardiac arrest is a field of expanding research in the modern era of critical care, as mounting evidence supports improvement in patient outcomes [40–44].

Outside of cardiac arrest-associated brain injury, fever has long been recognized as a contributor to secondary brain injury in varying primary pathologies, including ischemic and hemorrhagic stroke, subarachnoid hemorrhage, and traumatic brain injury [45–51]. Because of this, treatment of fever is considered a universal measure in the management of brain-injured patients along with standard airway, breathing, circulation assessment, according to the Emergency Neurological Life Support (ENLS) treatment algorithm for elevated ICP, and remains a staple of care for neurocritically ill patients during their ICU stay [50, 52].

Thermoregulatory Responses to Hypothermia and Fever in TTM

Core body temperature is normally tightly regulated by the hypothalamus and maintained between 36.5–37.5 °C. Below this temperature, peripheral vasoconstriction is activated to reduce heat loss in addition to eliciting behavioral responses to conserve heat. Shivering—involuntary oscillatory muscle movements which produce heat to increase core body temperature—commences at approximately 1 °C below the vasoconstriction threshold, activated at approximately 35.5 °C (Fig. 14.1) [53]. The shivering response ceases below temperatures of approximately 33.5 °C [51].

Fever, defined as an increase in core body temperature above normal which is triggered by a change in the hypothalamic set point, occurs commonly after acute brain injury. During fever, normal thermoregulatory responses (vasoconstriction and shivering) are also shifted to a higher value to maintain the elevated temperature. Thus, when TTM is used to actively lower core body temperature in a febrile patient, feedback pathways to the hypothalamus trigger these counter-regulatory mechanisms to induce shivering in an attempt to elevate core temperature back to the hypothalamic set point (Fig. 14.2) [50, 51]. For this reason, TTM for active fever control is often met with higher rates of shivering than therapeutic hypothermia after cardiac arrest [50, 51]. Shivering in the setting of both therapeutic hypothermia and controlled normothermia is associated with negative impacts on the patient, including increased metabolic rate and energy expenditure, oxygen consumption, and production of carbon dioxide as well as decreases in brain tissue oxygen levels [44, 54, 55].

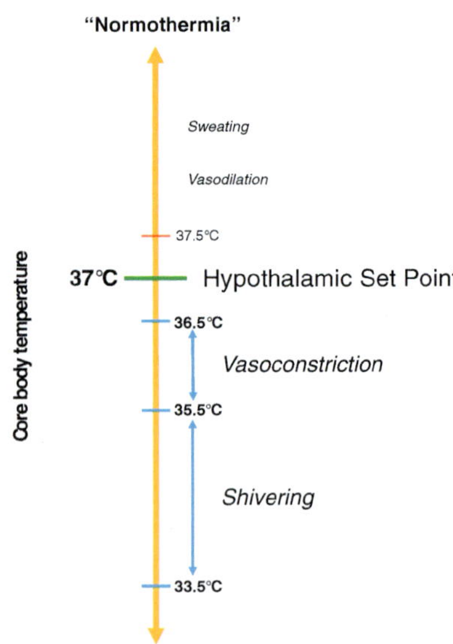

Fig. 14.1 Normal thermoregulatory responses to lowering core body temperature in hypothermia

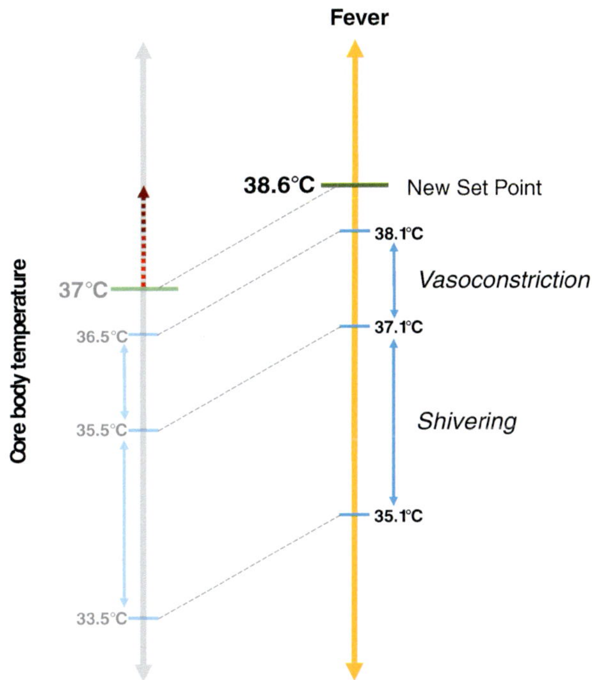

Fig. 14.2 Representation of thermoregulatory responses in fever; in this example where a patient's hypothalamic set point is raised to 38.6 °C, the normal counter-regulatory responses are also shifted upward, demonstrating the elevated risk of shivering when TTM is implemented even to maintain body temperatures in the normothermia range

Table 14.3 The Bedside Shivering Assessment Scale (BSAS)

Score	Interpretation	Definition
0	None	No shivering noted on palpation of the masseter, neck, or chest wall
1	Mild	Localized to the neck and/or thorax only
2	Moderate	Involves gross movement of the upper extremities (in addition to neck and thorax)
3	Severe	Involves gross movements of the trunk and upper and lower extremities

Adapted from [55]

The Bedside Shivering Assessment Scale (BSAS) is a widely used tool for shivering assessment (Table 14.3) [44, 55]. The BSAS was validated in neurocritical care patients with the assessment of the shivering score and indirect calorimetry to assess the metabolic impact of shivering severity. The authors found high inter-rater reliability of the scoring tool and demonstrated that each increased level of the BSAS score (0–3) was associated with an incremental rise and independent association with higher energy expenditure (Fig. 14.3) [55].

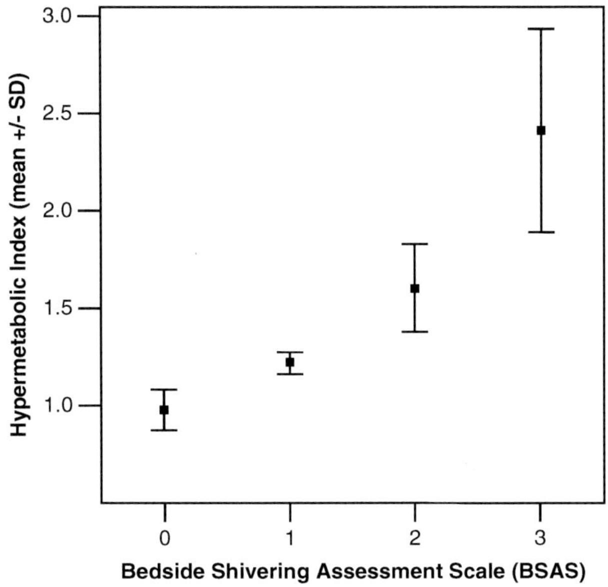

Fig. 14.3 Each increasing level of the BSAS score was found to be associated with a significant increase in each of the metabolic parameter outcomes, including hypermetabolic index (HMI), resting energy expenditure (REE), oxygen consumption, and carbon dioxide production. The BSAS was found to have the most significant association with the HMI, pictured here. The HMI was derived by dividing the REE (kcal/day) by the expected energy expenditure (calculated by Harris-Benedict equation × 1.2–1.3 to account for patient acuity) [55].

Younger age, male sex, higher body mass, and the presence of hypomagnesemia are factors consistently shown to increase the risk of shivering with TTM [51, 55, 56]. This may be considered when weighing the risk and benefit of inducing controlled normothermia in the febrile patient with acute brain injury.

Management of Shivering

In patients managed with therapeutic hypothermia after cardiac arrest, shivering must be aggressively controlled during the induction phase where body temperature is actively being lowered, as shivering can significantly prolong the time to reach goal temperature. In theory, if a lower temperature of 33 °C (TTM_{33}) is selected, then the shivering response is expected to abate once the patient reaches goal temperature, and will re-emerge upon re-warming when approaching normothermia. Conversely, patients managed with a target temperature of 36 °C (TTM_{36}) may be at risk for shivering for the entire duration of their hypothermia phase until rewarming [51]. Despite these theoretical concerns, however, there were no differences seen in the rate or severity of shivering between hypothermia doses in the recent TTM-trial, which compared outcomes after cardiac arrest in patients randomized to 24 hours of TTM at either 33° or 36 °C [42]. When utilizing normothermia for fever control, treatment of shivering is also necessary in order to obtain maximal benefit from implementation of TTM.

A number of pharmacologic and non-pharmacologic interventions have demonstrated beneficial effects in lowering of the vasoconstrictive and shivering thresholds (Table 14.4) [69]. This excludes the consideration of neuromuscular blocking agents, which exert direct actions on skeletal muscle to inhibit shivering.

Table 14.4 Selected therapies for the prevention and treatment of shivering in TTM

	Anti-Shivering Mechanism	Dosing	Reduction in Shivering Threshold
Opioids			
Meperidine (pethidine)	μ- and κ-opioid receptor agonist Central α_{2b}-receptor agonist	25–100 mg IV	1.2–2.3 °C
Tramadol	μ-receptor agonist Partial inhibition of norepinephrine and 5-HT uptake	125–250 mg IV[a]	0.6–0.9 °C
Other pure μ-opioid receptor agonists (fentanyl, alfentanil)	Activation of μ-opioid receptors	--	--
Dexmedetomidine	Central α_2-adrenergic agonist	0.2–1.5 mcg/kg/hr	0.7–2.4 °C
Buspirone	5-HT_{1A} partial agonist	30–60 mg	0.7–1 °C Synergistic effect in combination with meperidine
Propofol	General anesthetic ($GABA_A$ agonist)—vasodilator, blunts thermoregulatory responses	50–75 mcg/kg/min	1.3–2 °C
Skin counter-warming	Increases skin surface temperature (responsible for 20% of input to hypothalamic thermoregulatory center)	Forced air warming blanket (max temperature 43 °C)	1 °C for every 4 °C ↑ in skin temperature Synergistic effect in combination with meperidine
Magnesium sulfate	Cutaneous vasodilation and muscle relaxation	2–4 grams IV bolus or Infusion, 0.5–1 g/hr titrated to serum level 3–4 mg/dl	Minimal; improves rate of cooling, and has shown to improve patient comfort during induction

References [57–68]
[a]IV formulation not available in the United States

Meperidine is considered the most effective agent for the treatment of shivering, which is postulated to result from its effect on κ-opioid receptors as well as α_{2b}-receptors, potentially explaining its augmented anti-shivering activity as compared to other opioids [70–73]. Other pure μ-opioid receptor agonists also appear to be beneficial in the treatment of shivering, though to a lesser extent [70].

For most pharmacologic interventions, the impact on lowering of the shivering threshold is dose-dependent. For this reason, the use of combinations of therapies with synergistic effects is desirable to limit adverse effects related to individual medications, while optimizing efficacy. In particular, this has been demonstrated

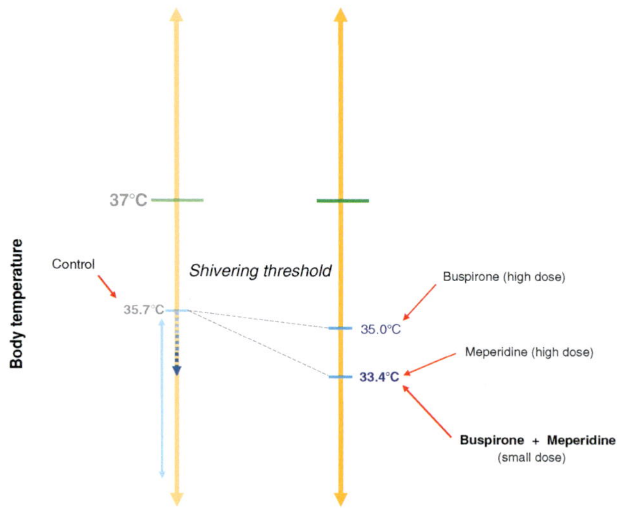

Fig. 14.4 This figure uses an example to demonstrate the use of anti-shivering medications to significantly lower the threshold temperature at which shivering occurs, highlighting the use of synergistic medication combinations. This example uses the reported change in shivering threshold demonstrated in one study (described in detail in the text), which found the combination of buspirone + meperidine to be synergistic in lowering the shivering threshold as compared to larger doses of either agent alone [57]

with the use of meperidine in combination with buspirone, as well as with the combined use of skin counter-warming (Fig. 14.4) [57, 58]. These findings are important, as they permit usage of lower doses of meperidine. Of particular concern in the brain-injured or post-cardiac arrest patient is the potential for accumulation of the neurotoxic active metabolite, normeperidine, which has impaired clearance in renal failure, and the potential increased risk of seizures due to lowering of the seizure threshold.

As an example of the synergistic potential with the use of combination of therapies, Mokhtarani and colleagues assessed the combination of meperidine with buspirone for the treatment of shivering (Fig. 14.4) [57]. This study was conducted in eight healthy volunteers treated with induction of hypothermia via administration of IV fluids (Lactated Ringer's solution) cooled to 4 °C. Each volunteer received each of four interventions on four separate days: (1) no therapy (control group), (2) high dose buspirone (60 mg), (3) high dose meperidine (0.8 mcg/mL), and (4) small-dose combination of buspirone 30 mg + meperidine 0.4 mcg/mL. Compared to the control group which had a baseline shivering threshold of 35.7 ± 0.2 °C, the combination of lower doses of buspirone plus meperidine lowered the shivering threshold by 2.3 °C (group 4), as compared to larger doses of either buspirone alone (group 2, shivering threshold lowered by 0.7 °C) or large dose meperidine (group 3, shivering threshold lowered by 2.3 °C). In this example, the combination produced a comparable lowering of the shivering threshold to that of large dose meperidine (shivering threshold lowered by 2.3 °C in both groups), with synergy demonstrated as the actual threshold in the small-dose combination group was significantly less than predicted for an additive response ($p = 0.0006$) [57].

Unfortunately, most of the evidence regarding efficacy of shivering therapies is derived from studies in healthy volunteers or in the post-anesthesia care environment [72]. The Columbia Anti-Shivering Protocol was the first comprehensive algorithm studied for the prevention and treatment of shivering in TTM and incorporated a multitude of therapies with varied mechanisms of actions and combinations effective for the treatment of shivering. These include antipyretics (namely acetaminophen), 5-HT agonists (buspirone), opioid agonists (meperidine and fentanyl), central α_2-agonists (dexmedetomidine), and propofol [74]. The protocol incorporates systematic assessment for the presence of shivering using the BSAS and recommends a stepwise approach for management (Table 14.5). Agents with the least sedating potential are preferred to reduce impact on neurologic examination. Synergistic combinations of less-sedating therapies are utilized first, with stepwise addition of more potent sedatives, and ultimately neuromuscular blockade. The Columbia Shivering Protocol is applicable regardless of mechanical ventilation status (with limitations on use of specific therapies such as propofol and paralytic agents in non-intubated patients) [44, 74, 75]. It remains the only systematically studied shivering protocol for use during TTM in the ICU and has been widely adapted for use for both normothermia and hypothermia [75].

Table 14.5 The Columbia Anti-Shivering Protocol

Step		Intervention	Dose
0	Baseline	Acetaminophen Buspirone Magnesium sulfate Skin counterwarming	650–1000 mg q4–6h 30 mg q8h 0.5–1 g/hr infusion (goal 3–4 mg/dL) Maximum 43 °C
1	Mild sedation	Dexmedetomidine *or* Opioid	0.2–1.5 mcg/kg/hr Fentanyl infusion[a] (25 mcg/hr+) Meperidine 50–100 mg IM/IV
2	Moderate sedation	Dexmedetomidine *plus* opioid	As above
3	Deep sedation	Propofol[a]	50–75 mcg/kg/min[a]
4	Neuromuscular blockade	Vecuronium[a]	0.1 mg/kg IV bolus[a]

The Columbia anti-shivering protocol included implementation of hourly assessments for shivering (using the Bedside Shivering Assessment Scale, BSAS) by the bedside nurse, with a target BSAS of 0–1. Prior to initiation of cooling, each of the Step 0 interventions are implemented for shivering prevention, and continued for the duration of TTM. If a BSAS of ≥2 is reported, then a Step 1 intervention is initiated. After maximizing a Step 1 intervention with failure to achieve a BSAS ≤1, the provider then proceeds to Step 2, and so on

Adapted from [74]

[a]Note: Patients receiving fentanyl or propofol infusions and neuromuscular blockade must be mechanically ventilated.

In publishing the results from implementation of the shivering protocol in their Neuro ICU over a period of approximately 4 years, a total of 213 patients were observed over a total of 289 hypothermia days and 1099 normothermia days; 124 of the 213 patients were initiated on TTM for normothermia goals only [74]. In total, 18% of all TTM patients (and 33% of patient days) received no intervention for the treatment of shivering. Beyond Step 0, the authors reported that 29% of patients required one agent, 35% received two agents, 15% received three, and 2.4% received four agents for the treatment of shivering. Thirty-six percent of Step 1 interventions included opioid administration, though these were not subdivided to account for the volume of use of meperidine as compared to fentanyl. However, dosages were recorded during the course of the study, with a median meperidine dose of 125 mg/24 hours, and fentanyl at a median dose of 47 mcg/hour [74].

Specific considerations for approach to the use of neuromuscular-blocking agents (NMBA) during therapeutic hypothermia are discussed below in relation to the use of sedation and analgesia during TTM after cardiac arrest.

Altered Metabolism and Pharmacodynamics of Medications in Hypothermia

Hypothermia is known to have a profound impact on the pharmacokinetic (PK) parameters of medications and largely results in higher serum levels due to reduced hepatic clearance. This is the result of both reduced hepatic blood flow and impaired metabolism of many drugs by cytochrome P450, in which the temperature-dependent enzymatic process is slowed and consequently reduces systemic drug clearance [76]. Additionally, impaired hepatic or renal function, either chronic or new-onset after cardiac arrest, further compounds this effect.

Few comprehensive pharmacokinetic studies have been performed to quantify the effects of hypothermia on medication clearance, with even fewer conducted in critically ill patients after cardiac arrest; however, estimates of the reduction in clearance in hypothermia are available (Table 14.6). One review analyzing existing PK studies in hypothermia prior to 2007 found that systemic clearance of drugs metabolized by CYP450 was overall reduced by 7–22% per degree below 37 °C, though the variation between patients in studies is understandingly wide, as many factors in an individual patient and setting can affect the PK parameters of specific drugs [76].

Sedation Practices in TTM and Considerations for Neuroprognostication

During hypothermia, sedation is routinely used primarily to prevent and treat shivering, ensure ventilator compliance, as well as to adequately prevent awareness in case use of neuromuscular blocking agents is required [83]. However, increasing recognition of the impact of hypothermia on prolonging the duration of action of sedative agents has called to question the influence these drugs may have on clinical

Table 14.6 Altered pharmacokinetic properties of common opioids used in therapeutic hypothermia

	Specific PK Changes Observed in TTM_{32-34}	Metabolism	Active Metabolites	Comments
Opioids				
Fentanyl	Cl_{total} ↓ 20–45%	Hepatic (CYP 3A4)	n/a	Risk for accumulation and prolonged effect with high doses
Morphine	Cl_{total} ↓ 29% t ½ ↑ 1.6-fold	Hepatic (glucuronidation)	Yes—renally cleared	Least optimal opiate in TTM, especially in hepatic and renal impairment
Remifentanil	Cl_{total} ↓ 27% *(↓6.7% per °C)*[a] Rewarming $C_{\Delta 33-37}$ ↑16%	Plasma and tissue esterases	n/a	Optimal agent where available—least variable PK

References [76–82]

Cl_{total} total clearance, *PK* pharmacokinetics, *PRN* as needed, *Rewarming* $C_{\Delta 33-37}$ Δ in serum concentration observed during rewarming period (from 33 → 37 °C), *t ½* half-life, TTM_{32-34} target temperature management with goal temperature between 32 and 34 °C

[a]Reduced clearance per each 1 °C below 37 °C

decision making after the completion of TTM [83, 84]. The underestimation of lingering sedation action and resultant late awakening can confound patient examination and neuroprognostic testing when performed too early after rewarming. Indeed, if not accounted for by the clinician, the most dire consequence of this would be resultant withdrawal of care in patients deemed to have a "poor prognosis" who may otherwise have been able to make a meaningful recovery [82, 83, 85, 86]. Nearly all components of the neurologic exam may be affected by sedative medications—including pupillary light reflex, corneal reflex, and motor responses. Electroencephalography (EEG) background rhythm is also known to be sensitive to residual sedative effects. Specific assessments which alternatively do not seem to be impacted by medications include brain imaging (loss of gray-white matter differentiation on head computed tomography, CT), interpretation of absent N20 potentials on somatosensory-evoked potentials (SSEPs), and serum biomarker levels such as neuron-specific enolase (NSE) [86–89].

Supporting this notion is a post-hoc analysis of the TTM-trial which assessed for factors related to time to awakening when comparing the TTM_{33} and TTM_{36} groups, with the aim of correlating this to long-term outcome in patients [90]. In this international multicenter study, sites were required to initiate sedation with TTM, but the specific regimens were left to local practice and provider decision. While no differences in cumulative analgesia or sedation doses were found within 48 hours between the study groups, randomization to the TTM_{33} arm was found to be an independent predictor of late awakening. As no differences in good neurologic outcome or prognostic factors were identified, the main hypothesis of the study authors was that the delay in awakening in the TTM_{33} group may have been related to delayed drug clearance occurring with deeper hypothermia [90].

Additionally, a recent study by May and colleagues aimed to address the issue of appropriate level of sedation needed in TTM [91]. At their center, patients were preemptively initiated on a predefined basal sedation dose prior to cooling to 33 °C, and shivering during TTM was instead treated largely with intermittent bolus doses of neuromuscular blocking agents (NMBA) rather than escalation of sedation doses. A total of 166 patients underwent TTM_{33}, and received fentanyl at a median dose of 25 mcg/hr. in addition to propofol at a median dose of 20 mcg/kg/min; a minority of patients (<15%) received alternative sedation, such as low-dose midazolam infusion. Ninety-five percent of patients were reported to experience shivering, and a median of five doses of NMBA were administered in the 24-hour cooling period. In their cohort, awakening occurred at a median of 3 hours after the end of rewarming, with extubation at a median of 28 hours after rewarming, in surviving patients. While this study has no comparator group, it suggests that implementing sedation doses sufficient to prevent awareness with NMB administration, but not unnecessarily deep so as to require an exaggerated period of time to clear after rewarming, is a safe and effective strategy. This is highlighted by comparison to the sedation doses reported in the TTM-trial, where patients received fentanyl and propofol at much higher doses (median ~175 mcg/hr and ~45 mcg/kg/min, respectively) [90]. While lower rates of shivering were reported in the TTM-trial (approximately 30% in both arms), awakening in the TTM_{33} group occurred at a median on day 4, which was likely a day later compared to the May study patients using estimated similar definitions [90, 92].

Lastly, a single-center PK study assessed the time to clearance after discontinuation of fentanyl in 23 patients after cardiac arrest treated with TTM_{36}. Patients received an average fentanyl dose of 119 mcg/hr for 24 hours of TTM, with a PK analysis showing that 68% of patients (15/22) would not have cleared at 24 hours, and 5/22 (23%) would have required >48 hours to achieve 95% clearance after discontinuation. These authors' findings emphasize the prolonged duration of effect these patients can experience and which may potentially interfere with prognostication assessments occurring soon after rewarming [91].

Cumulatively, these studies illustrate the impact of hypothermia on reduced clearance of analgesia and sedative agents, which is known to be proportional to the degree of hypothermia. While the precise cooling target to best optimize outcomes after cardiac arrest is still of considerable debate, the prolongation of effect when employing TTM_{33} as compared to TTM_{36} must be considered, since the lower target temperature has been shown to potentially result in longer time to awakening, especially when higher doses of analgesia and sedative agents are used [90]. The clinician must carefully consider the selection of agents and titration strategy to effectively prevent and treat shivering in patients undergoing TTM regardless of the temperature target.

Upon completion of the rewarming period, after the risk of shivering has abated, clinical assessment with minimization or discontinuation of sedation as soon as possible is important in order to allow for optimal prognostication conditions in patients who do not regain consciousness. Postponement of impacted prognostic assessments normally recommended at the 72-hour post-resuscitation point is highly recommended in patients receiving significant sedation and analgesia doses, as reasonable, in order to permit prolonged observation; consideration should be given to ordering non-impacted testing (SSEPs, brain imaging, NSE levels) first [88].

Paroxysmal Sympathetic Hyperactivity (PSH)

Pathophysiology and Clinical Presentation of PSH

Paroxysmal sympathetic hyperactivity (PSH) is a syndrome encountered in patients with various forms of severe acute neurologic injury who exhibit a constellation of symptoms with autonomic and motor features. This condition has historically been associated with severe TBI, which was noted to be the etiology of 79.4% of cases in a 2010 review. This was followed by hypoxic brain injury in 9.7%, hemorrhagic or ischemic stroke in 5.4% of cases, and the remaining associated with conditions such as hydrocephalus, tumor, and CNS infection [93].

This review also noted that over 30 terms have been used to describe PSH including "dysautonomia," "diencephalic seizures," and "sympathetic" or "autonomic storming" [93]. In 2014 a consensus group formed to address the definition and diagnosis of the syndrome and recommended the uniform term "paroxysmal sympathetic hyperactivity," and also created the first version of a unified diagnostic tool, which they termed the PSH Assessment Measure [94].

The pathophysiology of the condition is poorly understood, but impaired descending inhibitory control of excitatory spinal circuits, which then permits unregulated sympathetic outflow, is a commonly proposed mechanism [95]. Patients with PSH may display a number of autonomic features, including tachycardia, hypertension, tachypnea, fever, diaphoresis, and decerebrate posturing. Triggering of symptomatic episodes by both noxious and non-noxious stimuli also appears to be an important defining feature of PSH [95, 96]. Episodes may last several minutes to hours and recur several times per day [97–100]. Symptoms typically begin to manifest around one week after injury, often once sedation is weaned, and may persist for weeks to months, including into the rehabilitation period [101–103]. The degree of sympathetic overactivity and frequency of episodes varies widely across affected patients. Over time, episodes become less frequent and less pronounced in severity.

Pharmacologic Treatment of PSH

Numerous medications are used to treat PSH, but there is minimal strong evidence to guide therapy. The most common therapeutic classes employed in clinical practice include opioids, non-selective β-antagonists, α_2 agonists (e.g., clonidine),

Table 14.7 Selected opioids commonly used in the treatment of PSH

Medication	Mechanism in PSH	Suggested Initial Doses	Comments
Morphine	μ-opioid receptor agonists, modulate pain transmission and perception Target allodynia	IV: 2–4 mg q1–2h prn PO: 15–30 mg q4–6h[a]	IV morphine is the prototypical opiate studied in PSH (opiate of choice) Doses up to 10 mg IV have been used for treatment of PSH Histamine release with IV morphine is advantageous in PSH (BP and HR-lowering)
Fentanyl		25–100 mcg IV q1–2h prn	
Oxycodone		10–20 mg PO q4–6h[a]	

References [93, 104–106]
[a]Initial maintenance dosing based on current opiate requirements

GABA agonists (e.g., benzodiazepines and baclofen), and additional agents such as bromocriptine and gabapentin. Despite the preponderance of low quality evidence for therapeutic interventions in PSH, the majority of data support the use of opioids and β-blockers as the backbone of therapy. Beyond this, building a regimen may be guided by the patient's predominant symptoms and comorbidities, and by combining agents with varying mechanisms of action [93, 104–106].

The initial approach to treatment is two-fold. First, rapid-acting IV agents should be utilized to abort acute episodes. These agents may include morphine, β-blockers, or benzodiazepines, with trials necessary to establish the effective agent and dose. Second, maintenance medications should also be initiated with the goal of reducing the number and severity of paroxysms, while balancing efficacy with minimal adverse effects (Table 14.7).

Opioids, as well as nonselective β-blockers such as propranolol and labetalol, are typically considered first-line therapies for both the abortive and maintenance treatment of PSH, serving to combat the allodynic response that is thought to be central to the pathophysiology of PSH and the resultant sympathetic response. IV morphine is the prototypical agent used for treatment of PSH, and is particularly effective to abort symptomatic episodes, though other opiates may also be useful. Morphine can additionally be given on a scheduled basis orally or converted to an equivalent dosage of oxycodone or other preferred opiate [93, 104–107].

Once acceptable control of PSH has been achieved with pharmacotherapy, as indicated by the frequency, duration, and severity of episodes requiring abortive treatment, then therapeutic doses may be maintained for a period of time. Beyond this, attempts may be made to begin weaning agents carefully, while paying close attention to recrudescence of symptoms.

Conclusion

Opioid use in the neurocritical care population is similar in many ways to the general critical care population as it relates to sedation and treatment of pain. Specific disease states which rely on specific use of opioids include the prevention or treatment of shivering in TTM and the treatment of paroxysmal sympathetic hyperactivity. Influence of these medications on the assessment of the neurologic examination and neuroprognostication in acute brain injury require careful consideration by the critical care clinician.

References

1. Devlin JW, Skrobik Y, Gelinas C, et al. Clinical practice guidelines for the prevention and management of pain, agitation/sedation, delirium, immobility, and sleep disruption in adult patients in the ICU. Crit Care Med. 2018;46:e825–73.
2. Karabinis A, Mandragos K, Stergiopoulos S, et al. Safety and efficacy of analgesia-based sedation with remifentanil versus standard hypnotic-based regimens in intensive care unit patients with brain injuries: a randomised, controlled trial [ISRCTN50308308]. Crit Care. 2004;8:R268–80.
3. Egerod I, Jensen MB, Herling SF, Welling KL. Effect of an analgo-sedation protocol for neurointensive patients: a two-phase interventional non-randomized pilot study. Crit Care. 2010;14:R71.
4. Kress JP, Pohlman AS, O'Connor MF, Hall JB. Daily interruption of sedative infusions in critically ill patients undergoing mechanical ventilation. N Engl J Med. 2000;342:1471–7.
5. Girard TD, Kress JP, Fuchs BD, et al. Efficacy and safety of a paired sedation and ventilator weaning protocol for mechanically ventilated patients in intensive care (Awakening and Breathing Controlled trial): a randomised controlled trial. Lancet. 2008;371:126–34.
6. Strom T, Martinussen T, Toft P. A protocol of no sedation for critically ill patients receiving mechanical ventilation: a randomised trial. Lancet. 2010;375:475–80.
7. Mehta S, Burry L, Cook D, et al. Daily sedation interruption in mechanically ventilated critically ill patients cared for with a sedation protocol: a randomized controlled trial. JAMA. 2012;308:1985–92.
8. Makii JM, Mirski MA, Lewin JJ III. Sedation and analgesia in critically ill neurologic patients. J Pharm Pract. 2010;23(5):455–69.
9. Oddo M, Crippa IA, Mehta S, et al. Optimizing sedation in patients with acute brain injury. Crit Care. 2016;20:128–38.
10. Teitelbaum JS, Ayoub O, Skrobik Y. A critical appraisal of sedation, analgesia and delirium in neurocritical care. Can J Neurol Sci. 2011;38:815–25.
11. Payen JF, Bru O, Bosson JL, et al. Assessing pain in critically ill sedated patients by using a behavioral pain scale. Crit Care Med. 2001;29:2258–63.
12. Gelinas C, Fillion L, Puntillo KA, Viens C, Fortier M. Validation of the critical-care pain observation tool in adult patients. Am J Crit Care. 2006;15:420–7.
13. Riker RR, Fugate JE, Participants in the International Multi-disciplinary Consensus Conference on Multimodality Monitoring. Clinical monitoring scales in acute brain injury: assessment of coma, pain, agitation, and delirium. Neurocrit Care. 2014;21 Suppl 2:S27–37.
14. Yu A, Teitelbaum J, Scott J, et al. Evaluating pain, sedation, and delirium in the neurologically critically ill-feasibility and reliability of standardized tools: a multi-institutional study. Crit Care Med. 2013;41:2002–7.
15. Dehghani H, Tavangar H, Ghandehari A. Validity and reliability of Behavioral Pain Scale in patients with low level of consciousness due to head trauma hospitalized in intensive care unit. Arch Trauma Res. 2014;3:e18608.
16. Echegaray-Benites C, Kapoustina O, Gélinas C. Validation of the use of the Critical-Care Pain Observation Tool (CPOT) with brain surgery patients in the neurosurgical intensive care unit. Intensive Crit Care Nurs. 2014;30:257–65.
17. Joffe AM, McNulty B, Boitor M, Marsh R, Gélinas C. Validation of the Critical-Care Pain Observation Tool in brain-injured critically ill adults. J Crit Care. 2016;36:76–80.

18. Schnakers C, Chatelle C, Vanhaudenhuyse A, et al. The Nociception Coma Scale: a new tool to assess nociception in disorders of consciousness. Pain. 2010;148:215–9.
19. Chatelle C, Thibaut A, Whyte J, De Val MD, Laureys S, Schnakers C. Pain issues in disorders of consciousness. Brain Inj. 2014;28(9):1202–8.
20. Laureys S, Faymonville M, Peigneux P, et al. Cortical processing of noxious somatosensory stimuli in the persistent vegetative state. Neuroimage. 2002;17:732–41.
21. Boly M, Faymonville ME, Schnakers C, et al. Perception of pain in the minimally conscious state with PET activation: an observational study. Lancet Neurol. 2008;7:1013–20.
22. Kotchoubey B, Merz S, Lang S, Markl A, Muller F, Yu T, Schwarzbauer C. Global functional connectivity reveals highly significant differences between the vegetative and the minimally conscious state. J Neurol. 2013;260:975–83.
23. Chanques G, Payen JF, Mercier G, et al. Assessing pain in non-intubated critically ill patients unable to self report: an adaptation of the Behavioral Pain Scale. Intensive Care Med. 2009;35:2060–7.
24. Chatelle C, Majerus S, Whyte J, Laureys S, Schnakers C. A sensitive scale to assess nociceptive pain in patients with disorders of consciousness. J Neurol Neurosurg Psychiatry. 2012;83:1233–7.
25. Chatelle C, Hauger SL, Martial C, et al. Assessment of nociception and pain in participants in an unresponsive or minimally conscious state after acquired brain injury: the relation between the Coma Recovery Scale-Revised and the Nociception Coma Scale-Revised. Arch Phys Med Rehabil. 2018;99(9):1755–62.
26. Chugh C, Kofke WA. Cerebral blood flow physiology, pharmacology, and pathophysiology. In: Smith M, Kofke WA, Citerio G, editors. Oxford textbook of neurocritical care. Oxford: Oxford University Press; 2016.
27. Zacharia BE, Connolly SE. Principles of cerebral metabolism and blood flow. In: Le Roux PD, Levine JM, Kofke WA, editors. Monitoring in neurocritical care. Philadelphia: Saunders; 2013.
28. Roberts DJ, Hall RI, Kramer AH, Robertson HL, Gallagher CN, Zygun DA. Sedation for critically ill adults with severe traumatic brain injury: a systematic review of randomized controlled trials. Crit Care Med. 2011;39:2743–51.
29. Kelly DF, Goodale DB, Williams J, Herr DL, Chappell T, Rosner MJ. Propofol in the treatment of moderate and severe head injury: a randomized, prospective double-blinded pilot trial. J Neurosurg. 1999;90:1042–52.
30. Carney N, Totten AM, O'Reilly C, et al. Guidelines for the management of severe traumatic brain injury, fourth edition. Neurosurgery. 2017;80:6–15.
31. Albanese J, Arnaud S, Rey M, Thomachot L, Alliez B, Martin C. Ketamine decreases intracranial pressure and electroencephalographic activity in traumatic brain injury patients during propofol sedation. Anesthesiology. 1997;87:1328–34.
32. Bourgoin A, Albanèse J, Wereszcynski N, Charbit M, Vialet R, Martin C. Safety of sedation with ketamine in severe head injury patients: comparison with sufentanil. Crit Care Med. 2003;31:711–7.
33. Chang L, Raty S, Ortiz J, Bailard N, Mathew S. The emerging use of ketamine for anesthesia and sedation in traumatic brain injuries. CNS Neurosci Ther. 2013;19:390–5.
34. Pajoumand M, Kufera J, Bonds B, et al. Dexmedetomidine as an adjunct for sedation in patients with traumatic brain injury. J Trauma Acute Care Surg. 2016;81:345–52.
35. Sperry R, Bailey P, Reichman M, et al. Fentanyl and sufentanil increase intracranial pressure in head trauma patients. Anesthesiology. 1992;77:416–20.
36. Albanese J, Albanese J, Viviand X, et al. Sufentanil, fentanyl, and alfentanil in head trauma patients: a study on cerebral hemodynamics. Crit Care Med. 1999;27:407–11.
37. de Nadal M, Munar F, Poca M, Sahuquillo J, Garnacho A, Rossello J. Cerebral hemodynamic effects of morphine and fentanyl in patients with severe head injury: absence of correlation to cerebral autoregulation. Anesthesiology. 2000;92:11–9.
38. Lauer K, Connolly L, Schmeling W. Opioid sedation does not alter intracranial pressure in head injured patients. Can J Anaesth. 1997;44:929–33.

39. Werner C, Kochs E, Bause H, et al. Effects of sufentanil on cerebral hemodynamics and intracranial pressure in patients with brain injury. Anesthesiology. 1995;83:721–6.
40. Hypothermia after Cardiac Arrest Study Group. Mild therapeutic hypothermia to improve the neurologic outcome after cardiac arrest. N Engl J Med. 2002;346(8):549–56.
41. Bernard SA, Gray TW, Buist MD, et al. Treatment of comatose survivors of out-of-hospital cardiac arrest with induced hypothermia. N Engl J Med. 2002;346(8):557–63.
42. Nielsen N, Wetterslev J, Cronberg T, et al. Targeted temperature management at 33°C versus 36°C after cardiac arrest. N Engl J Med. 2013;369(23):2197–206.
43. Lascarrou JB, Merdji H, Le Gouge A, et al. The HYPERION trial. Targeted temperature management for cardiac arrest with nonshockable rhythm. N Engl J Med. 2019;381:2327–37.
44. Madden LK, Hill M, May TL, et al. The implementation of targeted temperature management: an evidence-based guideline from the Neurocritical Care Society. Neurocrit Care. 2017;27:468–87.
45. Hajat C, Hajat S, Sharma P. Effects of poststroke pyrexia on stroke outcome: a meta-analysis of studies in patients. Stroke. 2000;31:410–4.
46. Schwarz S, Hafner K, Aschoff A, et al. Incidence and prognostic significance of fever following intracerebral hemorrhage. Neurology. 2000;54:354–61.
47. Oliveira-Filho J, Ezzeddine MA, Segal AZ, et al. Fever in subarachnoid hemorrhage: relationship to vasospasm and outcome. Neurology. 2001;56:1299–304.
48. Fernandez A, Schmidt JM, Claassen J, et al. Fever after subarachnoid hemorrhage: risk factors and impact on outcome. Neurology. 2007;68:1013–9.
49. McHugh GS, Engel DC, Butcher I, et al. Prognostic value of secondary insults in traumatic brain injury: results from the IMPACT study. J Neurotrauma. 2007;24:287–93.
50. Badjatia N. Hyperthermia and fever control in brain injury. Crit Care Med. 2009;37 Suppl 1:S250–7.
51. Polderman KH, Herold I. Therapeutic hypothermia and controlled normothermia in the intensive care unit: practical considerations, side effects, and cooling methods. Crit Care Med. 2009;37(3):1101–20.
52. Cadena R, Shoykhe M, Ratcliff JJ. Emergency neurologic life support: intracranial hypertension and herniation. Neurocrit Care. 2017;27 Suppl 1:82–8.
53. Lopez M, Sessler DI, Walter K, et al. Rate and gender dependence of the sweating, vasoconstriction, and shivering thresholds in humans. Anesthesiology. 1994;80:780–8.
54. Frank SM, Higgins MS, Fleisher LA, et al. Adrenergic, respiratory, and cardiovascular effects of core cooling in humans. Am J Physiol. 1997;272:R557–62.
55. Badjatia N, Strongilis E, Gordon E, et al. Metabolic impact of shivering during therapeutic temperature modulation: the Bedside Shivering Assessment Scale. Stroke. 2008;39:3242–7.
56. Badjatia N, Kowalski RG, Schmidt JM, et al. Predictors and clinical implications of shivering during therapeutic normothermia. Neurocrit Care. 2007;6(3):186–91.
57. Mokhtarani M, Mahgoub AN, Morioka N, et al. Buspirone and meperidine synergistically reduce the shivering threshold. Anesth Analg. 2001;93:1233–9.
58. Kimberger O, Ali SZ, Markstaller M, et al. Meperidine and skin surface warming additively reduce the shivering threshold: a volunteer study. Crit Care. 2007;11:R29.
59. Doufas AG, Lin CM, Suleman MI, et al. Dexmedetomidine and meperidine additively reduce the shivering threshold in humans. Stroke. 2003;34:1218–23.
60. De Witte JL, Kim JS, Sessler DI, Bastanmehr H, Bjorksten AR. Tramadol reduces the sweating, vasoconstriction, and shivering thresholds. Anesth Analg. 1998;87:173–9.
61. Talke P, Tayefeh F, Sessler DI, Jeffrey R, Noursalehi M, Richardson C. Dexmedetomidine does not alter the sweating threshold, but comparably and linearly decreases the vasoconstriction and shivering thresholds. Anesthesiology. 1997;87:835–41.
62. Lenhardt R, Orhan-Sungur M, Komatsu R, Govinda R, Kasuya Y, Sessler DI, Wadhwa A. Suppression of shivering during hypothermia using a novel drug combination in healthy volunteers. Anesthesiology. 2009;111(1):110–5.
63. Matsukawa T, Kurz A, Sessler DI, Bjorksten AR, Merrifield B, Cheng C. Propofol linearly reduces the vasoconstriction and shivering thresholds. Anesthesiology. 1995;82:1169–80.

64. Zaza KJ, Hopf HW. Thermoregulation: Normal physiology, anesthetic effects, and perioperative considerations. In: Hemmings HC, Egan TD, editors. Pharmacology and physiology for anesthesia. Philadelphia: Elsevier; 2019. p. 300–10.
65. Cheng C, Matsukawa T, Sessler DI, et al. Increasing mean skin temperature linearly reduces the core-temperature thresholds for vasoconstriction and shivering in humans. Anesthesiology. 1995;82:1160–8.
66. Badjatia N, Strongilis E, Prescutti M, et al. Metabolic benefits of surface counter warming during therapeutic temperature modulation. Crit Care Med. 2009;37(6):1893–7.
67. Zweifler RM, Voorhees ME, Mahmood MA, Parnell M. Magnesium sulfate increases the rate of hypothermia via surface cooling and improves comfort. Stroke. 2004;35:2331–4.
68. Wadhwa A, Sengupta P, Durrani J, et al. Magnesium sulphate only slightly reduces the shivering threshold in humans. Br J Anaesth. 2005;94:756–62.
69. Weant KA, Martin JE, Humphries RL, Cook AM. Pharmacologic options for reducing the shivering response to therapeutic hypothermia. Pharmacotherapy. 2010;30(8):830–41.
70. Ikeda T, Kurz A, Sessler DI, et al. The effect of opioids on thermoregulatory responses in humans and the special antishivering action of meperidine. Ann N Y Acad Sci. 1997;813:792–8.
71. Kurz A, et al. Meperidine decreases the shivering threshold twice as much as the vasoconstriction threshold. Anesthesiology. 1997;86(5):1046.
72. Park SM, Mangat HS, Berger K, Rosengart AJ. Efficacy spectrum of antishivering medications: meta-analysis of randomized controlled trials. Crit Care Med. 2012;40:3070–82.
73. Takada K, Clark D, Davies F, et al. Meperidine exerts agonist activity at the alpha2b-adrenoceptor subtype. Anesthesiology. 2002;96:1420–6.
74. Choi HA, Ko SB, Presciutti M, et al. Prevention of shivering during therapeutic temperature modulation: the Columbia anti-shivering protocol. Neurocrit Care. 2011;14(3):389–94.
75. Brophy GM, Human T. Emergency neurologic life support: pharmacotherapy pearls. Neurocrit Care. 2017;27 Suppl 1:51–73.
76. Tortorici MA, Kochanek PM, Poloyac SM. Effects of hypothermia on drug disposition, metabolism, and response: a focus of hypothermia-mediated alterations on the cytochrome P450 enzyme system. Crit Care Med. 2007;35:2196–204.
77. Bjelland TW, Klepstad P, Haugen BO, Nilsen T, Dale O. Effects of hypothermia on the disposition of morphine, midazolam, fentanyl, and propofol in intensive care unit patients. Drug Metab Dispos. 2013;41:214–23.
78. Empey PE, Miller TM, Philbrick AH, Melick JA, Kochanek PM, Poloyac SM. Mild hypothermia decreases fentanyl and midazolam steady-state clearance in a rat model of cardiac arrest. Crit Care Med. 2012;40:1221–8.
79. Michelsen LG, Holford NH, Lu W, Hoke JF, Hug CC, Bailey JM. The pharmacokinetics of remifentanil in patients undergoing coronary artery bypass grafting with cardiopulmonary bypass. Anesth Analg. 2001;93:1100–5.
80. Bjelland T, Klepstad P, Haugen BO, Nilsen T, Salvesen O, Dale O. Concentrations of remifentanil, propofol, fentanyl, and midazolam during rewarming from therapeutic hypothermia. Acta Anaesthesiol Scand. 2014;58:709–15.
81. Riker RR, Gagnon DJ, May T, Seder DB, Fraser GL. Analgesia, sedation, and neuromuscular blockade during targeted temperature management after cardiac arrest. Best Pract Res Clin Anaesthesiol. 2015;29:435–50.
82. Perman SM, Kirkpatrick JN, Reitsma AM, et al. Timing of neuroprognostication in postcardiac arrest therapeutic hypothermia. Crit Care Med. 2012;40(3):719–24.
83. Samaniego EA, Mlynash M, Caulfield AF, Eyngorn I, Wijman CA. Sedation confounds outcome prediction in cardiac arrest survivors treated with hypothermia. Neurocrit Care. 2011;15(1):113–9.
84. Rey A, Rossetti RO, Miroz JP, Eckert P, Oddo M. Late awakening in survivors of postanoxic coma: early neurophysiologic predictors and association with ICU and long-term neurologic recovery. Crit Care Med. 2019;47:85–92.
85. Agarwal S, Morris N, Der-Nigoghossian C, May T, Brodie D. The influence of therapeutics on prognostication after cardiac arrest. Curr Treat Options Neurol. 2019;21:60–75.

86. Endisch C, Storm C, Ploner CJ, Leithner C. Amplitudes of SSEP and outcome in cardiac arrest survivors: a prospective cohort study. Neurology. 2015;85(20):1752–60.
87. Nolan JP, Soar J, Cariou A, et al. European Resuscitation Council and European Society of Intensive Care Medicine guidelines for post-resuscitation care 2015: section 5 of the European Resuscitation Council guidelines for resuscitation 2015. Resuscitation. 2015;95:202–22.
88. Lybeck A, Cronberg T, Aneman A, et al. Time to awakening after cardiac arrest and the association with target temperature management. Resuscitation. 2018;126:166–71.
89. Oddo M, Sandroni C, Citerio G, et al. Quantitative versus standard pupillary light reflex for early prognostication in comatose cardiac arrest patients: an international prospective multicenter double-blinded study. Intensive Care Med. 2018;44(12):2102–11.
90. May TL, Seder DB, Fraser GL, et al. Moderate-dose sedation and analgesia during targeted temperature management after cardiac arrest. Neurocrit Care. 2015;22:105–11.
91. May TL, Riker RR, Fraser GL, et al. Variation in sedation and neuromuscular blockade regimens on outcome after cardiac arrest. Crit Care Med. 2018;46:e975–80.
92. Baldwin F, Gray R, Boyd O, Waxman D, Patel B, Allen M, Scutt G. Safe prognostication following cardiac arrest: the role of the pharmacokinetics of fentanyl in patients treated with targeted temperature management. Resuscitation. 2020;149:10–6.
93. Perkes I, Baguley I, Nott M, Menon D. A review of paroxysmal sympathetic hyperactivity after acquired brain injury. Ann Neurol. 2010;68:126–35.
94. Baguley I, Perkes I, Fernandez-Ortega J, Rabinstein A, Dolce G, Hendricks H. For the Consensus Working Group. Paroxysmal sympathetic hyperactivity after acquired brain injury: consensus on conceptual definition, nomenclature, and diagnostic criteria. J Neurotrauma. 2014;31:1515–20.
95. Baguley I, Heriseanu R, Cameron I, Nott M, Slewa-Younan S. A critical review of the pathophysiology of dysautonomia following traumatic brain injury. Neurocrit Care. 2008;8:293–300.
96. Baguley I, Nott M, Slewa-Younan S, Heriseanu R, Perkes I. Diagnosing dysautonomia after acute traumatic brain injury: evidence for overresponsiveness to afferent stimuli. Arch Phys Med Rehabil. 2009;90:580–6.
97. Blackman J, Patrick P, Buck M, Rust R Jr. Paroxysmal autonomic instability with dystonia after brain injury. Arch Neurol. 2004;61:321–8.
98. Goddeau R Jr, Silverman S, Sims J. Dexmedetomidine for the treatment of paroxysmal autonomic instability with dystonia. Neurocrit Care. 2007;7:217–20.
99. Srinivasan S, Lim C, Thirugnanam U. Paroxysmal autonomic instability with dystonia. Clin Auton Res. 2007;17:378–81.
100. Fernandez-Ortega J, Prieto-Palomino M, Garcia-Caballero M, Galeas-Lopez J, Quesada-Garcia G, Baguley I. Paroxysmal sympathetic hyperactivity after traumatic brain injury: clinical and prognostic implications. J Neurotrauma. 2012;29:1364–70.
101. Rabinstein A. Paroxysmal sympathetic hyperactivity in the neurological intensive care unit. Neurol Res. 2007;29:680–2.
102. Baguley I. Autonomic complications following central nervous system injury. Semin Neurol. 2008;28:716–25.
103. Hughes J, Rabinstein A. Early diagnosis of paroxysmal sympathetic hyperactivity in the ICU. Neurocrit Care. 2014;20:454–9.
104. Baguley IJ, Cameron ID, Green AM, Slewa-Younan S, Marosszeky JE, Gurka JA. Pharmacological management of dysautonomia following traumatic brain injury. Brain Inj. 2004;18:409–17.
105. Rabinstein A, Benarroch E. Treatment of paroxysmal sympathetic hyperactivity. Curr Treat Options Neurol. 2008;10:151–7.
106. Samuel S, Allison T, Lee K, Choi H. Pharmacologic management of paroxysmal sympathetic hyperactivity after brain injury. J Neurosci Nurs. 2016;48:82–9.
107. Boeve BF, Wijdicks EF, Benarroch EE, Schmidt KD. Paroxysmal sympathetic storms ("diencephalic seizures") after severe diffuse axonal head injury. Mayo Clin Proc. 1998;73:148–52.

Chapter 15
Opioid Use in the Critically Ill Geriatric Patient

Marie-France Forget and Han Ting Wang

Epidemiology

Older Adults in Intensive Care Unit (ICU)

Most epidemiological studies show, with some variability, an increase in the proportion of older patients (65 years and older) in the ICU population [1]. A clinical review states that older adults represent 42–52% of all United States' ICU admissions and almost 60% of ICU-bed days [2]. The overall ICU admission rate is 0.72% for male and 0.47% for female patients and the highest peak in admission is seen for those between age 75 and 90 years (between 2.1 and 2.2%) [3].

Older Adults and Pre-ICU Opioid Exposure

Pre-ICU opioid use in geriatric ICU patients is prevalent and of great clinical importance. Clinic visits leading to opioid prescriptions for adults age 65 and older have more than doubled between 1999 and 2010 (from 4.1% to 9.0% ($p < 0.001$)) [4]. Opioids are among the most commonly used drugs in Canadian adults age 65 and

M.-F. Forget
Department of Medicine, Division of Geriatric Medicine, Centre hospitalier de l'Université de Montréal, Montréal, QC, Canada

Université de Montréal, Faculty of Montréal, Montréal, QC, Canada
e-mail: marie-france.forget@umontreal.ca

H. T. Wang (✉)
Department of Medicine, Division of Internal and Critical Care Medicine, Hôpital Maisonneuve-Rosemont, Montréal, QC, Canada

Faculty of Medecine, Université de Montréal, Montréal, QC, Canada

J. L. Pascual, T. G. Gaulton (eds.), *Opioid Use in Critical Care*,
https://doi.org/10.1007/978-3-030-77399-1_15

older (15.7% in 2016 and 16% in 2014) [5, 6]. The incidence of new opioid use in this population is also quite significant. In a study performed by the Canadian Institute for Health Information on all opioids dispensed from community pharmacies in three major provinces in Canada, 8.1% of the studied population filled a new opioid prescription, with the highest incidence in 65 years and older individuals (12.2%) [7]. Accordingly, once on opioids, older patients consume them more regularly and for a much longer period [7]. Among opioid users, older adults have the highest proportion of chronic opioid use (prescribed for a duration of 90 days out of 100 days), approximately 24.8% for patients 65 years and older compared to 21.7% for those between 45 and 64 years old and 8.7% for those between 25 and 44 years old [7].

The prevalence of pre-ICU opioids exposure in older adults admitted to ICU is not as well studied. In a retrospective population-based study in Ontario on 711,312 patients older than 65 years, 35% of older adults admitted to ICU were opioid users. Of those, 48,363 (6.8%) were chronic users and 200,149 (28.1%) were intermittent users [8]. Furthermore, between 2002 and 2014, the prevalence of pre-ICU chronic opioid use increased significantly from 5.3% to 8.1% [8]. Another Canadian study on chronic opioid use in older adults before ICU admission showed that 11.2% of all chronic users had at least two or more opioid prescriptions filled concomitantly before hospital admission and their median morphine equivalent (MEQ) daily dosing before hospital admission was 32.1 mg (IQR, 17.5–75.0 mg MEQ) [9].

Pre-ICU opioid use is not without consequences. In the United States, between 2009 and 2015, an average of 52.4/10,000 ICU admissions were related to opioid overdoses, of which older adults (70 years and older) represented approximately 29% of all admissions [10]. The ICU proportion is comparable to overall hospital admissions related to opioid overdoses, which increases with age (12% were 30–39 years, 13% were 40–49 years, 19% were 50–59 years, 19% were 60–69 years, and 25% of patients were 70 years or older) [10]. Older adults seem more vulnerable to overdoses than their younger counterparts. Furthermore, irrespective of overdose, pre-ICU opioid exposure is associated with increased mortality in geriatric patients. Between 2001 and 2016, the largest relative increases of mortality related to opioids in the United States occurred among adults aged 55 to 64 years (754% increase) and those aged 65 years and older (635% increase) [11]. According to the previous Ontario ICU study, chronic opioid users and intermittent users had higher in-hospital mortality compared to non-users (adjusted odds ratio (aOR): 1.12, 95% Confidence interval (CI), 1.09–1.15, $p < 0.0001$ for chronic users; aOR: 1.09, 95% CI, 1.07–1.11, $p < 0.0001$ for intermittent users) [8].

Older Adults and Opiate Use During and After ICU Stay

Opioid use is ubiquitous in the ICU setting. Most ICU patients receive some form of opioids as part of analgesia and sedation regimens. A Korean cross-sectional study on opioid use in ventilated ICU patients, between 2012 and 2016 showed an increase in median daily MEQ over time (21.6 in 2012 vs 30.0 mg in 2016, $p < 0.01$) [12]. The annual increase in daily MEDs paralleled the reduction of benzodiazepine use [12]. This might reflect compliance to new analgesia-sedation guidelines prioritizing optimal pain management through both opioids and other co-analgesics [13]. Just like pre-ICU opioid exposure in older patients, opioid use during an ICU stay is associated with adverse outcomes. Studies have reported a higher risk of longer delirium duration and respiratory depression [14, 15]. Adults aged between 71 and 80 had 5.4 times the risk of respiratory depression (95% CI, 2.4–11.8) and those 80 years and above had 8.7 times (95% CI, 3.8–20.0) when compared to younger adults (45 years and less) [15].

Opioid use after ICU discharge has not been extensively studied in older adults. The previous Canadian study revealed that among chronic opioid users who survived their ICU stay, 22.0% had filled prescriptions for a higher daily MEQ compared with prehospitalization at 6 months after hospital discharge, 19.8% were unchanged, 21.5% had a lower dose, and 36.7% had no prescriptions filled at all [9]. Being a medical patient (compared to a surgical one), having fentanyl as the primary opioid on hospital admission and a concurrent consumption of benzodiazepine on hospital admission were independently associated with an increased odd of continuing opioids at 6 months after discharge [9]. Interestingly, the overall median MEQ increased from 32.1 mg (IQR, 17.5–75.0 MEQ) to 39.8 mg (IQR, 20.0–93.1), $p < 0.0001$) for those who filled at least one opioid prescription at 6 months after discharge. This might reflect a change in opioid prescription patterns where higher potency medications are increasingly being prescribed. In the Ontario population study, the proportion of codeine prescriptions dropped from 42.8% before admission to 32.5% on 180-day after discharge, while hydromorphone and fentanyl prescriptions rose from 13.9% and 11.6% to 18.1% and 15.5%, respectively (Fig. 15.1) [9]. Similarly, the previous Korean study showed that during the 2012 and 2016 period, morphine use decreased, while fentanyl use increased [12].

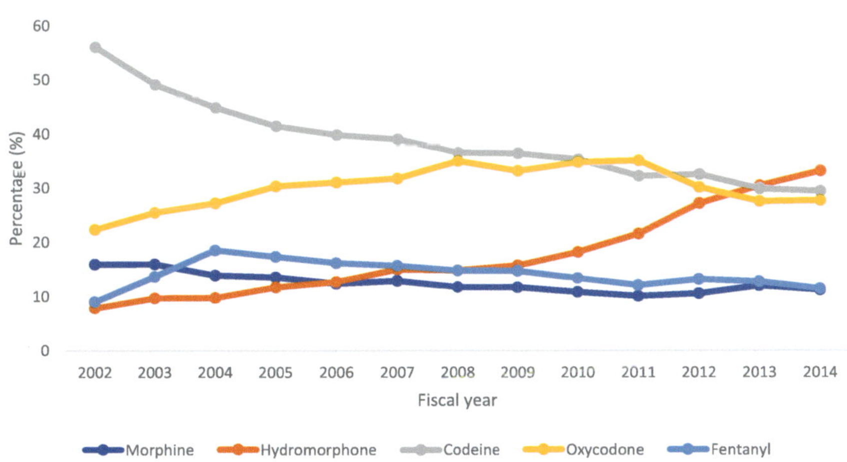

Fig. 15.1 Trends in opioid use before critical illness among 65 years and older patients in Ontario (2002–2015). (From Wang et al. [8]. With the authorization (pending) of Elsevier Inc.)

Judicious use of opioids in the ICU setting is critical considering the adverse effects they can cause. Higher opioids doses (64.6 ± 91.9 vs 32.9 ± 60.2 mg of morphine equivalents), independently of age, were associated with physical restraint use, in a retrospective study of 711 ICU mechanically ventilated patients with a mean age of 61 ± 16.7. Every 10 mg of morphine equivalents dose raised the risk of being physically restrained by 4% [16]. For reason, some authors have deemed opioid use as a potentially inappropriate medication when prescribed during ICU stay [17, 18]. Indeed, leaving a prescription active on ICU discharge when pain is no longer an issue might lead to overprescribing and inappropriate use. This does not mean opioids should be completely absent in ICU care but better, that adequate and regular pain assessment is instrumental for optimal patient management.

Pain Experience in Older Adults in Intensive Care Units

Managing pain and prescribing opioids in older ICU patients are challenging. There is a paucity of evidence and no trials specifically addressing this subgroup of patients. Nonetheless, clinical objectives are:

1. Titrating analgesia and lowering opioid doses
2. Improving analgesia quality by taking into consideration nociceptive and neuropathic pain
3. Reducing side effects

Pain in the ICU and Pain in Older Adults: Need for Monitoring

Guidelines for prevention and management of pain in ICU recommend routine pain assessment and treatment before considering sedative agents [13]. Treating older adults should not be any different. To that extent, adjunct medication to opioids for pain management has to also be considered in older ICU populations [19]. Individualizing treatment is a must since painful experiences seem to differ for the older adults compared to their younger counterparts.

Nociceptive and Neuropathic Pain in ICU

Nociceptive and neuropathic pain can coexist for ICU patients. Nociceptive pain is associated with nociceptor activation consequently to non-neural tissue damage. Neuropathic pain is due to central or peripheral somatosensory nervous system abnormalities or both. Normal aging is not associated with either nociceptive or neuropathic pain (e.g., diabetes-related neuropathic pain, chronic pain associated with osteoarthritis), but related comorbidities are more prevalent in older age [20]. For ICU patients, surgery, trauma, and invasive procedures induce additional pain.

Procedural pain (endotracheal suctioning or wound care pain) refers mostly to nociceptive pain, as long as neural tissue is not damaged. A prospective study on 3851 patients (median age of 62 (IQR 50–73)) undergoing 4812 procedures looked at pain intensity associated with 12 common ICU procedures [21]. Pain intensity during the procedure increased significantly from baseline ($p = 0.001$). Chest tube removal (pain evaluation of 5/10 (3–7) on the numeric rating scale), wound dressing removal (4.5 (2–7)), and arterial line insertion (4 (2–6)) were the three most painful procedures. A pre-intervention painful state and scheduled pre-intervention opioid exposure (preemptive analgesia) were associated with higher pain intensity [21]. Those results suggest the importance of basal pain evaluation and treatment *before* an ICU procedure. They highlight the concept of central sensitization. In either intense or repeated noxious stimuli, the subsequent stimuli can become amplified by sensitization of the nociceptive system [22, 23]. A review of the age effects on pain sensitivity supports that dorsal horn nociceptive neurons become sensitized with advancing age [22]. This enhances the theoretical pain vulnerability of older adults. The unexpected association with opioid use could be explained by an insufficient opioid dose or a lack of adequacy between time to peak effect and time of the procedure [21]. This leads to the important concept of preemptive analgesia, which aims to prevent central sensitization. Animal experiments demonstrated preemptive analgesia efficacy on initial and subsequent pain when analgesia was administered before the onset of the noxious stimulus [22]. Opioid-induced hyperalgesia, a phenomenon of increased sensitivity to painful and nonpainful stimuli secondary to high dose and high potency opioids, is another potential explanation [24]. This has been linked to opioid metabolites (morphine-3-glucuronide (M3G) or hydromorphone-3-glucuronide (H3G)) and activation of central nervous system N-methyl-D-aspartate (NMDA) receptors [25]. To our knowledge, it has not been studied in older adults.

Neuropathic pain can also be seen in some subgroups of ICU patients such as following cerebral ischemic stroke or post-surgery [26]. A cross-sectional survey of 2043 postsurgical patients (mean age 57 ± 12.37) reported a prevalence of persistent pain of 40.4% with an association between self-reported hypoesthesia or hyperesthesia (sensory abnormalities commonly seen in neuropathic pain) symptoms and the presence and intensity of persistent post-operative pain [26]. Neuropathic pain can occur after nerve damage secondary to procedural or surgical interventions. Age does not appear to be associated with an increase incidence of postsurgical neuropathic pain, although older age is associated with prolonged and increased thermal sensitivity, hyperalgesia, and allodynia [27]. Those results highlight the importance of evaluating and treating neuropathic pain, especially in older ICU patients.

Aging Pain Physiology and Homeostenosis

Emerging evidence suggests that efficient response to pain in older adults might be affected by homeostenosis, in opposition to homeostasis. Homeostasis is an adaptive response to internal and external variations, such as glucose levels or ambient temperature. With complex and dynamic physiologic mechanisms, such as insulin response and vasoconstriction, the organism tries to maintain normal physiologic constancy. Homeostenosis, the diminished capacity to face those challenges, is a well-known concept in geriatrics. It explains the vulnerability of many older adults in acute illness when compared to younger counterparts. An example of homeostenosis is the normal insulin resistance rise and longer time taken to reach a euglycemic state after hyperglycemia in older adults [28, 29]. Vulnerability in older adults comes from inherently diminished biological, psychological, and social reserve. A limited activation and feedback of the neuroendocrine, immune, and autonomic nervous system, altered opioid receptors, and modified pharmacokinetics diminish some older adult capacity to cope with pain [30]. Animal models have demonstrated a decrease in pain inhibition neurons in the dorsal horn region with aging. The loss of those inhibitory serotonin and noradrenaline neurons has been related to the increased nociceptive activity [31, 32]. Experimental studies have explored *offset analgesia*, defined as a disproportional pain reduction between older and younger adults caused by the slight pain of thermal stimulus. Older subjects demonstrated reduced offset which might reflect an age-related endogenous inhibitory system reduction, therefore adding complexity in the management of older patients [33, 34].

Variability in Pain Experience

Besides the possible change in pain physiology, the pain might be experienced differently for older adults. Atypical presentation of medical conditions is well described in geriatrics. The absence of pain, fever, or leucocytosis where one would expect, makes it harder to investigate and diagnose older adults [35]. For example, absence or difference in typical localization of pain in myocardial infarction has been associated with worst outcomes in older patients [36, 37]. In another retrospective study (15,670 charts), pain severity in the emergency department (on a scale of 1–10) was compared between older and younger adults. Reported pain was lower in older age patients for a diagnosis like appendicitis, migraine/headaches, and renal colic [38]. This variability can partly be explained by sex, education, or racial differences [39]. It also underlines the difficulty in pain assessment in the intensive care setting.

Pain Evaluation in Older Adults Able to Communicate and Unable to Communicate

There are no pain evaluation scales designed specifically for older ICU patients. Existing scales (Visual Analogue scale (VAS), Numerical Rating Scale (NRS), Verbal Rating Scale (VRS)) are used for all adult ICU patients, independent of their age. Few studies have looked at the reliability and validity of these scales in older patients. A psychometric study compared those three scales and other commonly used scales in 338 chronic pain patients, evenly distributed across different age brackets (<35, 35–44, 45–54, 55–64, 65–74, and 75 years and older). Difficulty in scoring pain (differentiation between weak, moderate, and strong pain scores) was associated with increasing age. Difficulty in scoring pain was mostly seen with VAS, with all scales deemed valid but the VRS preferred by the 75 years and older patients (VDS preference: 42.9%, NRS: 28.6%, horizontal VAS: 11.4%, and vertical VAS 17.1%) [40]. In a validity study of 75 chronic pain patients (mean age 49.8), difficulty in scoring pain with VAS was also related to increasing age ($r = 0.31$, $p < 0.01$) [41]. Those results favor the VRS scale for pain evaluation in older age ICU patients able to communicate.

For patients unable to communicate, it is even more challenging. Most tools are scales that take into account body movement, facial expressions, and ventilator compliance if applicable. The Behavioral Pain Scale (BPS) and Critical Care Pain Observation Tool (CPOT) are scales recommended and most frequently employed [42–44]. One must be careful when interpreting body movements for pain assessment, even in lightly sedated patients. Restlessness has been recognized as a significant pain sign in cognitively impaired older adults [45]. Moreover, the absence of movement can be a sign of undertreated pain. In a cohort of cognitively impaired older adults (mean age 83.2, SD7.7) who underwent surgical repair of a hip fracture, movement was found to correlate with a pain-free state [46]. Experiencing pain made patients more reluctant to move. Age, comorbidities, medication, critical illness, and pain itself might induce delirium [47–50], which brings even more complexity in pain recognition and evaluation.

Pain scales (BPS, VAS, and NRS) were compared in an ICU study of 113 critically ill patients (mean age 66 ± 15). In responsive patients, a high correlation between NRS and VAS was found ($r = 0.84$, $P < 0.001$). In ventilated patients, a moderate correlation was found between the NRS and the BPS ($r = 0.55$, $P < 0.001$) [51]. This suggests pain underestimation may occur in an observer-based evaluation. New pain assessment modalities integrating multiple physiological parameters are being developed and have shown efficacy and usefulness in monitoring pain in the perioperative setting [52]. But until it is validated for ICU patients, physicians must familiarize themselves with the existing scales and understand the potential pitfalls of their application in older ICU patients.

Pain Outcome for Elderly Adults in ICU

Undertreating pain is a risk factor for delirium. Among adults with a hip fracture, patients who received less than 10 mg of IV morphine equivalents per day had an increased risk of delirium, compared to patients who received a higher dose (RR 5.4, 95%CI 1.3–4.5) [53]. In another prospective study of 820 ICU patients, delirium incidence was higher in those who used a lower mean daily opioid dose (8.9 ± 24.3 mg morphine equivalents) compared to those using a higher mean of daily opioid dose (17–79 mg morphine equivalents) [54]. A systematic review of six observational studies in surgical settings concluded that meperidine was associated with an increased risk of delirium when compared to non-opioids. On the other hand, morphine, fentanyl, oxycodone, and codeine were not associated with delirium when compared to non-opioid and hydromorphone had the lowest association with delirium [55]. While the task is difficult, bedside providers must not underestimate the importance of pain in older ICU patients, have an adequate pharmacokinetic and dynamics of opioid medication, and use a personalized approach in managing each patient.

Opioid Analgesics, Non-opioid Analgesics, and Analgesic Alternatives

Age-Related Opioid Pharmacokinetics and Pharmacodynamics

Pharmacokinetics, which refers to absorption, distribution, metabolism, and drug elimination, and pharmacodynamics, which refer to the drug's effects, are subject to change in older adults. Generally speaking, opioids have a greater potency with age even after adjusting for age-related pharmacokinetic changes [56]. Therefore, starting with a lower dose is always a good rule of thumb [56]. More specifically, age, genetic polymorphisms, comorbidities, and concurrent medications contribute, independently and interdependently, to pharmacokinetics variability [57–59]. Some of those age-related modifications are well established while others report conflicting evidence. Therefore, predicting opioids effects and side effects in one individual is a daily reality for ICU providers. An acute illness or medical instability brings further complexity in the care of older adults. There is not one opioid that perfectly fits the wide variety of clinical situations. A network meta-analysis of 32 randomized controlled trials compared ten opioids in chronic pain analgesia. Patient satisfaction was similar with hydromorphone, oxycodone, and morphine [60].

Moreover, the vulnerability of older patients to the adverse effects of opioids strongly supports an individualized approach to care. Generating guidelines for clinical practice would be difficult and hazardous. In the following section, the most often seen and used opioids in the ICU setting will be discussed with some key concepts in pharmacokinetics and dynamics related to the older adult population (Table 15.1).

Table 15.1 Age-related opioid pharmacokinetics particularities and recommendations

Opioid	Distribution	Metabolism	Excretion	Recommendation
Fentanyl	Expected to ↗ [1, 2] ↗ intercompartmental clearance (faster redistribution between plasma and fat [3] compartment)	Phase I hepatic metabolism (CYP3A4) expected to be ↘ [4, 5]	Renal excretion ↘ [4] no active metabolite ↗ risk of tissue accumulation [6]	Use ↘ dose adequate to relieve pain or as intermittent boluses [6]
Hydromorphone	Expected to ↗ [1, 2]	Phase II hepatic metabolization glucuronidation [7], which is preserved through aging [5]	Renal excretion ↘ [4] Mostly excreted in active metabolite: H3G [8] ↗ risk of accumulation	Use ↘ dose and ↘ dose frequency adequate to relieve pain
Morphine	Expected to ↘ [9, 10]	Phase II hepatic metabolization glucuronidation [11], which is preserved through aging [5]	Renal excretion ↘ [11, 12] Mostly excreted in active metabolites: M3G and M6G [8, 13, 14] ↗ risk of accumulation	Use ↘ dose and ↘ dose frequency adequate to relieve pain Theoretical risk of higher clinical neurotoxicity: morphine is less potent than hydromorphone. requested higher dose raise active metabolites level

Refs. [59, 61–63, 65, 72–79, 81]
CYP3A4 cytochrome P450 3A4, *HG3* hydromorphone-3-glucuronide, *M3G* morphine-3-glucuronide, *M6G* morphine-6-glucuronide

Fentanyl

Intravenous fentanyl is often used to achieve analgesia in the critically ill. It is a highly lipophilic molecule [61, 62]. Age-associated reduced lean body mass and total body water leads to a proportionally higher fat mass percentage. Consequently, fentanyl is expected to have a higher volume of distribution in older adults [61, 62]. Also, fentanyl has a higher intercompartmental clearance (faster redistribution between plasma and fat compartment) in older adults when compared to younger ones. One study on 337 adults 57 years (± 15 (range 19 to 87)) reported an approximately four- to fivefold faster distribution in tissues (14.59 ± 5.64 L/kg/h vs. 3.18 ± 4.93 L/kg/h, $p < 0.05$) [63], which could suggest a faster nervous system penetration. Nonetheless, in a prospective study of 337 ICU patients, age was not associated with volume of distribution or intercompartmental clearance. Weight, the occurrence of severe liver disease, and heart failure accounted for much more interindividual variability than age in this study, suggesting that the effects of chronic and acute organ dysfunction may have a much larger effect than age [64]. Fentanyl is metabolized by the liver through the cytochrome P450 (CYP) 3A4 and has no active metabolites [59]. The P450 pathway is part of phase I hepatic metabolism and is known to be attenuated by aging [65] in opposition to phase II hepatic metabolism, which is not significantly affected by age [66]. One of the hypotheses for this phase I change is a lower hepatic blood flow (1015 ± 163 ml/min for 75 years and older vs. 1514 ± 250 ml/min for the 45 years and less group, $p = 0.00223$ [67]) and liver volume reduction with age [68–70]. Moreover, drug interactions are to be taken into consideration with all other medications dependent on CYP3A4 due to potential drug-drug interactions [59]. For example, most anticonvulsant agents (carbamazepine, phenytoin) [71] are CYP3A4 inducers, and fluoxetine, haloperidol, nortriptyline, and sertraline are inhibitors. Ultimately, fentanyl is eliminated almost exclusively by the kidney. Renal elimination is involved in all types of opioid pharmacokinetics [59]. Aging is associated with a reduced renal excretion, hence prolongation of elimination half-life due to a reduced renal mass and renal blood flow [58]. Therefore, fentanyl does offer the advantage of no active metabolite, but physicians need to take into consideration the risk of tissue accumulation and use the lowest perfusion dose adequate to relieve pain or as intermittent boluses [72].

Hydromorphone

Hydromorphone is another highly lipophilic opioid. It can be administered intravenously, as subcutaneous injections or it can be given orally. It is extensively metabolized by glucuronidation (hepatic phase II) [73], which is preserved through aging [65]. It does not use the CYP3A4, as fentanyl does, and therefore has a low risk of interactions. The main active metabolite is hydromorphone-3-glucuronide (H3G). H3G intracerebral infusion in rats induces neuroexcitatory side effects (allodynia, myoclonus, and seizure) [74] but no human studies have reported clinical safety issues [73]. No data on adverse effects in ICU patients were found, but some were reported in the context of chronic pain management. In the previously cited network meta-analysis of 32 non-ICU randomized controlled trials, there was no significant difference in adverse events or study withdrawal when hydromorphone was compared to other opioids [60]. Most of the hydromorphone is renally excreted in H3G. Because of its pharmacokinetic properties, hydromorphone might be a safer opioid for intermittent use. Due to its distribution in fat tissues and because of its renal clearance, HG3 can still accumulate and requires vigilance, especially in those suffering from acute kidney failure.

Morphine

Unlike the above two drugs, morphine is a hydrophilic molecule [75]. Therefore, a lower volume distribution is expected because of the lean body mass reduction in older age. Studies on healthy participants comparing older to younger adults showed either no difference or a trend to a smaller volume of distribution for morphine [76, 77]. Morphine's hepatic metabolism depends on a glucuronidation reaction (phase II) and is age-independent [75]. Morphine is metabolized into two active metabolites: Morphine-3-glucuronide (M3G) and morphine-6-glucuronide (M6G). M3G has no analgesic activity but is assumed to have a dose-dependent excitatory behavior (allodynia, hyperalgesia, myoclonus, and seizures) [74, 78, 79]. These effects have been suggested in animal models but have not been well elucidated in humans [79]. The other metabolite, M6G, is responsible for the analgesic effect [80]. Morphine and its active metabolites are excreted by the kidneys [75] and are at higher risk of accumulation because of reduced renal function with age [81]. Morphine clearance is lower in older than in younger adults (1.33 ± 0.12 vs 2.05 ± 0.08 ml/kg/min, $p = 0.01$). Some studies support an increased opioid pharmacodynamic effect with morphine and increased receptor affinity [66, 82, 83]. Glomerular filtration rate decreases and raises the risk for opioids or opioid metabolite toxicity. All considered, morphine is a safe choice among older ICU patients without renal failure. With renal impairment, studies have shown a level of H3G approximately 100 times that of normal plasma concentrations, although without showing clinical neurotoxicity [84]. Because morphine is less potent than hydromorphone, the neurotoxic effects might occur more frequently than with hydromorphone, although this remains speculative.

Codeine

Codeine, a pro-drug of morphine, is mostly known in its oral formulation and is not often used in the ICU setting. Codeine is metabolized by phase I hepatic enzymes, CYP2D6 [85]. CYP2D6 polymorphism produces unpredictable effects [57] in older as in younger adults. With morphine as the active metabolite and because of the known polymorphisms, there is little use of codeine in the adult ICU setting.

Oxycodone

Oxycodone has a low lipophilic profile that resembles that of morphine [86]. It has a low "first-pass" metabolism [87] and is only accessible for the enteral route in Canada and in the United States. CYP 3A4 (and partly CYP2D6) metabolizes oxycodone in oxymorphone and noroxycodone [59] and is thus affected with reduced hepatic flow associated with advancing age [65]. Oxymorphone is responsible for the analgesic activity and as with fentanyl, drug interactions are to be considered with all other drugs that are CYP3A4 inhibitors and inducers. Oxycodone's phase I metabolites have to undergo phase II glucuronidation [59]. Oxycodone and its metabolites are excreted by the kidney [73] and their use in the ICU is limited due to its formulations (tablets and suppositories) and the risk of interactions with other drugs (if intolerance or allergy).

Non-opioid Analgesics and Analgesic Alternatives

Nonpharmacological adjuncts, including optimizing sleep, limiting catheters, tubes, and IV access, thermal therapy (cold and heat), are important to opioid-based pain management. Listening to music and sounds, simple massage, distraction, passive exercises, and emotional support are other types of nonpharmacological interventions. There is a need for more studies on the effect of those interventions in the ICU, but their simplicity and limited evidence support their use [88, 89]. Similarly, non-opioid analgesics and nonchemical approaches can lower opioid requirements and improve overall pain control. The most common ones will be described below.

Paracetamol/Acetaminophen

Paracetamol, or acetaminophen as it is known in the United States, is widely used as the first-line treatment of mild to moderate pain. Its hydrophilic properties provide a decreased distribution volume in older adults. Hepatic metabolism is mainly achieved by conjugation reactions (Phase II preserved through aging) with 5–10% metabolized by CYP450 2E1 to a toxic metabolite [90]. Because of the lower proportion of lean mass in older adults, weight-based paracetamol should be prescribed based on lean weight (15 mg/kg every 6 hours) to prevent hepatotoxicity [91]. More recently, in a randomized controlled study on 120 cardiac surgery patients, 60 years and older, IV acetaminophen (1 g/h every 6 hours for 8 doses) was compared to placebo and combined with dexmedetomidine or propofol. There were significant differences favoring acetaminophen vs. placebo in delirium duration (median, 1 vs. 2 days; difference, −1 [95% CI, −2 to 0]), ICU length of stay (median, 29.5 vs. 46.7 hours; difference, −16.7 [95% CI, −20.3 to −0.8]), and breakthrough analgesia requirement (median, 322.5 vs. 405.3 μg morphine equivalents; difference, −83 [95% CI, −154 to −14]) [92]. This study clearly demonstrates the beneficial effect of non-opioid analgesics as adjunctive therapy in an acute care setting.

Nonsteroidal Anti-Inflammatory Drugs (NSAIDs)

NSAIDs are often not recommended in critical illness because of bleeding risk, renal impairment risk, or vulnerability to renal failure in older adults. NSAIDs are also highly protein-bound drugs [93] which raises the risk of drug-drug interaction. Guidelines usually are cautious and do not suggest routine use of COX-1 selective NSAIDs [13]. This rationale is even more pertinent in older adults. Nonetheless, NSAID COX-1 selective can be an option for some older adults, with caution for the potential renal or bleeding risk mentioned. For example, it could have an adjunctive pain managing benefit in post-surgical pain. Some clinicians will add proton-pump inhibitors to reduce upper-gastrointestinal events [18]. Selective COX2 inhibitors are more effective in preventing gastrointestinal events but are associated with cardiovascular events in older adults [94]. If NSAID is chosen as a non-opioid analgesic, a limited and definite time of trial is recommended.

Sodium Channel Blocker/Gabapentinoids

Sodium channel blockers are recommended for lowering the required opioid dose and for improving analgesia, especially in the setting of neuropathic pain [13]. Pregabalin has been associated with reduced total oxycodone consumption and with significantly lower postoperative pain incidence at 3 months in the cardiovascular surgery population (mean age 79.5 (75–91)) [95]. Pregabalin and gabapentin are the preferred agents for older adults. Caution on potential side effects is necessary. Dizziness, somnolence, and fatigue are common (>10%) [96, 97]. The 2019 American Geriatric Society Beers Criteria for older adults recommend avoiding the combination of pregabalin or gabapentin with opioids because of an increased risk of sedation-related adverse events [18]. However, when the combination aims to reduce the opioid dose, caution remains but the rationale supports the intervention. Carbamazepine, another sodium channel blocker, is a strong hepatic inducer CYP2C9 and CYP3A4 (auto-induction) and is implicated in numerous drug-drug interactions and therefore is less ideal [98].

Alpha 2 Agonists

Dexmedetomidine and clonidine have analgesic, anxiolytic, and sedative effects [99]. The pharmacokinetics and dynamics of dexmedetomidine in older adults have not been well documented. Dexmedetomidine, a highly protein-bound drug, is metabolized by the liver via glucuronidation (hepatic phase II) to inactive metabolites and is not influenced by renal impairment [100, 101]. In a cohort study of older post-abdominal surgery adults, use of dexmedetomidine reduced morphine consumption in the 72 hours following surgery (median difference – 9.0 mg [95% CI −10.0, −6.0], $P < 0.001$), lowered the perception of pain on the NRS scale (the median difference between −1 and −2 at time 4, 24, 48, and 72 hours after surgery, $p < 0.01$) and subjective quality of sleep was improved for the first night after surgery ($p = 0.031$) and for the night after, $p < 0.001$) [102]. Although the associated side effects, bradycardia, and hypotension [101] are to be considered before use [103], dexmedetomidine requires a continuous IV infusion which limits its clinical application.

Conclusion

Individualizing pain management approaches for the older adult ICU patient is key. Older adults' presence in the ICU and their generous exposure to opioids is rising, emphasizing the importance of a rationale for safe opioid use in that population. Individualizing opioid utilization is particularly necessary in elder individuals due to important differences between young and older adults and because of growing interindividual variability with aging. While opioid medication can definitely lead to adverse effects in ICU patients, judicious choices based on pharmacokinetics and dynamics can make them safe for older adults in ICU.

References

1. Flaatten H, et al. The status of intensive care medicine research and a future agenda for very old patients in the ICU. Intensive Care Med. 2017;43(9):1319–28.
2. Marik PE. Management of the critically ill geriatric patient. Crit Care Med. 2006;34 (9 Suppl):S176–82.
3. Garland A, et al. Epidemiology of critically ill patients in intensive care units: a population-based observational study. Crit Care. 2013;17(5):R212.
4. Steinman MA, et al. Use of opioids and other analgesics by older adults in the United States, 1999–2010. Pain Med. 2015;16(2):319–27.
5. Canadian Institute For Health Information. Drug use among seniors on public drug programs in Canada. Ottawa: Cihi; 2014.
6. Canadian Institute For Health Information. Drug use among seniors in Canada, 2016. Ottawa: Cihi; 2018.

7. Canadian Institute For Health Information. Opioid prescribing in Canada: how are practices changing? Ottawa: Cihi; 2019., Canadian Institute For Health Information.
8. Wang HT, et al. Trends in opioid use before critical illness among elderly patients in Ontario. J Crit Care. 2020;55:128–33.
9. Wang HT, et al. Opioid use after ICU admission among elderly chronic opioid users in Ontario: a population-based cohort study. Crit Care Med. 2018;46(12):1934–42.
10. Stevens JP, et al. The critical care crisis of opioid overdoses in the United States. Ann Am Thorac Soc. 2017;14(12):1803–9.
11. Gomes T, et al. The burden of opioid-related mortality in the United States. JAMA Netw Open. 2018;1(2):E180217.
12. Jung SY, Lee HJ. Utilisation of medications among elderly patients in intensive care units: a cross-sectional study using a nationwide claims database. BMJ Open. 2019;9(7):E026605.
13. Devlin JW, et al. Clinical practice guidelines for the prevention and management of pain, agitation/sedation, delirium, immobility, and sleep disruption in adult patients in the ICU. Crit Care Med. 2018;46(9):E825–73.
14. Pisani MA, et al. Benzodiazepine and opioid use and the duration of intensive care unit delirium in an older population. Crit Care Med. 2009;37(1):177–83.
15. Cepeda MS, et al. Side effects of opioids during short-term administration: effect of age, gender, and race. Clin Pharmacol Ther. 2003;74(2):102–12.
16. Luk E, et al. Predictors of physical restraint use in Canadian intensive care units. Crit Care. 2014;18(2):R46.
17. Morandi A, et al. Inappropriate medication prescriptions in elderly adults surviving an intensive care unit hospitalization. J Am Geriatr Soc. 2013;61(7):1128–34.
18. American Geriatrics Society. Beers Criteria Update Expert Panel, American Geriatrics Society 2019 updated AGS Beers Criteria for potentially inappropriate medication use in older adults. J Am Geriatr Soc. 2019;67(4):674–94.
19. Erstad BL. Implications of the opioid epidemic for critical care practice. J Am Coll Clin Pharm. 2019;2:161–6.
20. Reid MC, Eccleston C, Pillemer K, Management of chronic pain in older adults. BMJ. 2015;350:H532.
21. Puntillo KA, et al. Determinants of procedural pain intensity in the intensive care unit. The Europain(R) study. Am J Respir Crit Care Med. 2014;189(1):39–47.
22. Woolf CJ. Central sensitization: implications for the diagnosis and treatment of pain. Pain. 2011;152(3 Suppl):S2–15.
23. Latremoliere A, Woolf CJ. Central sensitization: a generator of pain hypersensitivity by central neural plasticity. J Pain. 2009;10(9):895–926.
24. Rivat C, Ballantyne J. The dark side of opioids in pain management: basic science explains clinical observation. Pain Rep. 2016;1(2):E570.
25. Chau DL, et al. Opiates and elderly: use and side effects. Clin Interv Aging. 2008;3(2):273–8.
26. Johansen A, et al. Persistent postsurgical pain in a general population: prevalence and predictors in the Tromso study. Pain. 2012;153(7):1390–6.
27. Yezierski RP. The effects of age on pain sensitivity: preclinical studies. Pain Med. 2012;13 Suppl 2:S27–36.
28. Defronzo RA. Glucose intolerance and aging: evidence for tissue insensitivity to insulin. Diabetes. 1979;28(12):1095–101.
29. Kalyani RR, Egan JM. Diabetes and altered glucose metabolism with aging. Endocrinol Metab Clin North Am. 2013;42(2):333–47.
30. Karp JF, et al. Advances in understanding the mechanisms and management of persistent pain in older adults. Br J Anaesth. 2008;101(1):111–20.
31. Ko ML, et al. The effects of aging on spinal neurochemistry in the rat. Brain Res Bull. 1997;42(2):95–8.
32. Iwata K, et al. Plastic changes in nociceptive transmission of the rat spinal cord with advancing age. J Neurophysiol. 2002;87(2):1086–93.

33. Naugle KM, et al. Offset analgesia is reduced in older adults. Pain. 2013;154(11):2381–7.
34. Naugle KM, et al. Loss of temporal inhibition of nociceptive information is associated with aging and bodily pain. J Pain. 2017;18(12):1496–504.
35. Limpawattana P, et al. Atypical presentations of older adults at the emergency department and associated factors. Arch Gerontol Geriatr. 2016;62:97–102.
36. Grosmaitre P, et al. Significance of atypical symptoms for the diagnosis and management of myocardial infarction in elderly patients admitted to emergency departments. Arch Cardiovasc Dis. 2013;106(11):586–92.
37. Breining A, et al. Determinants of clinical presentation on outcomes in older patients with myocardial infarction. Geriatr Gerontol Int. 2018;18(12):1591–6.
38. Daoust R, et al. Impact of age on pain perception for typical painful diagnoses in the emergency department. J Emerg Med. 2016;50(1):14–20.
39. Crimmins EM, Saito Y. Trends in healthy life expectancy in the United States, 1970–1990: gender, racial, and educational differences. Soc Sci Med. 2001;52(11):1629–41.
40. Peters ML, Patijn J, Lame I. Pain assessment in younger and older pain patients: psychometric properties and patient preference of five commonly used measures of pain intensity. Pain Med. 2007;8(7):601–10.
41. Jensen MP, Karoly P, Braver S. The measurement of clinical pain intensity: a comparison of six methods. Pain. 1986;27(1):117–26.
42. Young J, et al. Use of a behavioural pain scale to assess pain in ventilated, unconscious and/or sedated patients. Intensive Crit Care Nurs. 2006;22(1):32–9.
43. Gelinas C, et al. Validation of the critical-care pain observation tool in adult patients. Am J Crit Care. 2006;15(4):420–7.
44. Dale CM, et al. Validation of the critical-care pain observation tool (Cpot) for the detection of oral-pharyngeal pain in critically ill adults. J Crit Care. 2018;48:334–8.
45. Nygaard HA, Jarland M. The checklist of nonverbal pain indicators (CNPI): testing of reliability and validity in Norwegian nursing homes. Age Ageing. 2006;35(1):79–81.
46. Feldt KS. The checklist of nonverbal pain indicators (CNPI). Pain Manag Nurs. 2000;1(1):13–21.
47. Van Rompaey B, et al. Risk factors for delirium in intensive care patients: a prospective cohort study. Crit Care. 2009;13(3):R77.
48. Inouye SK, et al. A predictive model for delirium in hospitalized elderly medical patients based on admission characteristics. Ann Intern Med. 1993;119(6):474–81.
49. Inouye SK. Delirium in hospitalized elderly patients: recognition, evaluation, and management. Conn Med. 1993;57(5):309–15.
50. Van Rompaey B, et al. Risk factors for intensive care delirium: a systematic review. Intensive Crit Care Nurs. 2008;24(2):98–107.
51. Ahlers SJ, et al. Comparison of different pain scoring systems in critically ill patients in a general ICU. Crit Care. 2008;12(1):R15.
52. Bollag L, et al. The nociception level index (Nol) response to intubation and incision in patients undergoing video-assisted thoracoscopic surgery (Vats) with and without thoracic epidural analgesia. A pilot study. F1000Res. 2018;7:875.
53. Morrison RS, et al. Relationship between pain and opioid analgesics on the development of delirium following hip fracture. J Gerontol A Biol Sci Med Sci. 2003;58(1):76–81.
54. Ouimet S, et al. Incidence, risk factors and consequences of ICU delirium. Intensive Care Med. 2007;33(1):66–73.
55. Swart LM, et al. The comparative risk of delirium with different opioids: a systematic review. Drugs Aging. 2017;34(6):437–43.
56. Gupta DK, Avram MJ. Rational opioid dosing in the elderly: dose and dosing interval when initiating opioid therapy. Clin Pharmacol Ther. 2012;91(2):339–43.
57. Somogyi AA, Coller JK, Barratt DT. Pharmacogenetics of opioid response. Clin Pharmacol Ther. 2015;97(2):125–7.

58. Klotz U. Pharmacokinetics and drug metabolism in the elderly. Drug Metab Rev. 2009;41(2):67–76.
59. Smith HS. Opioid metabolism. Mayo Clin Proc. 2009;84(7):613–24.
60. Meng Z, et al. Tolerability of opioid analgesia for chronic pain: a network meta-analysis. Sci Rep. 2017;7(1):1995.
61. Narayanan M, Venkataraju A, Jennings J. Analgesia in intensive care: part 1. BJA Edu. 2016;16(2):72–8.
62. Mclachlan AJ, et al. Clinical pharmacology of analgesic medicines in older people: impact of frailty and cognitive impairment. Br J Clin Pharmacol. 2011;71(3):351–64.
63. Ariano RE, Duke PC, Sitar DS. Population pharmacokinetics of fentanyl in healthy volunteers. J Clin Pharmacol. 2001;41(7):757–63.
64. Choi L, et al. Population pharmacokinetics of fentanyl in the critically ill. Crit Care Med. 2016;44(1):64–72.
65. Mclachlan AJ, Pont LG. Drug metabolism in older people--a key consideration in achieving optimal outcomes with medicines. J Gerontol A Biol Sci Med Sci. 2012;67(2):175–80.
66. Mangoni AA, Jackson SH. Age-related changes in pharmacokinetics and pharmacodynamics: basic principles and practical applications. Br J Clin Pharmacol. 2004;57(1):6–14.
67. Zoli M, et al. Total and functional hepatic blood flow decrease in parallel with ageing. Age Ageing. 1999;28(1):29–33.
68. Wynne HA, et al. The effect of age upon liver volume and apparent liver blood flow in healthy man. Hepatology. 1989;9(2):297–301.
69. Schmucker DL. Aging and the liver: an update. J Gerontol A Biol Sci Med Sci. 1998;53(5):B315–20.
70. Schmucker DL. Liver function and phase I drug metabolism in the elderly: a paradox. Drugs Aging. 2001;18(11):837–51.
71. Wilkinson GR. Drug metabolism and variability among patients in drug response. N Engl J Med. 2005;352(21):2211–21.
72. Pergolizzi J, et al. Opioids and the management of chronic severe pain in the elderly: consensus statement of an International Expert Panel with focus on the six clinically most often used World Health Organization Step III opioids (buprenorphine, fentanyl, hydromorphone, methadone, morphine, oxycodone). Pain Pract. 2008;8(4):287–313.
73. Lotsch J. Opioid metabolites. J Pain Symptom Manage. 2005;29(5 Suppl):S10–24.
74. Smith MT. Neuroexcitatory effects of morphine and hydromorphone: evidence implicating the 3-glucuronide metabolites. Clin Exp Pharmacol Physiol. 2000;27(7):524–8.
75. Hospira. Morphine Sulfate injection label, Solution for Intravenous Use: U.S Food & Drug Administration. https://www.accessdata.fda.gov/drugsatfda_docs/label/2019/019916s019,019917s012lbl.pdf. Accessed Nov 2019.
76. Baillie SP, et al. Age and the pharmacokinetics of morphine. Age Ageing. 1989;18(4):258–62.
77. Villesen HH, et al. Pharmacokinetics of morphine and oxycodone following intravenous administration in elderly patients. Ther Clin Risk Manag. 2007;3(5):961–7.
78. Labella FS, Pinsky C, Havlicek V. Morphine derivatives with diminished opiate receptor potency show enhanced central excitatory activity. Brain Res. 1979;174(2):263–71.
79. Andersen G, Christrup L, Sjogren P. Relationships among morphine metabolism, pain and side effects during long-term treatment: an update. J Pain Symptom Manage. 2003;25(1):74–91.
80. Hoskin PJ, et al. The bioavailability and pharmacokinetics of morphine after intravenous, oral and buccal administration in healthy volunteers. Br J Clin Pharmacol. 1989;27(4):499–505.
81. King S, et al. A systematic review of the use of opioid medication for those with moderate to severe cancer pain and renal impairment: a European palliative care research collaborative opioid guidelines project. Palliat Med. 2011;25(5):525–52.
82. Aymanns C, et al. Review on pharmacokinetics and pharmacodynamics and the aging kidney. Clin J Am Soc Nephrol. 2010;5(2):314–27.
83. Wilder-Smith OH. Opioid use in the elderly. Eur J Pain. 2005;9(2):137–40.

84. Wright AW, Mather LE, Smith MT. Hydromorphone-3-glucuronide: a more potent neuro-excitant than its structural analogue, morphine-3-glucuronide. Life Sci. 2001;69(4):409–20.
85. Naples JG, Gellad WF, Hanlon JT. The role of opioid analgesics in geriatric pain management. Clin Geriatr Med. 2016;32(4):725–35.
86. Poyhia R, Seppala T. Liposolubility and protein binding of oxycodone in vitro. Pharmacol Toxicol. 1994;74(1):23–7.
87. Purdue Pharma L.P. Oxycodone hydrochloride extended-release tablets, for oral use : U.S Food & Drug Administration. 2018. https://www.fda.gov/media/131026/download. Accessed Nov 2019.
88. Sandvik RK, et al. Pain relief from nonpharmacological interventions in the intensive care unit: a scoping review. J Clin Nurs. 2020;29(9–10):1488–98.
89. Martorella G. Characteristics of nonpharmacological interventions for pain management in the ICU: a scoping review. AACN Adv Crit Care. 2019;30(4):388–97.
90. Rumack BH. Acetaminophen hepatotoxicity: the first 35 years. J Toxicol Clin Toxicol. 2002;40(1):3–20.
91. Mian P, et al. Paracetamol in older people: towards evidence-based dosing? Drugs Aging. 2018;35(7):603–24.
92. Subramaniam B, et al. Effect of intravenous acetaminophen vs placebo combined with propofol or dexmedetomidine on postoperative delirium among older patients following cardiac surgery: the dexacet randomized clinical trial. JAMA. 2019;321(7):686–96.
93. Verbeeck RK, Blackburn JL, Loewen GR. Clinical pharmacokinetics of non-steroidal anti-inflammatory drugs. Clin Pharmacokinet. 1983;8(4):297–331.
94. Solomon DH, et al. Relationship between selective cyclooxygenase-2 inhibitors and acute myocardial infarction in older adults. Circulation. 2004;109(17):2068–73.
95. Pesonen A, et al. Pregabalin has an opioid-sparing effect in elderly patients after cardiac surgery: a randomized placebo-controlled trial. Br J Anaesth. 2011;106(6):873–81.
96. Ulc UC. Product monograph: prlyrica®, pregabalin capsules. 2020.
97. Ulc UC. Product monograph: prneurontin®, gabapentin. 2020.
98. Punyawudho B, et al. Population pharmacokinetics of carbamazepine in elderly patients. Ther Drug Monit. 2012;34(2):176–81.
99. Belleville JP, et al. Effects of intravenous dexmedetomidine in humans. I. Sedation, ventilation, and metabolic rate. Anesthesiology. 1992;77(6):1125–33.
100. De Wolf AM, et al. The pharmacokinetics of dexmedetomidine in volunteers with severe renal impairment. Anesth Analg. 2001;93(5):1205–9.
101. Weerink MAS, et al. Clinical pharmacokinetics and pharmacodynamics of dexmedetomidine. Clin Pharmacokinet. 2017;56(8):893–913.
102. Li HJ, et al. Dexmedetomidine in combination with morphine improves postoperative analgesia and sleep quality in elderly patients after open abdominal surgery: a pilot randomized control trial. PLoS One. 2018;13(8):E0202008.
103. Stamenkovic DM, et al. Chronic pain and chronic opioid use after intensive care discharge - is it time to change practice? Front Pharmacol. 2019;10:23.

Chapter 16
Opioid Use in the Critically Ill Obstetric Patient

Charles Prior and Anthony Chau

Introduction

Opioids were first introduced into regular obstetric practice in the early twentieth century in the form of "twilight sleep," a technique that combined the use of subcutaneously administered morphine and scopolamine for their amnesic and analgesic effects during labor [1]. Subsequently, revolutions in medical education and practice ensued, through which obstetrics came to be perceived as one of the most scientifically advanced specialties of the time [2]. Since then, our basic science knowledge and clinical awareness of opioid pharmacology and placental transfer as well as complications affecting both the mother and newborn have advanced. The desire to deliver safe and effective anesthesia and analgesia for the mother-baby dyad prompted a growing popularity in regional techniques, but opioids continue to play a key role. In fact, opioids remain a mainstay for analgesia in many critically ill parturients in the intensive care unit, as antinociception is most commonly targeted via a central mechanism. In this chapter, we aim to outline the considerations and approach for using opioids in a critically ill obstetric patient and to highlight the importance of a coordinated and multidisciplinary team to optimize outcomes for both the mother and her baby.

C. Prior
Department of Anesthesia, BC Women's Hospital, Vancouver, BC, Canada

A. Chau (✉)
Department of Anesthesia, BC Women's Hospital, Vancouver, BC, Canada

Department of Anesthesiology, Pharmacology & Therapeutics, University of British Columbia, Vancouver, BC, Canada
e-mail: Anton.Chau@ubc.ca

J. L. Pascual, T. G. Gaulton (eds.), *Opioid Use in Critical Care*,
https://doi.org/10.1007/978-3-030-77399-1_16

Opioid Use in Obstetric Patients: Maternal Considerations

The Impact of Maternal Physiology on Opioid Pharmacology

During pregnancy, hormonal stimulation invokes significant maternal physiological changes with the ultimate purpose of adapting to fetal growth and development. Many of these physiological alterations can influence opioid pharmacodynamics and pharmacokinetics [3] (see Table 16.1). Although some changes (e.g., decreased

Table. 16.1 Physiological changes in pregnancy and the impact on opioid pharmacodynamics and pharmacokinetics [3, 4]

Physiological changes in Pregnancy	Opioid Pharmacodynamics	Opioid Pharmacokinetics
Respiratory		
↑O_2 consumption (by 20% at term) ↓Functional residual capacity (by 25% at term) Compensated respiratory acidosis	Poor tolerance of respiratory depressive effects Rapid desaturation during periods of hypopnea/ apnea	May affect protein binding
Cardiovascular		
↑plasma volume (by up to 50% at term) ↑total body water and ↑extra-cellular space ↑cardiac output (by up to 40% at term) ↑uteroplacental blood flow (up to 17% of cardiac output at term)	↓sympathetic drive and histamine release ↓heart rate and SVR ↓mean arterial pressure: (May be significant, e.g., during hemorrhage)	↑volume of distribution ↓circulating drug concentration ↑delivery to fetal circulation
Gastrointestinal		
↓gastric pH during labor ↓GI transit time during labor	Exacerbated ↓GI transit time ↑nausea and vomiting (stimulation of chemoreceptor trigger zone)	↓enteral absorption
Hepatic		
↓plasma albumin concentration Variable changes in phase I microsomal CYP enzymes ↓hepatic blood flow relative to cardiac output		↑bioavailability of unbound drug Variable metabolism ↑CYP3A4 metabolism of fentanyl ↑CYP2D6 metabolism of codeine and hydrocodone ↓first-pass metabolism
Renal		
↑GFR ↑renal plasma flow ↑creatinine clearance		↑renal excretion of active metabolites

enteric absorption, higher volume of distribution, and enhanced renal excretion) would suggest an increased requirement for opioid dosing and frequency of administration, these effects are offset by other changes (e.g., decrease in protein binding, increased bioavailability, and decreased first pass metabolism) and the overall impact is difficult to predict, especially given interindividual differences in pharmacodynamic responses [4]. Further changes in maternal physiology could occur secondary to the underlying critical illness, thus the clinical context for both mother and fetus should be individually considered and evaluated by a multidisciplinary team.

Common Opioids Encountered in Parturients

Opioids for Labor Analgesia

Since the 1940s, meperidine has been administered intramuscularly for early labor analgesia and remains in use in some countries [5]. However, in contemporary obstetric anesthesia practice, the use of meperidine in labor has largely been abandoned in North America, due to a high incidence of nausea and vomiting as well as concerns regarding its association with serotonergic syndrome and the toxic metabolite, norpethidine [6]. Intramuscular morphine is now more commonly used for analgesia in the latent and early active stages of labor. Intravenous fentanyl is more effective in the late active and second stages but has greater risk of maternal respiratory depression [6]. Parental opioids given in labor have been associated with a delay in gastric emptying and increased gastric acidity, increasing the risk of aspiration [7]. This risk should be considered and caution taken for patients at high risk of requiring emergency operative delivery.

Administration of a solution consisted of a local anesthetic and opioid is the contemporary gold standard for epidural labor analgesia. The purpose of adding an opioid into the epidural space is to augment the block quality so that a more dilute concentration of local anesthetic solution can be used to minimize motor block. Different initiation techniques have evolved with the most common being standard epidural, and combined spinal epidural (CSE) techniques. In a standard epidural procedure, an epidural catheter is sited into the epidural space and remains in place for the duration of labor. The CSE has all the elements of the standard epidural, with the additional administration of intrathecal local anesthetic with or without opioid, immediately prior to epidural catheter insertion. The intended benefit of the CSE is a more rapid onset and a more reliable spread of analgesic block. Once epidural analgesia is initiated, a combined local anesthetic and opioid solution (e.g., bupivacaine or ropivacaine, plus fentanyl) is administered through the epidural catheter to maintain the block throughout labor. Methods of epidural analgesia maintenance include continuous infusion, patient-controlled epidural analgesia (PCEA), and most recently programmed intermittent epidural bolus (PIEB) [8].

Opioids administered via the epidural space confer their analgesic effect by simple diffusion and subsequent binding to opioid receptors within the spinal cord. This process is dependent on the physicochemical properties of the opioid, particularly lipophilicity [9]. The spinal bioavailability of hydrophilic opioids (e.g., morphine, hydromorphone or diamorphine) is increased compared to more lipophilic opioids (e.g., fentanyl, sufentanil) because less drug is taken up by surrounding tissues. In general, the degree of lipid solubility of an opioid will confer its potency and speed of onset. Latency and duration of action of an opioid are related to pKa and protein binding [10]. Lipophilic opioids have a synergistic effect with local anesthetic drugs when given via the neuraxis, producing profound visceral and somatic analgesia. Systemic side effects are limited due to the mechanism of action on localized receptors, although the incidence of pruritus remains significant.

In cases where epidural analgesia for labor is contraindicated, for example, in a patient with coagulopathy or sepsis, intravenous opioids administered via patient-controlled analgesia (PCA) systems can be considered. At present, the two opioids established for PCA use in labor are fentanyl and remifentanil. The use of fentanyl PCA for labor is associated with lower rates of maternal sedation and respiratory depression compared with remifentanil, which is associated with a lower risk of neonatal respiratory depression [11, 12]. The higher rate of maternal respiratory depression, desaturation, and apnea with remifentanil PCA necessitate continuous monitoring and meticulous safety protocols.

Opioids for Operative Delivery

Neuraxial anesthesia, typically consisting of a combination of local anesthetic and opioid, is the most common anesthetic technique for operative delivery. A short-acting, lipid-soluble opioid, such as fentanyl or sufentanil, is added to improve the quality of visceral anesthesia. Longer acting, hydrophilic opioids, such as morphine is usually added to extend post-operative analgesia. Compared with systemically administered opioids, a profound analgesic effect from spinal or epidural opioids can be achieved at lower doses. This effect is conferred by a dense concentration of pre and post-synaptic opioid receptor sites in Rexed laminae I, II, and V within the dorsal horn of the spinal cord [10]. Neuraxially administered opioids also have a more favorable side effect profile, as well as preserving sensation and proprioception [13].

Cesarean deliveries are performed under general anesthesia in cases when time is limited to perform neuraxial block due to clinical urgency, or when neuraxial techniques are contraindicated. In these scenarios, opioids are generally withheld or minimized until after delivery to prevent uptake by the fetus.

Opioids in the Postpartum Period

Ongoing pain relief may be required postpartum, usually following cesarean delivery or a significant perineal tear. A multimodal analgesic approach consisting of neuraxial long-acting opioid as well as regular acetaminophen and nonsteroidal inflammatory drugs is the current gold standard. Neuraxial preservative-free morphine is the most effective element of this regimen [14], treating both static and dynamic pain and lasting for up to 36 hours post administration [15]. Common side effects include pruritus, nausea, and vomiting, which are dose related. Low doses of spinal morphine (e.g., 50–150 mcg) or epidural morphine (1.5–3 mg) are generally selected to offer the greatest balance of efficacy and minimal side effects [16]. The risk of respiratory depression following neuraxial opioids is recognized and appropriate monitoring is essential. The Society for Obstetric Anesthesia and Perinatology (SOAP) recommends that for the majority of healthy parturients receiving low dose neuraxial opioids, monitoring of respiratory rate and sedation scores every 2 hours for the first 12 hours is adequate. However, for higher doses and for patients with additional risk factors, an increased duration, frequency, and intensity of monitoring should be considered [17].

Opioid Use in Obstetric Patients: Fetal and Neonatal Considerations

Opioid Transfer Across the Placenta

The placenta is a complex and dynamic organ with important metabolic, nutritional, and hormonal regulatory functions. Approximately 12% of maternal cardiac output flows through the uterine arteries at term and 80–90% of this blood supplies the placenta. The utero-placental circulation is a low resistance, dilated vascular system with a limited capacity for autoregulation. The rate of opioid transfer between the two circulations depends on concentration gradients, permeability, and mechanisms that restrict movement. Other influential factors include maternal and fetal blood flow, placental binding, maternal and fetal protein binding, placental metabolism, and diffusion capacity [18].

In general, opioids readily cross the placenta. A comparison of pharmacokinetics and in vitro placental transfer characteristics between commonly used opioids is shown in Table 16.2. Morphine is hydrophilic and has low lipid solubility in comparison with other opioids. Although it rapidly crosses the placenta (owing in part to its high unionized fraction), the subsequent placental tissue content is low and washout is fast. When administered intramuscularly, the mean fetal-to-maternal concentration ratio (F/M ratio) is 0.61 and there is a reduction in fetal breathing movements and heart rate accelerations within 20–30 minutes. In contrast, when administered intrathecally, the F/M ratio is 0.92. However, due to the low intrathecal dose requirement, the absolute fetal concentration is well below the threshold associated with fetal and neonatal side effects [18].

Fentanyl has high lipid solubility and albumin binding (as opposed to alpha$_1$-acid glycoprotein), and therefore has a relatively high F/M ratio. When administered via the epidural route for labor analgesia in combination with local anesthetic, it has not been found to significantly depress neonatal respiration or neurobehavioral function [19].

Table 16.2 Opioid transfer during in vitro perfusion of the human placenta[a]. Adapted from Chestnut's Obstetric Anesthesia, Principles and Practice [18]

	Morphine	Fentanyl	Sufentanil	Alfentanil
Lipid solubility	1.4	816	1727	129
Percentage unionized at pH 7.4	23%	8.5%	20%	89%
Percent protein binding	30%	84%	93%	93%
Placenta drug ratio	0.1	3.4	7.2	0.53
F/M ratio (maternal to fetal direction of perfusion)	0.08	0.19	0.14	0.22
Minutes to steady state	30	40–60	40–60	20

[a]Data from non-recirculated experiments, using perfusate Media 199 without protein, with maternal flow 12 mL/min and fetal flow 6 mL/min

For comparison, in vivo animal studies of remifentanil have demonstrated an F/M ratio of 0.1 at a fixed maternal infusion rate of 0.33 mcg/kg/minute [20]. However, due to dose-dependent vasoactivity, the F/M ratio is likely to vary significantly according to maternal plasma concentration. Clinically, remifentanil used in labor is associated with a lower incidence for neonatal resuscitation requirement in comparison with other opioids [21]. This is likely due to rapid metabolism by non-specific esterases and very short context-sensitive half-time in the mother and neonate.

Impact of Routine Maternal Opioid Use on the Fetus and Neonate

Systemic and Neuraxial Opioids

Compared with neuraxial opioids, adverse effects of maternal systemic opioids have a greater impact on the fetus including central nervous system and respiratory depression, decreased heart rate variability, increased fetal acidosis, abnormal behavioral patterns, and decreased sucking reflex [22]. As a general rule, pediatricians regard the administration of systemic maternal opioids within 4 hours of delivery as a risk factor suggesting a greater need for neonatal resuscitation [23]. Effective communication with the pediatric team regarding maternal opioids used in labor is always warranted in order to allow appropriate and timely neonatal risk assessment.

Occasionally, opioids such as fentanyl or sufentanil are given intrathecally in labor as part of a CSE technique, in order to achieve rapid analgesia. Intrathecal opioids have been implicated in causing fetal bradycardia when compared with non-intrathecal routes [24]. The mechanism behind this phenomenon is not fully understood but one proposed theory is that rapid onset of analgesia results in catecholamine imbalance, leading to uterine tachysystole and subsequent decreased utero-placental blood flow and impaired oxygen delivery to the fetus.

Opioids and Breastfeeding

Neonates can be exposed to opioids through breast milk. The absolute infant drug dose is determined by the average breast milk intake multiplied by the average concentration of drug in the milk. A dose of less than 10% of the therapeutic plasma concentration is generally regarded as safe [25]. As these figures cannot be feasibly calculated accurately in normal clinical practice, a pragmatic approach must be taken. The fact that effective postpartum analgesia is associated with ongoing breastfeeding success should also be taken into account. The American College of Obstetricians and Gynecologists recommends that women be counseled regarding the risk of central nervous system depression in the woman and infant. Particular caution should be taken when prescribing codeine, meperidine, and tramadol, as there are significant interindividual variations in metabolism [26].

Long-Term Neurodevelopmental Effects of Opioids

The long-term effects of peripartum maternal opioid administration on the neurodevelopment of the infant are not fully understood due to lack of robust clinical studies [27]. It is likely endogenous opioid systems are important in early development, as receptors have been found within critical sites of the fetal brain [28]. It has also been shown that hippocampal development of rats is affected when the mother is exposed to opioids for the entire second trimester [29]. The applicability of this evidence to humans receiving peripartum clinical doses of opioid is currently unknown but not thought to be clinically significant.

Implications of Maternal Critical Illness

Scope of Critical Illness in the Obstetric Population

In the United States, up to 10 obstetric patients in every 1000 deliveries require critical care admission [30]. Most of these cases involve parturients admitted for intensive monitoring only, with fewer requiring lifesaving organ support. Of those obstetric patients requiring critical care, approximately two-thirds are postpartum admissions. The median maternal death rate in developed countries following admission to ICU is approximately 3.3% [30].

The leading causes of critical illness requiring ICU admission in obstetrics are major obstetric hemorrhage and severe hypertensive disorders in the peripartum period. Recently, opioid use disorder (OUD) in pregnancy has become an increasingly encountered problem. Other implicated conditions include cardiovascular disease and cardiomyopathy, sepsis, acute respiratory distress syndrome (ARDS), Coronavirus Disease 2019, trauma, amniotic fluid embolism, pulmonary thromboembolism, diabetic ketoacidosis, and neurological diseases [31]. Ultimately, any disease that can complicate pregnancy or the postpartum period, if severe enough, can lead to significant maternal morbidity and mortality.

General Considerations for Critical Care of the Obstetric Patient

A multidisciplinary approach to managing the obstetric patient on ICU is essential. Obstetricians and obstetric anesthesiologists should work with the intensivist to interpret laboratory and physiological parameters affected by pregnancy. Together with neonatologists, optimal strategies for fetal monitoring and timing for delivery can be planned. Maternal stabilization is the first priority when managing obstetric critical illness. While consideration should be given to limit exposure to teratogenic medications and ionizing radiation whenever possible, medications and diagnostic imaging critical for the parturient should not be withheld due to fetal concerns as fetal outcome often depends on maternal outcome [32].

Opioid Pharmacology in the Critically Ill Obstetric Patient

Changes in organ function associated with critical illness can significantly affect opioid pharmacology. Opioids are complex three-dimensional compounds and their analgesic effect is dependent on their stereochemical structure. They often exist as two isomers with the levorotatory isomer usually bearing the intrinsic activity of the drug; pharmacological activity can be altered by even minor changes in acid-base status and ionization. Therefore, acidosis in critical illness can influence opioid pharmacology and pharmacodynamics [10]. The decreased respiratory reserve secondary to reduced functional residual capacity and increased metabolic demand in pregnancy may be exacerbated by critical illness, rendering the patient particularly susceptible to the respiratory depressive effects of opioids. Shock states that lead to reduced intravascular volume will lead to a reduced volume of distribution. Impaired hepatic function and associated low serum albumin level are common in obstetric critical illness, for example in preeclampsia. This may affect metabolism and protein binding. Renal failure associated with hemorrhagic shock or preeclampsia may also affect opioid elimination. Changes in opioid pharmacology during critical illness are dynamic as physiological function changes according to disease process and therapeutic interventions. It is therefore important to titrate doses of opioid to clinical effect, in order to maximize analgesic efficacy and minimize side effects.

Opioids for Induction of Anesthesia and Intubation of the Critically Ill Obstetric Patient

Traditionally, systemic opioids are avoided until after delivery in order to minimize neonatal exposure. However, in some cases, maternal benefit of intravenous opioid may outweigh the risk to the neonate. For example, in those with severe hypertensive diseases of pregnancy, short-acting opioids such as remifentanil or fentanyl used during induction of anesthesia are effective for obtunding the hypertensive response to laryngoscopy and airway manipulation. Similarly, in patients who are in shock states due to sepsis or major hemorrhage, an opioid-based anesthesia induction with fentanyl may confer greater hemodynamic stability. A recent study suggests that remifentanil 0.5–1 mcg/kg and alfentanil 7.5–10 mcg/kg are both effective, with no difference in 1- and 5-minute Apgar scores when compared with placebo. However, the use of fentanyl 0.5–1 mcg/kg was associated with significantly reduced Apgar scores at 5 minutes [33].

Opioid Use Disorder

Opioid use disorder (OUD) in pregnancy is a growing problem in North America in all socioeconomic groups [34]. These patients may be encountered in the critical care setting following an overdose or infectious complication. OUD is also associated with adverse obstetric outcomes including fetal demise and neonatal opioid withdrawal [35]. Caring for obstetric patients with OUD requires a multidisciplinary approach and where possible, consultation with specialist OUD teams to ensure appropriate management. This includes holistic care that is patient-centered, non-judgmental, and sensitive to a vulnerable patient group with a high prevalence of domestic, sexual, emotional, and physical abuse. Pharmacologically, patients should have access to individualized care plans, which usually consist of opioid agonist treatment (OAT) such as methadone or buprenorphine/naloxone. Slow-release oral morphine or injectable OAT may also be considered as second- and third-line therapies under specialist guidance. In the peripartum period, OUD patients should have access to all necessary analgesics in addition to established doses of OAT. Concerns regarding adverse fetal side effects should not prevent the adequate dosing of OAT for OUD patients. The long-term benefits to the mother and baby of appropriate maternal OAT have been shown to far outweigh the short-term risks of neonatal respiratory depression or withdrawal. The onset of neonatal withdrawal depends on the half-life and amount used during pregnancy and when the last maternal dose was taken. For example, while heroin withdrawal can occur within 1–3 days following birth, methadone withdrawal can take over a week to manifest.

Impact of Maternal Critical Care on the Fetus

When maternal critical care is required, fetal mortality is high. Specific factors associated with increased mortality include absent prenatal care, early gestational age, maternal shock, and organ failure and the need for maternal blood transfusion [36]. Utero-placental blood flow is poorly autoregulated and therefore requires a well-maintained maternal mean arterial pressure. Therefore, maternal shock states are poorly tolerated. Systemic vasopressors constrict uterine blood vessels, which may also decrease flow to the fetus [37]. Optimizing fluid resuscitation and maximizing aortocaval flows are therefore essential for reducing vasopressor requirement where possible. Balancing optimal management for the mother and fetus during critical illness is complex and multidisciplinary care is vital [32].

Maternal Critical Illness and Placental Transfer of Opioids

Placental transfer of opioids may be altered in critical illness, most commonly due to impaired utero-placental blood flow. Impaired fetal perfusion leads to changes in pH gradients between maternal and fetal circulations. Basic drugs including opioids are subject to "ion trapping" within the fetal circulation if the fetal environment becomes more acidic. Alterations in protein binding in critical illness states, such as severe pre-eclampsia, may also alter rates of placental opioid transfer. Severe intrauterine infection may also have a significant impact on drug transfer. Most of these effects will tend to increase opioid concentration in the neonate relative to the situation in normal health. It is therefore prudent to consider the neonate of a critically ill mother at a relatively higher risk of adverse opioid effects for a given maternal dose. When delivery is planned in the context of maternal critical illness, it is important to liaise with the neonatal team regarding maternal opioid administration to facilitate optimal risk assessment, preparation for resuscitation, and allocation of neonatal critical care resources.

Non-opioid Analgesic Adjuncts and Regional Techniques in Obstetrics

Non-opioid Analgesic Adjuncts

Entonox is an inhaled analgesic consisting of a 50/50 mixture of oxygen and nitrous oxide commonly used for labor. It provides consistent, moderate analgesia but is also associated with nausea and vomiting, dizziness, and amnesia [38].

Ketamine is a noncompetitive, reversible inhibitor of the N-methyl-D-aspartate (NMDA) receptor and acts as an agonist at mu-opioid receptors, monoaminergic receptors, gamma aminobutyric acid receptors, and others at high doses. Acceptable labor analgesia using infusion of intravenous ketamine (bolus 0.1 mg/kg followed by infusion of 0.2 mg/kg/h) has been reported [39]. It has also been used as an adjunctive agent during general anesthesia (bolus 0.5 mg/kg followed by infusion of 0.25 mg/kg/h) when neuraxial technique is contraindicated or unsatisfactory [40]. It can reduce opioid consumption and is particularly useful in parturients who are at increased risk of opioid-related respiratory depression (e.g., obstructive sleep apnea), history of chronic pain, or those with high tolerance to opioids (e.g., OUD).

Dexmedetomidine is a highly selective α2-agonist with several desirable pharmacologic properties including sedation, anxiolysis, sympatholysis, analgesia, and a smooth emergence profile. It has been used in obstetrics as a sedative and analgesic adjunct for both labor and cesarean delivery [41]. Minimal adverse affects on the fetus and neonate have been observed in case reports [42]. This is in keeping with recent studies demonstrating that fetal transfer of dexmedetomidine is limited by high placental retention and lipophilicity [43]. However, caution is required in patients with bradyarrhythmias, ventricular impairment, and hypovolemic states [44]. Further studies are required to be carried out within the critically ill obstetric population.

Acetaminophen is used universally post cesarean delivery unless contraindicated, providing an opioid-sparing effect of up to 20% [45]. The use of a nonsteroidal anti-inflammatory drug (NSAID) has been shown to reduce opioid requirement by up to 50%, which confers a reduction in opioid side effects of 30% [46]. There is an additive opioid-sparing effect when acetaminophen and NSAIDs are administered together, especially when both are given regularly in a scheduled manner [47]. Common NSAIDs given in obstetric practice postpartum include ibuprofen, diclofenac, and ketorolac. Contraindications to NSAIDs are as for the general population but also include renal impairment secondary to preeclampsia. NSAIDs are generally considered safe in breastfeeding mothers at regular doses [48].

Use of sedative agents for critically unwell pregnant patients requiring intubation and ventilation should take into account the potential effect on the fetus. Again, there is a paucity of data evaluating individual agents due to practical and ethical considerations for randomized controlled trials in this population. Therefore, available evidence is largely based on case reports and animal studies, which may not be directly applicable. Benzodiazepines should be used with caution in the first trimester, as there has been some association with congenital malformation such as cleft palate as well as a risk of spontaneous miscarriage [49]. When used in the late third trimester, they may cause floppy infant syndrome and neonatal withdrawal [50]. There is, however, no substantial evidence at present to suggest any association of benzodiazepines with long-term neurodevelopmental impairment [51].

Truncal Blocks and Peripheral Nerve Blocks

When neuraxial techniques are contraindicated, achieving effective analgesia post cesarean delivery can be challenging. In such cases, there are several alternative regional techniques that have been used to provide analgesia. Of course, non-neuraxial regional techniques may also be contraindicated in some cases, for example, in severe coagulopathy [52].

The most common regional analgesic technique used in this scenario is the bilateral transversus abdominis plane (TAP) block. As part of a multimodal postoperative analgesic regimen, TAP blocks have been shown to reduce opioid requirements for up to 48 hours when administered in the absence of intrathecal opioid [53]. There is also evidence that they are effective in treating breakthrough pain following administration of neuraxial morphine [54]. TAP blocks are usually performed using an in-plane, ultrasound-guided technique. A radio-opaque needle is passed through the skin between the level of the anterior superior iliac spine and the lower costal margin. The needle tip is visualized on ultrasound and advanced through subcutaneous tissue, external oblique, and internal oblique muscles until it reaches the fascial plane between internal oblique and transversus abdominis muscles. Within this plane lie the terminal nerve branches arising from the anterior primary rami of thoracic nerve roots T7 to T12 and lumbar nerve root L1. Here, long-acting, dilute local anesthetic such as ropivacaine 0.25% or bupivacaine 0.25% is injected to provide analgesia. Spread of the local anesthetic and reliable blockade depends on having a large volume of injectate to dissect the TAP plane; a minimum of 15 mL is recommended but typically 20 mL is injected on each side. As such, the weight of the patient should be considered to ensure that a maximum safe dose is not exceeded.

The quadratus lumborum (QL) block has also been used for analgesia post cesarean delivery. It involves ultrasound-guided injection of local anesthetic into the fascial plane between QL and psoas major muscles. This may have an advantage over the TAP block, as the QL facial plane is in continuum with the paravertebral space [55]. This allows spread of local anesthetic to the sympathetic chain, which may help to block visceral pain. Trials have shown that QL blocks may be useful in the absence of intrathecal morphine but add no benefit in conjunction with it [56].

Local anesthetic wound infiltration, including peritoneal instillation of lidocaine or subfascial wound infiltration, has also been investigated. These techniques may be of benefit improving dynamic pain and reducing systemic opioid use, especially for women undergoing general anesthesia without a long-acting neuraxial opioid [57]. However, wound leakage associated with the high infusion volumes required have limited its use. Field blocks of the iliohypogastric and ilioinguinal nerves have shown some benefit for treating breakthrough pain. However, they are inferior when compared to neuraxial morphine [58].

Summary

Key Considerations

- Management of critically unwell obstetric patients requires a multidisciplinary approach involving intensivists, obstetricians, anesthesiologists, and neonatologists.
- Physiological changes in pregnancy and critical illness have variable and complex effects on opioid pharmacology. Opioid administration should be titrated according to efficacy and side effects.

- All opioids are generally regarded as safe to use in the critically ill obstetric patient when indicated and used appropriately at the minimum required dose.
- Neuraxial techniques are the mainstay of analgesia and anesthesia in obstetric practice but they are often contraindicated in critical illness.
- Systemic opioids readily cross the placenta but can be given safely during labor and delivery. However, standardized safety and monitoring protocols are required to monitor the risk of maternal respiratory depression. The neonatal team should be informed for all opioid administration close to delivery.
- Post cesarean delivery, multimodal analgesic regimens including regional techniques should be used unless contraindicated, for their opioid sparing effects.
- Critically ill obstetric patients suffering from opioid use disorder require specialist management and individualized care plans including the use of adequate opioid agonist treatment.

References

1. Von Steinbüchel R. Vorläufige Mittheilung über die Anwendung von Skopolamin-Morphium-injektionen in der Geburtshilfe. Centralblatt Gyn. 1902;30:1304–6.
2. Kaufman M. American medical education: the formative years, 1765–1910. Westport: Greenwood Press; 1976.
3. Frederiksen MC. Physiologic changes in pregnancy and their effect on drug disposition. Semin Perinatol. 2001;25(3):120–3.
4. Ward RM, Varner WV. Principles of pharmacokinetics in the pregnant woman and fetus. Clin Perinatol. 2019;46:383–98.
5. Tuckey JP, Prout RE, Wee MY. Prescribing intramuscular opioids for labour analgesia in consultant-led maternity units: a survey of UK practice. Int J Obstet Anesth. 2008;17:3–8.
6. Elbourne E, Wiseman R.A. Types of intramuscular opioids for maternal pain relief in labour. Cochrane Database Syst Rev. 2006;(4):CD001237.
7. Cheek TG, Gutsche BB. Pulmonary aspiration of gastric contents. In: Hughes SC, Levinson G, Rosen MA, editors. Shnider and Levinson's anesthesia for obstetrics. 4th ed. Lippincott Williams & Wilkins: Philadelphia; 2001. p. 391–4.
8. Lim G, Facco FL, Nathan N, Waters JH, Wong CA, Eltzschig HK. A review of the impact of obstetric anesthesia on maternal and neonatal outcomes. Anesthesiology. 2018;129(1):192–215.
9. Bernards CM. Understanding the physiology and pharmacology of epidural and intrathecal opioids. Best Pract Res Clin Anaesthesiol. 2002;16:489–505.
10. Bucklin BA, Santos AC. Local anesthetics and opioids. In: Chestnut DH, Wong CA, Tsen LC, Ngan Kee WD, Beilin Y, Mhyre JM, editors. Chestnut's obstetric anesthesia principles and practice. 5th ed. Philadelphia: Saunders; 2014. p. 268–306.
11. Douma MR, Verwey RA, Kam-Endtz CE, van der Linden PD, Stienstra R. Obstetric analgesia: a comparison of patient-controlled meperidine, remifentanil, and fentanyl in labour. Br J Anaesth. 2010;104:209–15.
12. Marwah R, Hassan S, Carvalho JC, Balki M. Remifentanil versus fentanyl for intravenous patient-controlled labour analgesia: an observational study. Can J Anaesth. 2012;59:246–54.
13. Dahlgren G, Hultstrand C, Jakobsson J, Norman M, Eriksson EW, Martin H. Intrathecal sufentanil, fentanyl, or placebo added to bupivacaine for caesarean section. Anesth Analg. 1997;85:1288–93.
14. Lim Y, Jha S, Sia AT, Rawal N. Morphine for post-caesarean section analgesia: intrathecal, epidural or intravenous? Singapore Med J. 2005;46:392–6.

15. Palmer CM, Emerson S, Volgoropolous D, Alves D. Dose-response relationship of intrathecal morphine for postcesarean analgesia. Anesthesiology. 1999;90:437–44.
16. Yurashevich M, Habib AS. Monitoring, prevention and treatment of side effects of long-acting neuraxial opioids for post-cesarean analgesia. Int J Obstet Anesth. 2019;39:117–28.
17. Bauchat JR, Weiniger CF, Sultan P, Habib AS, Ando K, Kowalczyk JJ, et al. Society for obstetric anesthesia and perinatology consensus statement: monitoring recommendations for prevention and detection of respiratory depression associated with administration of neuraxial morphine for cesarean delivery analgesia. Anesth Analg. 2019;129(2):458–74.
18. Zakowski MI, Geller A. The placenta: anatomy, physiology, and transfer of drugs. In: Chestnut DH, Wong CA, Tsen LC, Ngan Kee WD, Beilin Y, Mhyre JM, eds. Chestnut's obstetric anesthesia principles and practice. 5th ed. Philadelphia: Saunders; 2014. P.55–84.
19. Porter J, Bonello E, Reynolds F. Effect of epidural fentanyl on neonatal respiration. Anesthesiology. 1998;89(1):79–85.
20. Sato M, Masui K, Sarentonglaga B, Yamaguchi M, Fukumori R, Nagao Y, et al. Influence of maternal remifentanil concentration on fetal-to-maternal ratio in pregnant ewes. J Anesth. 2017;31(4):517–22.
21. Van de Velde M, Carvalho B. Remifentanil for labor analgesia: an evidence-based narrative review. Int J Obstet Anesth. 2016;25:66–74.
22. Kopecky EA, Ryan ML, Barrett JF, et al. Fetal response to maternally administered morphine. Am J Obstet Gynecol. 2000;183:424–30.
23. Yi Wen P, Broom E, Flatley C, Kumar S: Maternal demographic and intrapartum antecedents of severe neonatal outcomes at term. J Matern Fetal Neonatal Med. 2020;33(12):2103–8.
24. Abrão KC, Francisco RP, Miyadahira S, Cicarelli DD, Zugaib M. Elevation of uterine basal tone and fetal heart rate abnormalities after labor analgesia: a randomized controlled trial. Obstet Gynecol. 2009;113:41–7.
25. Flood P, Aleshi P. Postoperative and chronic pain: systemic and regional analgesic techniques. In: Chestnut DH, Wong CA, Tsen LC, Ngan Kee WD, Beilin Y, Mhyre JM, editors. Chestnut's obstetric anesthesia principles and practice. 5th ed. Philadelphia: Saunders; 2014. p. P604–22.
26. ACOG Committee Opinion No. 742 Summary: postpartum pain management. Obstet Gynecol. 132(1):252–3.
27. Conradt E, Flannery T, Aschner J, Annett RD, Croen LA, Duarte CS, et al. Prenatal opioid exposure: neurodevelopmental consequences and future research priorities. Pediatrics. 2019;144(3):e20190128. https://doi.org/10.1542/peds.2019-0128.
28. Tripathi A, Khurshid N, Kumar P, Iyengar S. Expression of deltaand mu-opioid receptors in the ventricular and subventricular zones of the developing human neocortex. Neurosci Res. 2008;61:257–70.
29. Niu L, Cao B, Zhu H, et al. Impaired in vivo synaptic plasticity in dentate gyrus and spatial memory in juvenile rats induced by prenatal morphine exposure. Hippocampus. 2009;19:649–57.
30. Pollock W, Rose L, Dennis CL. Pregnant and postpartum admissions to the intensive care unit: a systematic review. Intensive Care Med. 2010;36:1465–74.
31. Callaghan WM. Overview of maternal mortality in the United States. Semin Perinatol. 2012;36:2.
32. ACOG Practice Bulletin No. 211: critical care in pregnancy. Obstet Gynecol 2019;133(5):e303–e319.
33. White LD, Hodsdon A, An GH, Thang C, Melhuish TM, Vlok R. Induction opioids for caesarean section under general anaesthesia: a systematic review and meta-analysis of randomised controlled trials. Int J Obstet Anesth. 2019;40:4–13.
34. Martins F, Oppolzer D, Santos C, Barroso M, Gallardo E. Opioid use in pregnant women and neonatal abstinence syndrome—a review of the literature. Toxics. 2019;7(1):9.
35. British Columbia Centre on Substance Use, B.C. Ministry of Health, B.C. Ministry of Mental Health and Addictions & Perinatal Services BC. A guideline for the clinical management of opioid use disorder - pregnancy supplement. Published June 1, 2018. Available at: http://www.bccsu.ca/care-guidance-publications/.

36. Aoyama K, Seaward PG, Lapinsky SE. Fetal outcome in the critically ill pregnant woman. Crit Care. 2014;18:307.
37. Van Nimwegen D, Dyer DC. The action of vasopressors on isolated uterine arteries. Am J Obstet Gynecol. 1974;118:1099.
38. Rosen MA. Nitrous oxide for relief of labor pain: a systematic review. Am J Obstet Gynecol. 2002;186(Suppl 5):S110–26.
39. Joselyn AS, Cherian VT, Joel S. Ketamine for labour analgesia. Int J Obstet Anesth. 2010;19(1):122–3.
40. Halilogu M, Ozdemir M, Uzture N, Cenksoy PO, Bakan N. Perioperative low-dose ketamine improves postoperative analgesia following Cesarean delivery with general anesthesia. J Matern Fetal Neonatal Med. 2016;29(6):962–6.
41. Sng BL, Dabas R, Sia AT. Intravenous dexmedetomidine use in obstetric anaesthesia: a weapon in our armoury? Int J Obstet Anesth. 2018;36:1–2.
42. Palanisamy A, Klickovich RJ, Ramsay M, Ouyang DW, Tsen LC. Intravenous dexmedetomidine as an adjunct for labor analgesia and cesarean delivery anesthesia in a parturient with a tethered spinal cord. Int J Obstet Anesth. 2009;18:258–61.
43. Nair AS, Sriprakash K. Dexmedetomidine in pregnancy: review of literature and possible use. Journal of Obstetric Anaesthesia and Critical Care. 2013;3:3.
44. Nair AS, Sriprakash K. Dexmedetomidine in pregnancy: review of literature and possible use. J Obstet Anaesth Crit Care. 2013;3(1):3–6.
45. Ong CK, Seymour RA, Lirk P, Merry AF. Combining paracetamol (acetaminophen) with nonsteroidal anti-inflammatory drugs: a qualitative systematic review of analgesic efficacy for acute postoperative pain. Anesth Analg. 2010;110:1170–9.
46. Marret E, Kurdi O, Zufferey P, Bonnet F. Effects of nonsteroidal anti-inflammatory drugs on patient-controlled analgesia morphine side effects: meta-analysis of randomized controlled trials. Anesthesiology. 2005;102:1249–60.
47. Valentine AR, Carvalho B, Lazo TA, Riley ET. Scheduled acetaminophen with as-needed opioids compared to as needed acetaminophen plus opioids for post-cesarean pain management. Int J Obstet Anesth. 2015;24:210–6.
48. American Academy of Pediatrics Committee on Drugs. Transfer of drugs and other chemicals into human milk. Pediatrics. 2001;108:776–89.
49. Sheehy O, Zhao JP, Bérard A. Association between incident exposure to benzodiazepines in early pregnancy and risk of spontaneous abortion. JAMA Psychiat. 2019;15. https://doi.org/10.1001/jamapsychiatry.2019.0963.
50. McElhatton PR. The effects of benzodiazepine use during pregnancy and lactation. Reprod Toxicol. 1994;8(6):461–75.
51. Lupatelli A, Chambers CD, Bandoli G, Handal M, Skurtveit S, Nordeng H. Association of maternal use of benzodiazepines and Z-hypnotics during pregnancy with motor and communication skills and attention-deficit/hyperactivity disorder symptoms in preschoolers. JAMA Netw Open. 2019;2(4):e191435. https://doi.org/10.1001/jamanetworkopen.2019.1435.
52. Horlocker TT, Vandermeulen E, Kopp SL, Gogarten W, Leffert LR, Benzon HT. Regional anesthesia in the patient receiving antithrombotic or thrombolytic therapy: American Society of Regional Anesthesia and Pain Medicine Evidence-Based Guidelines(fourth edition). Reg Anesth Pain Med. 2018;43(3):263–309.
53. Abdallah FW, Halpern SH, Margarido CB. Transversus abdominis plane block for postoperative analgesia after caesarean delivery performed under spinal anaesthesia ? A systematic review and meta-analysis. Br J Anaesth. 2012;109:679–87.
54. Mirza F, Carvalho B. Transversus abdominis plane blocks for rescue analgesia following Cesarean delivery: a case series. Can J Anaesth. 2013;60:299–303.
55. Blanco R, Ansari T, Riad W, Shetty N. Quadratus lumborum block versus transversus abdominis plane block for postoperative pain after caesarean delivery: a randomized controlled trial. Reg Anesth Pain Med. 2016;41:757–62.

56. Irwin R, Stanescu S, Buzaianu C, Rademan M, Roddy J, Gormley C, Tan T: Quadratus lumborum block for analgesia after caesarean section: a randomised controlled trial. Anaesthesia. 2019. https://doi.org/10.1111/anae.14852.
57. Bamigboye AA, Hofmeyr GJ. Local anaesthetic wound infiltration and abdominal nerves block during caesarean section for postoperative pain relief. Cochrane Database Syst Rev. 2009:CD006954.
58. Coffman JC, Fiorini K, Small RH. Ilioinguinal-iliohypogastric block used to rescue ineffective transversus plane block after caesarean delivery. Int J Obstet Anesth. 2015;24:394–5.

Index

J. L. Pascual, T. G. Gaulton (eds.), *Opioid Use in Critical Care*,
https://doi.org/10.1007/978-3-030-77399-1

D

E

F

G

Printed by Printforce, the Netherlands